Microbial
Ecology
and
Infectious
Disease

Microbial
Ecology
and
Infectious
Disease

Edited by
Eugene Rosenberg

Department of Molecular Microbiology and Biotechnology
Tel Aviv University, Ramat Aviv 69978, Israel

ASM
PRESS

Washington, DC

39700782

12-10-02

Cover: detail from an interpretation in chalk pastel of interacting cells, by Edra London

Copyright © 1999 American Society for Microbiology
1325 Massachusetts Ave., N.W.
Washington, DC 20005-4171

Library of Congress Cataloging-in-Publication Data

Microbial ecology and infectious disease / edited by Eugene Rosenberg.
    p.   cm.
    Includes bibliographical references and index.
    ISBN 1-55581-148-5
    1. Medical microbiology. 2. Microbial ecology. I. Rosenberg,
Eugene.
    QR46.M5383   1998
    616'.01—DC21

98-30758
CIP
Rev

All Rights Reserved
Printed in the United States of America

This book is dedicated to my scientific mentor and close friend, the late Stephen Zamenhof

CONTENTS

CONTRIBUTORS

Frans W. J. Albers
Department of Otorhinolaryngology, University Hospital Groningen, Hanzeplein 1, 9713 EZ Groningen, The Netherlands

Rom T. Altstock
Department of Human Microbiology, Sackler School of Medicine, Tel Aviv University, Tel Aviv 69978, Israel

Serge Ankri
Department of Biological Chemistry, The Weizmann Institute of Science, Rehovot 76100, Israel

M. Baetens
Department of Microbiology and Immunology, Stanford University School of Medicine, Sherman Fairchild Science Building, Stanford, California 94305

E. Banin
Department of Molecular Microbiology and Biotechnology, Tel Aviv University, Ramat Aviv 69978, Israel

Oded Béjà
Department of Biological Chemistry, Weizmann Institute of Science, Rehovot 76100, Israel

Shimshon Belkin
Environmental Sciences, The Fredy & Nadine Herrmann Graduate School of Applied Science, The Hebrew University of Jerusalem, Jerusalem 91904, Israel

Y. Ben-Haim
Department of Molecular Microbiology and Biotechnology, Tel Aviv University, Ramat Aviv 69978, Israel

Eshel Ben-Jacob
School of Physics and Astronomy, Raymond and Beverly Sackler Faculty of Exact Sciences, Tel Aviv University, Tel Aviv 69978, Israel

Ericka L. Benson
Department of Microbiology and Molecular Genetics, Harvard Medical School, Boston, Massachusetts 02115

Hervé Bercovier
Department of Clinical Microbiology, The Hebrew University-Hadassah Medical School, Ein Karem, Jerusalem 91120, Israel

Eitan Bibi
Department of Biological Chemistry, Weizmann Institute of Science, Rehovot 76100, Israel

Eva M. Busch
Institute for Medical Microbiology, University of Giessen, Frankfurterstrasse 107, D-35392 Giessen, Germany

Henk J. Busscher
Laboratory for Materia Technica, University of Groningen, Bloemsingel 10, 9712 KZ Groningen, The Netherlands

Trinad Chakraborty
Institute for Medical Microbiology, University of Giessen, Frankfurterstrasse 107, D-35392 Giessen, Germany

Su L. Chiang
Department of Microbiology and Molecular Genetics and Shipley Institute of Medicine, Harvard Medical School, 200 Longwood Avenue, Boston, Massachusetts 02115

R. John Collier
Department of Microbiology and Molecular Genetics, Harvard Medical School, Boston, Massachusetts 02115

Eugen Domann
Institute for Medical Microbiology, University of Giessen, Frankfurterstrasse 107, D-35392 Giessen, Germany

Sam Dukan
Institut Jacques Monod, CNRS-Université Paris 7 and Université Paris-6, 2, place Jussieu, 75251 Paris Cedex 05, France

Martin Dworkin
Department of Microbiology, University of Minnesota, Minneapolis, Minnesota 55445-0312

Rotem Edgar
Department of Biological Chemistry, Weizmann Institute of Science, Rehovot 76100, Israel

Ina Fabian
Department of Cell Biology and Histology, Sackler School of Medicine, Tel Aviv University, Tel Aviv 69978, Israel

Yuan Fang
Department of Molecular Genetics and Biotechnology, The Hebrew University Faculty of Medicine, P.O. Box 12272, Jerusalem 91120, Israel

M. Fine
Department of Zoology, Tel Aviv University, Ramat Aviv 69978, Israel

Alan Finkelstein
Department of Physiology and Biophysics, Albert Einstein College of Medicine, Bronx, New York 10461

Dan Graur
Department of Zoology, George S. Wise Faculty of Life Sciences, Tel Aviv University, Tel Aviv 69978, Israel

E. Peter Greenberg
Department of Microbiology, University of Iowa, Iowa City, Iowa 52242-1109

David L. Gutnick
Department of Molecular Microbiology and Biotechnology, George S. Wise Faculty of Life Sciences, Tel Aviv University, Tel Aviv 69978, Israel

Emanuel Hanski
Clinical Microbiology, Hadassah Medical School, Hebrew University, Ein Karem, Jerusalem 91120, Israel

Iris Hillel
Department of Biological Chemistry, Weizmann Institute of Science, Rehovot 76100, Israel

Paul D. Huynh
Department of Physiology and Biophysics, Albert Einstein College of Medicine, Bronx, New York 10461

Jeries Jadoun
Department of Human Microbiology, Sackler School of Medicine, Tel Aviv University, Tel Aviv 69978, Israel

A. Kushmaro
Department of Zoology, Tel Aviv University, Ramat Aviv 69978, Israel

Yves Levi
Faculté de Pharmacie, Laboratoire Santé Publique-Environnement, Université Paris-Sud, 5 rue J. B. Clément, 92296 Chatenay-Malabry Cedex, France

Jack London
National Institute of Dental Research, National Institutes of Health, Bethesda, Maryland 20892

Y. Loya
Department of Zoology, Tel Aviv University, Ramat Aviv 69978, Israel

A. Matin
Department of Microbiology and Immunology, Stanford University School of Medicine, Sherman Fairchild Science Building, Stanford, California 94305

Ann G. Matthysse
Department of Biology, University of North Carolina, Chapel Hill, North Carolina 27599-3280

John J. Mekalanos
Department of Microbiology and Molecular Genetics and Shipley Institute of Medicine, Harvard Medical School, 200 Longwood Avenue, Boston, Massachusetts 02115

Yael Meller-Harel
Department of Biological Chemistry, Weizmann Institute of Science, Rehovot 76100, Israel

David Mirelman
Department of Biological Chemistry, The Weizmann Institute of Science, Rehovot 76100, Israel

Leonid Mittelman
Interdepartmental Core Facility, Sackler School of Medicine, Tel Aviv University, Tel Aviv 69978, Israel

Itzhak Ofek
Department of Human Microbiology, Sackler Faculty of Medicine, Tel Aviv University, Ramat Aviv 69978, Israel

Elisha Orr
Department of Molecular Microbiology and Biotechnology, Tel Aviv University, Ramat Aviv 69978, Israel

S. Pandža
Department of Microbiology and Immunology, Stanford University School of Medicine, Sherman Fairchild Science Building, Stanford, California 94305

C. H. Park
Department of Microbiology and Immunology, Stanford University School of Medicine, Sherman Fairchild Science Building, Stanford, California 94305

Marc Robinson
Department of Zoology, George S. Wise Faculty of Life Sciences, Tel Aviv University, Tel Aviv 69978, Israel

Eliora Z. Ron
Department of Molecular Microbiology and Biotechnology, George S. Wise Faculty of Life Sciences, Tel Aviv University, Tel Aviv 69978, Israel

E. Rosenberg
Department of Molecular Microbiology and Biotechnology, Tel Aviv University, Ramat Aviv 69978, Israel

Ilan Rosenshine
Department of Molecular Genetics and Biotechnology, The Hebrew University Faculty of Medicine, P.O. Box 12272, Jerusalem 91120, Israel

Edward G. Ruby
Pacific Biomedical Research Center, University of Hawaii, Manoa, Honolulu, Hawaii 96813

Hana Sandovsky-Losica
Department of Human Microbiology, Sackler School of Medicine, Tel Aviv University, Tel Aviv 69978, Israel

Ester Segal
Department of Human Microbiology, Sackler School of Medicine, Tel Aviv University, Tel Aviv 69978, Israel

Gil Segal
Department of Microbiology, College of Physicians and Surgeons, Columbia University, 701 West 168th Street, New York, New York 10032

Shlomo Sela
Department of Human Microbiology, Sackler School of Medicine, Tel Aviv University, Tel Aviv 69978, Israel

James A. Shapiro
Department of Biochemistry and Molecular Biology, University of Chicago, Cummings Life Sciences Center, 920 East 58th Street, Chicago, Illinois 60637-4931

Howard A. Shuman
Department of Microbiology, College of Physicians and Surgeons, Columbia University, 701 West 168th Street, New York, New York 10032

Albert Taraboulos
Department of Molecular Biology, The Hebrew University-Hadassah Medical School, P.O. Box 12272, Jerusalem 91120, Israel

A. Toren
Department of Molecular Microbiology and Biotechnology, Tel Aviv University, Ramat Aviv 69978, Israel

Danièle Touati
Institut Jacques Monod, CNRS-Université Paris 7 and Université Paris-6, 2, place Jussieu, 75251 Paris Cedex 05, France

Ilan Tsarfaty
Department of Human Microbiology, Sackler School of Medicine, Tel Aviv University, Tel Aviv 69978, Israel

S. Ulitzur
Department of Food Engineering and Biotechnology, Technion, Haifa 32000, Israel

Betsy van de Belt–Gritter
Laboratory for Materia Technica, University of Groningen, Bloemsingel 10, 9712 KZ Groningen, The Netherlands

Henny C. van der Mei
Laboratory for Materia Technica, University of Groningen, Bloemsingel 10, 9712 KZ Groningen, The Netherlands

Ranny van Weissenbruch
Department of Otorhinolaryngology, University Hospital Groningen, Hanzeplein 1, 9713 EZ Groningen, The Netherlands

S. Waggoner
Department of Microbiology and Immunology, Stanford University School of Medicine, Sherman Fairchild Science Building, Stanford, California 94305

Ronald Weiner
Department of Cell Biology and Molecular Genetics, University of Maryland, College Park, Maryland 20742

Minca Westerhof
Laboratory for Materia Technica, University of Groningen, Bloemsingel 10, 9712 KZ Groningen, The Netherlands

PREFACE

The major objective of this book is to demonstrate, using current research projects, how microbial ecology and medical microbiology are interrelated subjects. Although each of these two fields of microbiology has developed independently throughout most of this century, they are now converging in a way that makes it imperative for scientists in either of the fields to become familiar with the techniques and concepts of the other field. Each field has much to offer the other. Some of the most elegant research in microbial ecology has come from medical microbiologists who have studied the mechanisms by which bacteria are able to adhere to tissues, invade, survive, and multiply in their hosts. On the other hand, microbial ecologists have made dramatic progress in the last few years in understanding how bacteria grow in Nature, such as the importance of biofilms, cell-to-cell interactions, quorum sensing, and the molecular and genetic mechanisms for adapting to starvation and other stress conditions.

The chapters in this book were derived from two international meetings on Microbial Ecology and Infectious Disease. The first one was held at the National Institutes of Health (NIH), Bethesda, Md., in July 1996. The second one, sponsored by the Israel Center for Emerging Diseases, was held in April 1998 at Ma'ale Hachamisha, Israel. At both meetings, participants commented on the scientific stimulation they received by considering the relationships between microbial ecology and infectious disease. A representative of the ASM Press, present at the NIH meeting, suggested that the symposia form the basis for a book.

I thank Jeff Holtmeier for encouraging me to proceed with the book and providing me with interesting comments from several microbiologists. It was a pleasure to work with Karen R. Jones at the ASM Press, who made my job much easier by providing all the necessary instructions. Finally, to the authors and participants in both symposia, thank you all.

BACTERIAL ECOPHYSIOLOGY

I

INTRODUCTION

James A. Shapiro

The first section of this volume is devoted to considerations of how bacteria operate metabolically and behaviorally in complex and variable ecosystems. Ecophysiology is relevant to pathogenesis in two fundamental ways. First, survival in the general environment is a primary factor in the spread of disease organisms. Second, the host organism comprises a challenging and changeable environment for the invading pathogen. Thus, understanding how bacteria adapt to new environments makes a significant contribution to our appreciation of the mechanisms pathogens can use as they migrate from host to host and proliferate within an infected host. This ecological perspective is very much in keeping with recent discoveries in bacterial molecular genetics that show how fundamental cellular systems, such as surface appendages and membrane transport systems, have been specifically adapted for interactions with mammalian target cells.

James A. Shapiro, Department of Biochemistry and Molecular Biology, University of Chicago, Cummings Life Sciences Center, 920 East 58th Street, Chicago, IL 60637-4931.

This section focuses on four different case studies. Martin Dworkin recounts the multiple interactions that occur during the development of *Myxococcus xanthus* populations. He describes the importance of cellular sensing and intercellular signaling, especially that based on direct cell-cell contact, during myxococcal fruiting body morphogenesis. He also makes the intriguing proposal that extracellular fibrils with auto-ADP-ribosylation activity may serve as tactile antennae. Ronald Weiner discusses survival of marine bacteria, emphasizing the morphological plasticity of the bacterial cells. He describes how *Hyphomonas* species undergo striking changes in shape and behavior between planktonic and attached forms, which correlate with growth in impoverished pelagic zones and nutrient-rich biofilms, and how an *Alteromonas* strain is able to transform itself from a normal gram-negative bacillus into a miniscule resting ultraform when carbon sources are depleted. Finally, A. Matin and colleagues discuss the molecular biology of starvation responses in *E. coli*. They point out that there is a special set of starvation genes that are activated at the end of exponential growth and show how expression of these functions can protect *E. coli* cells from a wide variety of different stress conditions.

They also describe the role of the RpoS stationary-phase sigma factor in expression of starvation-specific functions and the significance of posttranscriptional proteolytic regulation of RpoS activity by the ClpXP protease.

COMMON THEMES IN PATHOGENESIS AND DEVELOPMENT IN *MYXOCOCCUS XANTHUS*

Martin Dworkin

I

The emphasis of this chapter is on those aspects of myxobacterial development and cell-cell interactions that overlap with some familiar themes in pathogenesis.

MYXOCOCCUS XANTHUS

The myxobacteria are a group of gram-negative prokaryotes that go through a complex life cycle that culminates in the formation of a macroscopic, multicellular fruiting body. Figure 1 is a photo of the fruiting body of *Chondromyces crocatus*, the most complex of all the myxobacteria. Even though it is not the favorite experimental organism among the myxobacteria, it exemplifies the complexity and multicellularity of this group. Most myxobacteriologists work with *Myxococcus xanthus*, which forms a substantially simpler fruiting body (Fig. 2).

The life cycle of *M. xanthus* is illustrated in Fig. 3. Fruiting body formation is an alternative to growth and is induced by three conditions. First, the cells must see a nutritional shiftdown. A reduction in the level of any of the required amino acids is sufficient to induce

a stringent response, mediated by the elevation of the intracellular levels of (p)ppGpp (29). Second, the cells must be on a substratum that permits their characteristic gliding motility. Third, they must be present at an extremely high cell density (28). The cells then aggregate by means of a peculiar gliding motility, in response to directional signals that are not well understood, and form a simple, elevated mound comprising about 10^5 resting cells called myxospores.

PATHOGENESIS AND DEVELOPMENT

A number of aspects of the developmental physiology of *M. xanthus* coincide with common themes in pathogenesis: (i) Dependence on contact-mediated cell-cell interactions via pili and/or fibrils, (ii) ADP-ribosylation, (iii) mechanisms for density sensing, (iv) tyrosine kinase, and (v) cell-cell signaling.

Density-sensing mechanisms and cell-cell signaling have been studied by other laboratories and are not covered in this chapter. Readers interested in a description of the role of the A signal as a cell density sensor in *M. xanthus* are directed to a recent review (21); for a detailed and recent description of intercellular signaling in *M. xanthus*, the reader is directed to the chapter on the subject in

Martin Dworkin, Department of Microbiology, University of Minnesota, Minneapolis, MN 55445-0312.

Microbial Ecology and Infectious Disease, Edited by Eugene Rosenberg
©1999 American Society for Microbiology, Washington, D.C.

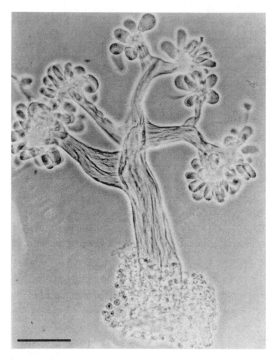

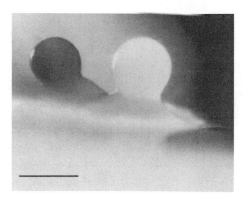

FIGURE 2 *Myxococcus fulvus* fruiting bodies. Phase contrast. Bar, 50 μm. Courtesy of Hans Reichenbach.

Myxobacteria II (20) or to the most recent review on the myxobacteria (7).

Contact-Mediated Cell–Cell Interactions in *M. xanthus*

Explicit evidence for contact-mediated cell-cell interactions in *M. xanthus* comes from two directions.

FIGURE 1 *Chondromyces crocatus* fruiting body. Slide mount, phase contrast. Bar, 100 μm. Courtesy of Hans Reichenbach.

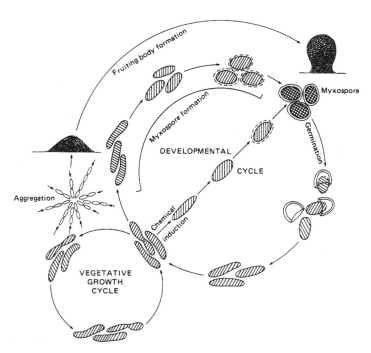

FIGURE 3 Diagram of the life cycle of *M. xanthus* (6). The fruiting body is not drawn to scale but is a few hundredths of a millimeter in diameter. The vegetative cells are about 5–7 by 0.7 μm.

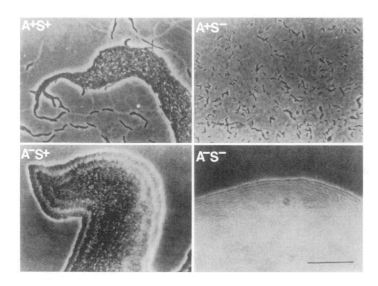

FIGURE 4   Effect of A (adventurous) and S (social) motility mutations on *M. xanthus* cell behavior (26).

ROLE OF PILI IN SOCIAL MOTILITY

In 1977 Hodgkin and Kaiser (17) showed that there were two modes of gliding motility in *M. xanthus*. In one of these, so-called A (adventurous) motility, cells moved individually. In the second, the so-called S (social) motility, cells moved as groups. Each of these is regulated by a separate genetic system; mutants in the "S" system can move only as individual cells, and conversely, mutants in the "A" system can move only as groups of cells (Fig. 4). "S" mutants were subsequently shown to lack the polar pili characteristic of wild-type cells (18). Hodgkin and Kaiser also showed that there was a set of conditional "S" mutants, whose group motility could be restored by the close physical proximity of wild-type cells (16). This complementation was mediated by the wild-type pili and the rescued "S" motility mutants temporarily regained the ability to make their own pili. Thus, it seemed clear that the pili were physically mediating some aspect of social motility.

FIBRILS AND SOCIAL BEHAVIOR

The second clue was the finding by Arnold and Shimkets in 1988 (1) that wild-type cells of *M. xanthus* possessed a set of peritrichous, epicellular appendages they called fibrils. A dispersed-growing mutant, designated *dsp*, lacked fibrils and was unable to undergo development or to manifest characteristic social behavior such as cohesion or social motility. Behmlander and Dworkin (2) subsequently studied and characterized these fibrils. A scanning electron micrograph (SEM) of vegetative cells and their fibrils is shown in Fig. 5.

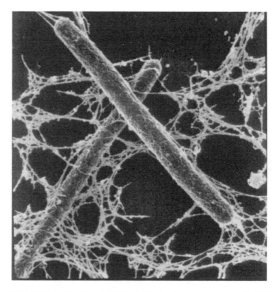

FIGURE 5   LV-SEM images of vegetative cells of *M. xanthus* with extensive fibrillar interconnections. Photo supplied by R. M. Behmlander.

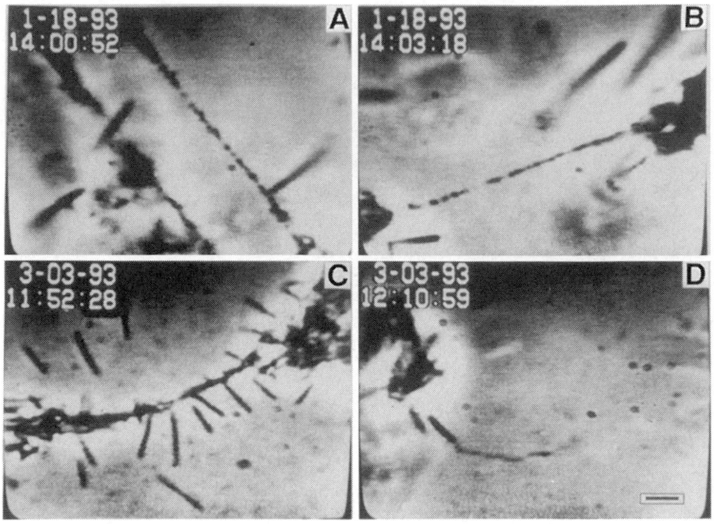

FIGURE 6 Phase-contrast micrographs of *M. xanthus* stained with India ink to observe hydrated fibrils on living cells. The still images were taken from video-recorded originals. Bar in panel D, 5 μm (3).

The fibrils are structurally polysaccharide with a set of adhering integral fibril proteins (IFP). The average diameter of the fibrils is 30 nm, and thus they are beneath the resolving power of the light microscope. However, by coating the fibrils with carbon particles, Behmlander and Dworkin (3) were able to view them on living cells by using phase-contrast microscopy (Fig. 6). Thus, they are present on living cells and not a preparational artifact. The fibrils could be isolated and purified by repeated washing with sodium dodecyl sulfate (Fig. 7).

The role of these fibrils in mediating cell-cell contact is indicated by the fact that addition of isolated, purified fibrils will temporarily restore development and social behavior to the *dsp* mutant (5). It became clear at this point that the fibrils were bona fide organelles of the cell and that they participated in the social and developmental behavior of the organism. To try to understand the role of one or more of the associated proteins in the process, our laboratory took both a molecular and a biochemical approach.

We had generated a set of monoclonal antibodies directed against a variety of the cell surface antigens of *M. xanthus*, present during either growth or development (11–13). Monoclonal antibody (MAb) 2105 was found to be directed against one of the fibril proteins, IFP-20 (Fig. 8). We decided to use this antibody to assist in cloning the gene for the protein, in the hope that in so doing, a sequence homology comparison would give us a clue as to the function of the fibril protein and a mutation in the gene would also help to reveal its function.

Behmlander and Dworkin (4) isolated one of the isoforms of the protein and determined

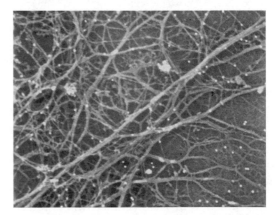

FIGURE 7 Field-emission SEM of isolated *M. xanthus* fibrils probed with MAb 2105 and a gold-conjugated secondary antibody (3).

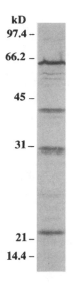

FIGURE 8 Western blot of whole cells of *M. xanthus* probed with MAb 2105 (4).

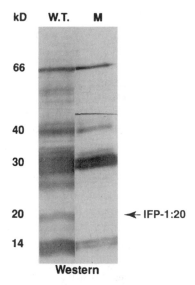

Western

FIGURE 9 Western blot analysis of wild-type (WT) and mutant (M) fibrils of *M. xanthus* with MAb 2105 (30).

its N-terminal sequence. Smith and Dworkin (30) constructed a corresponding oligonucleotide probe and cloned and sequenced the gene. The cloned fragment contained 993 bp and one open reading frame coding for 164 amino acids with a collective molecular mass of 19 kDa. To our initial disappointment, however, a homology search revealed no significant hits. Thus, this did not provide a clue as to the function of IFP-20. On the other hand, it did suggest the possibility of a novel and therefore interesting protein.

Smith and Dworkin (30) generated a site-directed mutation in the gene and did thereby obtain a clue as to the function of the fibril protein. The mutant had a number of interesting properties. The isolated mutant fibrils when examined by Western blot (immunobot) were totally lacking the 20-kDa band present as one of the components of the wild-type fibril proteins (Fig. 9). This was consistent with the fact that the cloned gene has a molecular mass of 19 kDa. Not unexpectedly, the fibril mutation interfered with normal development as measured by fruiting body formation (Fig. 10). The cells were delayed in aggregation and never formed fully mature

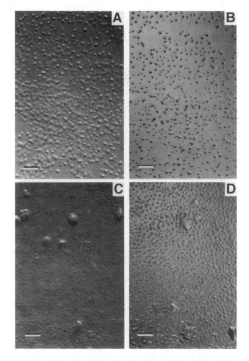

FIGURE 10 Fruiting body formation in wild-type cells of *M. xanthus* at 12 (A) and 48 h (B) compared with mutant cells at 12 (C) and 48 h (D). Bars, 500 μm (30).

fruiting bodies. In addition, the cells made only 14% of the normal complement of myxospores.

We then sought to determine whether the mutated protein generated any sort of morphological aberration in the fibrils. When cells bearing the IFP-20 mutation were viewed under the scanning electron microscope, however, the cells were devoid of fibrils, despite the fact that fibrils had been isolated from the mutant for the Western blot analysis. Apparently, during the critical point drying (part of the preparation for electron microscopy), the rapid flow of liquid CO_2 across the cells ripped the fibrils off the cell. Under these conditions, wild-type cells, in contrast, were able to retain their fibrils. Clearly, the IFP-20 mutation affected the stability of the cell-fibril interaction.

One of the aspects of social behavior in *M. xanthus* is what is referred to as *cohesion*. That is the ability of cells in liquid suspension to clump out of suspension in response to the presence of high levels of Mg^{2+}. This behavior is a laboratory mimic of the normal adhesive property that is a part of developmental aggregation. Recall that Chang and Dworkin (5) were able to rescue cohesion in the *dsp* mutant by addition of wild-type fibrils. Fibrils from the IFP-20 mutant, on the other hand, were completely unable to rescue cohesion of *dsp* (30).

When the kinetics of cohesion of cells with the IFP-20 mutation were compared with those of wild-type cells, there was, to our surprise, no difference. But, when the cohered cells were examined microscopically, a substantial difference did indeed appear (Fig. 11). Whereas wild-type cells cohered in a three-dimensional side-by-side fashion, the cells with the mutant fibrils cohered in a one-dimensional, end-to-end linear fashion. This may reflect a functional distinction that occurs during different stages of aggregation and indicate different modes of cell-to-cell signal exchange.

Søgaard-Andersen and Kaiser (31) have proposed that the exchange of the C signal,

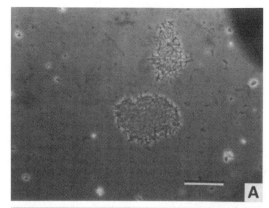
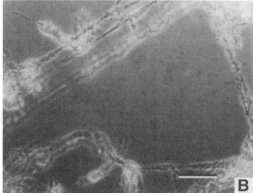

FIGURE 11 Phase contrast observation of wild-type (A) and mutant cells (B) under cohesion conditions. Bars, 50 μm (30).

which occurs at least 6 h after the initiation of development, takes place as a result of the end-to-end orientation of the cells. They have demonstrated (31) that exchange of the C signal induces an increase in methylation of FrzCD, a signal-transducing protein that regulates the rate of reversal of movement (23). The result of this sequence of events is that the characteristic back-and-forth movement of individual cells is transformed by the methylation to a more unidirectional movement.

We propose that this is preceded by an earlier side-by-side orientation, during which the A signal, which monitors early cell density, is exchanged. This side-by-side orientation is mediated by the peritrichous fibrils and has been disrupted by the mutation in the IFP-20 fibril protein. Consistent with this interpretation, the expression of an early Tn*5-lac* reporter gene Ω*4521* is inhibited by the IFP-20 mutation, while that of a later expressed gene Ω*4500* is unaffected (Fig. 12).

ADP-Ribosylation by the Fibrils

Our biochemical approach to understanding the role of fibrils focused on the ability of *M. xanthus* to carry out ADP-ribosylation. Cholera, diphtheria, and pertussis toxins, among others, exert their effects by ADP-ribosylating various critical host proteins such as G proteins and EF-2 (22). In addition, ADP-ribosylation has been shown to play a role in the normal regulation of some prokaryotic processes such as dinitrogen fixation in the genus *Rhodospirillum* (10), and Reich and Schoolnik (25) have demonstrated the presence of an ADP-ribosyltransferase in *Vibrio fischeri*, the symbi-

otic partner of the squid *Euprymna scolopes*, and have suggested that it functions as a signaling molecule.

Eastman and Dworkin (8) had shown earlier that *M. xanthus* could carry out ADP-ribosylation and that the pattern of ADP-ribosylation changed during development. Preliminary results indicated that a substantial fraction of the activity was in the particulate fraction. Upon further examination, it turned out that isolated, purified fibrils (Fig. 7) were capable of carrying out ADP-ribosylation. The fibrils were exposed to ^{32}P-labeled NAD, the substrate for ADP-ribosyl transferase, and then examined on a two-dimensional gel by Western blot and autoradiography (Fig. 13). A 30-kDa protein was labeled as the presumptive substrate for the ADP-ribosyltransferase. The protein was subjected to mild alkaline hydrolysis to release the ADP-ribose, which was then identified as such by high-pressure liquid chromotagraphy.

To rationalize the ability of an extracellular appendage such as the fibril to contain both the ADP-ribosyltransferase as well as its protein substrate, we propose that the fibrils may be acting as tactile antennae and that the ADP-ribosylation is part of the signal-transduction mechanism that perceives the presence of a solid surface, presumably a closely juxtaposed cell (Fig. 14). It will now be interesting to see which of the fibrillar proteins are identified with the ADP-ribosyltransferase, which correspond to its substrate, which (if any) to a corresponding esterase, and their possible role in the proposed transduction of a physical signal.

Reich and Schoolnik (25) have demonstrated that *V. fischeri* excreted ADP-ribosyltransferase as part of the interactive mechanism between it and its host, the squid *E. scolopes*. They proposed that the ADP-ribosyltransferase may function as a signaling molecule in that symbiosis. In addition, Ginnochio et al. (14) have presented SEM photos of *Salmonella typhimurium* with fibrils that are remarkably similar to the fibrils we are discussing (Fig. 15). They showed that contact

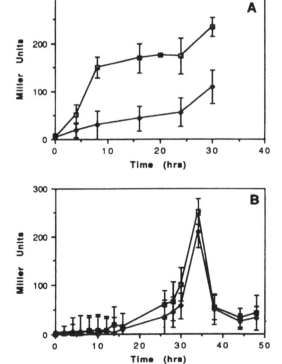

FIGURE 12 Effects of the IFP-20 mutation on expression of Ω*4521* (A) and Ω*4500* (B). □, expression in the parent strain; ◆, expression in IFP-20 (30).

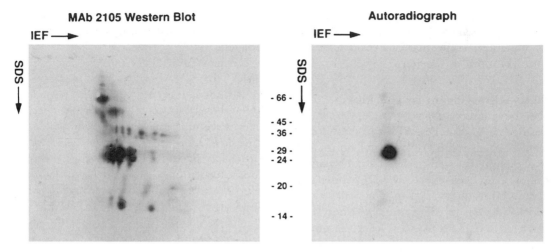

FIGURE 13 Two-dimensional sodium dodecyl sulfate-polyacrylamide gel electrophoresis of the ADP-ribosylated fibrillar proteins showing that the same protein was both ADP-ribosylated and immunoreactive with MAb 2105. The ^{32}P-labeled ADP-ribosylated proteins were separated by two-dimensional gel electrophoresis, blotted to nitrocellulose, and subjected to autoradiography. (A) Western immunoblot of fibrillar proteins probed with MAb 2105. The arrow points to the spot that is equivalent to the radioactively labeled spot in Fig. 2B. (B) Autoradiograph of immunoblot (15).

between the *Salmonella* and host epithelial cells induced formation of the fibrils. It seems clear that these sorts of fibrils may be more widespread among those bacteria that need to perceive the physical presence of another cell.

Tyrosine Kinase in *M. xanthus*

The last point of intersection between myxobacterial behavior and pathogenic mechanisms that I wish to mention focuses on tyrosine kinase. Tyrosine kinase has been shown to play a role as part of the host defense mechanisms against bacterial pathogens. YopH, coding for tyrosine phosphatase and part of the pathogenicity island in *Yersinia pseudotuberculosis* and *Yersinia enterocolitica* is transported across cell membranes via a type III secretion system and mediates dephosphorylation of tyrosine residues in host cells, thus compromising the host defense. Activation of the system depends on cell-cell contact between the bacterial pathogen and its eukaryotic host (24).

While tyrosine kinase is characteristically associated with eukaryotic systems, the dividing line has become increasingly blurred with tyrosine phosphorylation shown to be present in *M. xanthus* (9) and *Pseudomonas*, *Acinetobacter*, *Clostridium*, *Rhodomicrobium*, and *Streptomyces* spp. (32). Frasch and Dworkin (9) have shown not only that tyrosine kinase is present in *M. xanthus*, but also that it seems to be involved in development.

The first clue that there might be a protein tyrosine kinase came with the finding of an effect of 100-μM sodium vanadate, a specific inhibitor of protein tyrosine phosphatase on the general pattern of protein phosphorylation. An antiphosphotyrosine MAb and Western blot analysis was then used to demonstrate the presence of phosphorylated tyrosine in cells (Fig. 16). The specificity of the recognition was demonstrated by showing that the phosphorylation could be blocked with free phosphotyrosine but not with either phosphoserine or phosphothreonine (Fig. 16).

The relevance of the process to myxobacterial development was demonstrated by tracking the patterns of tyrosine phosphorylation during development and in different

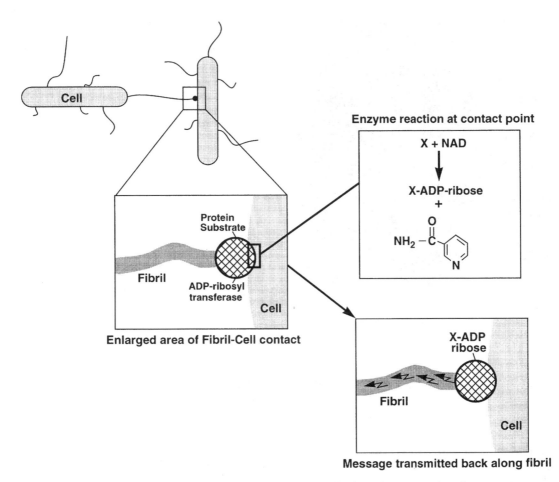

FIGURE 14 Model for the role of ADP-ribosylation by fibrils as the sensor of tactile interaction.

signaling mutants (Fig. 17). Phosphorylation of the 83-kDa protein disappeared almost immediately after the initiation of development, the 40-kDa band disappeared shortly thereafter, and a new band at 20 kDa appeared at the time of myxosporulation, i.e., 18 to 24 h. When the pattern of tyrosine phosphorylation was examined in a set of signaling mutants blocked at different times during development, the 83-kDa band, which disappeared early during normal development, persisted in all the mutants for at least 24 h, the 20-kDa band never appeared, and the 40-kDa band varied from one mutant to the other. Thus, protein tyrosine kinase joins protein serine and threonine kinases (32) as typical eukaryotic protein kinases present in *M. xanthus*.

The presence of a tyrosine kinase and its cognate tyrosine phosphatase in *M. xanthus* raises questions about the evolutionary origin of tyrosine phosphorylation. Tyrosine phosphorylation was first associated with transforming retroviruses. It was assumed that tyrosine kinases evolved at the time of eukaryotic multicellularity and that the viruses acquired the kinase by lateral transmission from their eukaryotic hosts and later adapted the enzyme for their own use. The presence of tyrosine kinase in bacteria suggests that tyrosine phosphorylation may have evolved much earlier. It has been calculated that the myxobacteria emerged between 650–800 million years ago (27) and approximately 1.5 billion years ago (19) and thus probably preceded the

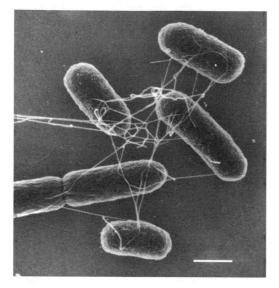

FIGURE 15 High-resolution SEM of *Salmonella ty-phimurium* 30 min after infecting a culture of MDCK cells. Bar, 0.5 μm (14).

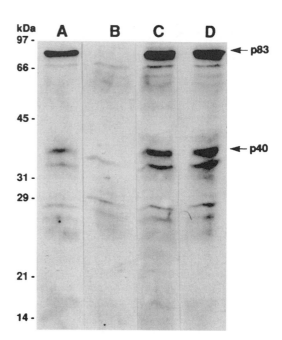

FIGURE 16 Tyrosine phosphorylation in *M. xanthus*. Demonstrated by antiphosphotyrosine monoclonal antibody and Western blot analysis (lane A). Blocking by free phosphotyrosine (lane B). No effect of free phosphoserine (lane C) or phosphothreonine (lane D) (9).

emergence of multicellular eukaryotes, whose appearance has been estimated to have taken place 700 million years ago.

UNRESOLVED QUESTIONS AND DIRECTIONS FOR FUTURE RESEARCH

It has become increasingly clear that extracellular fibrils of bacteria in general play a role in cell-cell interactions. These have been dem-onstrated in pathogenesis, biofilm interactions, and bacterial-plant interactions. In particular, they play a role in the social behavior of *M. xanthus*. Is their role that of physically maintaining close juxtaposition of cells? Do the fi-

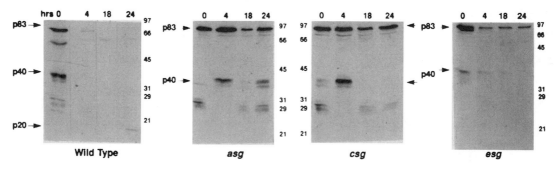

FIGURE 17 Tyrosine phosphorylation during development of *M. xanthus* and the effects of various developmental mutations. Changes in tyrosine phosphorylation during development were examined by antiphosphotyrosine monoclonal antibody and Western blot analysis of membrane preparations from 0-, 4-, 18-, and 24-h developmental cells of wild type and the *asg*, *csg*, and *esg* developmental signaling mutants (9).

brils also participate in detection of cell proximity? Do the fibrils serve as tactile antennae?

The most pressing questions pertain to the mechanisms whereby the fibril is able to perceive the presence of an apposing surface and how that perception is transduced into a cellular response. Hildebrandt et al. (15) have proposed that ADP-ribosylation plays a role in that process. Whether that is so and, if so, how it happens remain to be determined. In that context, how *M. xanthus* makes NAD, the substrate for the ADP-ribosylation, available outside the cell is an interesting problem. Behmlander and Dworkin (2) have previously shown that the formation of the fibrils is a density-dependent process and have suggested that the density-sensing process may be mediated by the polar pili of the cells. Whether or not that is the case remains to be determined. How the fibrils are synthesized and assembled outside the cells remains to be examined.

Smith and Dworkin (30) have proposed that at least two cell-cell cohesion mechanisms play a role in signal exchange during development. It needs to be determined whether or not the fibrils indeed play a role in one of these and whether or not the cell-cell contact mediated by the fibrils facilitates exchange of one or more of the developmental signals.

It is now clear that tyrosine kinase is present in cells of *M. xanthus* and that the pattern of protein tyrosine phosphorylation changes during development (9). Whether or not it is part of a kinase cascade and of the complex of signal-transducing mechanisms during development remains to be determined.

CONCLUSION

The unique social behavior of *M. xanthus* during its life cycle and the fact that it exists much of the time as a rudimentary multicellular organism has led to the hypothesis that the myxobacteria may have been one of Nature's earliest experiments with multicellularity. The cell-cell interactions characteristic of myxobacterial multicellularity may have been a

necessary precursor to the development of equivalent interactions required for symbiotic associations as well as for the kinds of cell-cell interactions required for pathogenesis.

REVIEWS AND KEY PAPERS

Arnold, J. W., and L. J. Shimkets. 1988. Cell surface properties correlated with cohesion in *Myxococcus xanthus*. *J. Bacteriol.* **170:**5771–5777.

Behmlander, R. M., and M. Dworkin. 1991. Extracellular fibrils and contact-mediated interactions in *Myxococcus xanthus*. *J. Bacteriol.* **173:**7810–7821.

Dworkin, M. 1996. Recent advances in the social and developmental biology of the myxobacteria. *Microbiol. Rev.* **60:**70–102.

Frasch, S. C., and M. Dworkin. 1996. Tyrosine phosphorylation in *Myxococcus xanthus*, a multicellular prokaryote. *J. Bacteriol.* **178:**4084–4088.

Hildebrandt, K., D. Eastman, and M. Dworkin. 1997. ADP-ribosylation by the extracellular fibrils of *Myxococcus xanthus*. *Mol. Microbiol.* **23:**231–235.

REFERENCES

1. **Arnold, J. W., and L. J. Shimkets.** 1988. Cell surface properties correlated with cohesion in *Myxococcus xanthus*. *J. Bacteriol.* **170:**5771–5777.
2. **Behmlander, R. M., and M. Dworkin.** 1991. Extracellular fibrils and contact mediated interactions in *Myxococcus xanthus*. *J. Bacteriol.* **173:** 7810–7821.
3. **Behmlander, R. M., and M. Dworkin.** 1994. Biochemical and structural analyses of the extracellular matrix fibrils of *Myxococcus xanthus*. *J. Bacteriol.* **176:**6295–6303.
4. **Behmlander, R. M., and M. Dworkin.** 1994. Integral proteins of the extracellular matrix fibrils of *Myxococcus xanthus*. *J. Bacteriol.* **176:**6304–6311.
5. **Chang, B.-Y., and M. Dworkin.** 1994. Isolated fibrils rescue cohesion and development in the *dsp* mutant of *Myxococcus xanthus*. *J. Bacteriol.* **176:**7190–7196.
6. **Dworkin, M.** 1986. *Developmental Biology of the Bacteria*. The Benjamin/Cummings Publishing Co., Inc., Menlo Park, Calif.
7. **Dworkin, M.** 1996. Recent advances in the social and developmental biology of the myxobacteria. *Microbiol. Rev.* **60:**70–102.
8. **Eastman, D., and M. Dworkin.** 1994. Endogenous ADP-ribosylation during development of the prokaryote *Myxococcus xanthus*. *Microbiology* **140:**3167–3176.
9. **Frasch, S. C., and M. Dworkin.** 1996. Tyrosine phosphorylation in *Myxococcus xanthus*, a

multicellular prokaryote. *J. Bacteriol.* **178:**4084–4088.

10. **Fu, H. R., H. Burris, and G. P. Roberts.** 1990. Reversible ADP-ribosylation is demonstrated to be a regulatory mechanism in prokaryotes by heterologous expression. *Proc. Natl. Acad. Sci. USA* **87:**1720–1724.

11. **Gill, J. S., and M. Dworkin.** 1986. Cell surface antigens during submerged development of *Myxococcus xanthus* examined with monoclonal antibodies. *J. Bacteriol.* **168:**505–511.

12. **Gill, J. S., and M. Dworkin.** 1988. Isolation of additional antibodies directed against cell surface antigens of *Myxococcus xanthus* cells undergoing submerged development. *J. Bacteriol.* **170:**5953–5955.

13. **Gill, J. E., E. Stellwag, and M. Dworkin.** 1985. Monoclonal antibodies against cell surface antigens of developing cells of *Myxococcus xanthus. Ann. Inst. Pasteur/Microbiol.* (Paris) **136A:**11–18.

14. **Ginnocchio, C. C., S. B. Olmsted, C. L. Wells, and J. Galan.** 1994. Contact with epithelial cells induces the formation of surface appendages on *Salmonella typhimurium. Cell* **76:**717–724.

15. **Hildebrandt, K., D. Eastman, and M. Dworkin.** 1997. ADP-ribosylation by the extracellular fibrils of *Myxococcus xanthus. Mol. Microbiol.* **23:**231–235.

16. **Hodgkin, J., and D. Kaiser.** 1977. Cell-to-cell stimulation of movement in nonmotile mutants of *Myxococcus. Proc. Natl. Acad. Sci. USA* **74:**2938–2942.

17. **Hodgkin, J., and D. Kaiser.** 1979. Genetics of gliding motility in *Myxococcus xanthus*: two gene systems control movement. *Mol. Gen. Genet.* **171:**177–191.

18. **Kaiser, D.** 1979. Social gliding is correlated with the presence of pili in *Myxococcus xanthus. Proc. Natl. Acad. Sci. USA* **76:**5952–5956.

19. **Kaiser, D.** 1986. Control of multicellular development: *Dictyostelium* and *Myxococcus. Ann. Rev. Genet.* **20:** 539–566.

20. **Kaiser, D., and L. Kroos.** 1993. Intercellular signaling, p. 257–284. *In* M. Dworkin and D. Kaiser (ed.), *Myxobacteria II.* American Society for Microbiology, Washington, D.C.

21. **Kaplan, H. B., and L. Plamann.** 1996. A *Myxococcus xanthus* cell density-sensing system required for multicellular development. *FEMS Microbiol. Lett.* **139:**89–95.

22. **Krueger, K. M., and J. T. Barbieri.** 1995. The family of bacterial ADP-ribosylating exotoxins. *Clin. Microbiol. Rev.* **8:**34–47.

23. **McBride, M. J., T. Köhler, and D. R. Zusman.** 1992. Methylation of FrzCD, a methyl-accepting taxis protein of *Myxococcus xanthus*, is correlated with factors affecting cell behavior. *J. Bacteriol.* **174:**4246–4257.

24. **Pettersson, J., R. Nordfelth, E. Dubinina, T. Bergman, M. Gustafsson, K. E. Magnusson, and H. Wolf-Watz.** 1996. Modulation of virulence factor expression by pathogen target cell contact. *Science* **272:**1231–1233.

25. **Reich, K. A., and G. K. Schoolnik.** 1996. Halovibrin, secreted from the light organ symbiont *Vibrio fischeri*, is a member of a new class of ADP-ribosyltransferases. *J. Bacteriol.* **178:**209–215.

26. **Shimkets, L. J.** 1986. Correlation of energy-dependent cell cohesion with social motility in *Myxococcus xanthus. J. Bacteriol.* **166:**837–841.

27. **Shimkets, L. J.** 1993. The myxobacterial genome, p. 85–107. *In* M. Dworkin and D. Kaiser (ed.), *Myxobacteria II.* American Society for Microbiology, Washington, D.C.

28. **Shimkets, L. J., and M. Dworkin.** 1981. Excreted adenosine is a cell density signal for the initiation of fruiting body formation in *Myxococcus xanthus. Dev. Biol.* **84:**51–60.

29. **Singer, M., and D. Kaiser.** 1995. Ectopic production of guanosine penta- and tetraphosphate can initiate early developmental gene expression in *Myxococcus xanthus. Genes Dev.* **9:**1633–1644.

30. **Smith, D. R., and M. Dworkin.** 1997. A mutation that affects fibril protein, development, cohesion and gene expression in *Myxococcus xanthus. Microbiology* **143:**3683–3692.

31. **Søgaard-Andersen, L., and D. Kaiser.** 1996. C factor, a cell-surface-associated intercellular signaling protein, stimulates the cytoplasmic Frz signal transduction system in *Myxococcus xanthus. Proc. Natl. Acad. Sci. USA* **93:**2675–2679.

32. **Zhang, C.-C.** 1996. Bacterial signalling involving eukaryotic-type protein kinases. *Mol. Microbiol.* **20:**9–15.

THE PLASTICITY OF MARINE BACTERIA: ADAPTATIONS TO HIGH- AND LOW-NUTRIENT HABITATS

Ronald Weiner

2

Microorganisms are highly regulated to accommodate changing environments. Adaptations to extreme physical environments have been well documented, and most of the biota adapted to these niches have become inflexible specialists. However, environmental extremes also include the shift between natural ecosystems and eucaryotic hosts and ecosystems in which nutrients are plentiful versus those in which nutrient levels are scarce. When an organism travels from one niche to another, it may undergo substantial transformation. The morphology may change, and after morphogenesis, the emerged form may hardly resemble its progenitor. The synthesis of entire organelles—such as flagella, capsules, and fimbriae—may be turned on or off. Multiple membrane proteins or enzyme systems can be down- or upregulated. Each adaptation can make the organism a survival specialist in the new environment.

The cell changes may be temporally regulated—as an insect is preprogramed to enter into a complex life cycle—or occur in response to environmental stimuli—as melanin synthesis by animals—or a combination of both. In the marine environment particularly, the developmental cycle of much biota is directed primarily toward finding nutrients in a relatively carbon-poor ecosystem. Among the eucaryotes, the oyster exemplifies this theorem. Its larval stage is motile and directed toward the search for a suitable surface upon which to set (33). If it does not encounter a substratum coated with a suitable biofilm (64) within approximately 15 days, it dies while searching (67). Only after being cued by some property of the biofilm and cementing down (set) can it metamorphose into a young adult (spat). This behavior favors placing the sessile adult on a fertile substratum, which is scarcer in the ocean than in terrestrial soil. Such adaptations have been long associated with higher organisms; however, only recently has the magnitude of changes associated with microorganisms been recognized. This adaptability may also have a profound influence on disease processes and on emerging diseases (14).

Among the eucaryotic microorganisms, one cogent example that has affected the Chesapeake Bay, near my institution in the United States, is the sudden emergence (or recognition) of a dinoflagellate, *Pfiesteria* sp., which produces toxins that destroy tissue and

Ronald Weiner, Department of Cell Biology and Molecular Genetics, University of Maryland, College Park, MD 20742.

Microbial Ecology and Infectious Disease, Edited by Eugene Rosenberg
©1999 American Society for Microbiology, Washington, D.C.

affect the nervous system of animals. Its free-living form is enriched to ever-greater numbers by increased runoff of nutrients from farms and other human activities that abut the bay. *Pfiesteria* has a complex life cycle encompassing some 24 flagellated, ameboid, and encysted stages, the motile and a few other stages being toxic to fish or other animals (10). Some excretion from an animal induces toxicity, as the dinoflagellate becomes a predator, taking advantage of the presence of fish. The rest of the time it is a benign autotroph, saprophyte, or cyst.

Pfiesteria is, by no means, the only example. Other eucaryotic microorganisms have recently been highly visible in terms of their impact on the Chesapeake Bay region. To cite one, *Perkinsus marinus*, which has ravaged the once abundant oyster population, has two different life cycles, one in the oyster, where it causes Dermo, and the other a resting form in the less nutrient rich water column (22).

Showing that procaryotes also have complex developmental cycles, we now turn to the focus of this paper, two examples of gram-negative, marine bacteria that exemplify different types of development. *Hyphomonas* sp. has swarm and reproductive phases (Fig. 1). Each follows in obligate temporal sequence. The former is suited to low-nutrient regimens, the latter to high-nutrient regimens. Species 2-40 has one cell cycle when it is grown in glucose and another environmentally induced program when complex polysaccharides are the only available carbon. In both types of bacteria, there are significant morphological and physiological contrasts between the high and low available-nutrient specialists.

NUTRIENTS AND NUTRIENT-UTILIZING BACTERIA IN NATURAL WATERS

The offshore marine habitat is generally more stable than other ecosystems. With rare but notable exceptions such as the hydrothermal vents, there are relatively few major fluctuations in salinity, temperature, predation, oxygen concentration, and other factors. Pressure changes are constant. Therefore, as is true for many econiches but even more so in marine environments, the greatest challenge to marine bacteria is to obtain food. Much of the bacterial plasticity is involved with surviving famine, establishment in oases that offer feast, and special utilization of compounds and biopolymers recalcitrant to, unavailable to, or toxic to higher biota.

Nutrient concentrations in lakes, ponds, rivers, estuaries, and inshore ocean are generally high (copious), although not all sources are readily accessible. (As is discussed below, procaryotes have evolved ingenious morphological and physiological strategies to utilize insoluble and/or recalcitrant nutrients there.) Organisms autochthonous to nutrient-rich environments have been termed *copiotrophs* (47) or *eutrophs*.

In the open ocean (pelagic zone), nutrients are scarce (oligoconcentrations) with <0.1 mg of carbon per liter of seawater (0.000001%; [29]). This includes measurements ranging from 2 to 80 μg (0.002–0.08 mg) and usually below 10 μg of glucose per liter of seawater. In the euphotic zone (surface waters where photosynthesis occurs), there are approximately 50 μg of glucose, 50 μg of other sugars, 60 μg of amino acids, and 50 μg of other usable carbon (total of 0.21 mg of carbon per liter of seawater [29]). Species that can heterotrophically metabolize exogenous nutrients in these waters have been termed *oligotrophs*. A proposed working definition of oligotrophs is those organisms that can be cultivated in the laboratory at concentrations of 1 to 15 mg of carbon per liter (47). While this concentration range is 10–>150-fold greater than that measured in the pelagic zone and >5-fold greater than that measured in the euphotic zone, it is also approximately 1,000-fold lower than that used to cultivate copiotrophs in the laboratory.

Obviously, the bacterial species that can both flourish in feast and thrive in famine will have very different phenotypes when it is in the pelagic zone than when it is in nutrient-rich zones. The special properties of oligo-

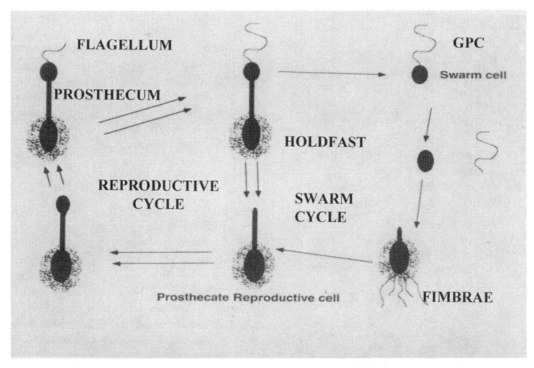

FIGURE 1 Representation of the biphasic life cycle of *Hyphomonas* MHS-3. The swarm cycle is shown with a single arrow; the reproductive cycle with double arrows. Temporalities of the syntheses of adhesive structures are represented.

trophs that tailor them to such low-nutrient habitats are listed in Table 1. They all logically entail physiological and morphological adaptations that bring more nutrients into the cell, enable more-efficient nutrient utilization, provide more flexibility as to which nutrients can be used, and channel utilization toward cellular maintenance.

On surfaces, especially those supporting biofilms (37), and on small, floating, condensed particles of organic matter ("marine snow"), nutrient concentrations are often considerably higher and represent the main nonsymbiotic "oasis" in the "pelagic desert" (59). Biofilms consist of adherent microorganisms (15), exopolymeric substances (EPS; often composed primarily of capsular exopolysaccharide [11]) and, sometimes, higher organisms including algae, fungi, and invertebrates. The EPS is a nutrient sink, sequestering ions and macromolecules (18, 33).

TABLE 1 Selected general characteristics of oliogotrophic bacteria

Class	Property
Morphological	Small cell size (high surface/ volume ratio)
	Storage bodies, adhesive envelopes, and flagella
Physiological	Catabolize more than one carbon source simultaneously
	Low anabolic rates
	Low energy charge
Macromolecular	High-affinity transporters
	More unsaturated membrane fatty acids
	Lower turnover
	More transporters

SURVIVAL STRATEGIES OF MARINE BACTERIA

Many marine bacteria are motile, arguably to seek out nutrient-richer surfaces. To adhere to these surfaces and participate in biofilm formation, a number of different organelles can be synthesized, especially including fimbriae, capsules, flagella (dual purpose), and sticky envelopes or S-layers (11, 30, 56). Like the oyster (noted above) that has a larval stage with one injunction, namely to find a fertile home, many species of bacteria seek nutrient-rich surfaces where they can reproduce (9, 72). As discussed elsewhere in this volume, others form some symbiosis with biota, ranging from mutualistic to parasitic (disease causing). Others, still, are chemo- or photo-autotrophic.

Perhaps the more challenging problem, however, remains survival in the "pelagic desert" (24). Bacteria can utilize endogenous metabolites including polyalkanoates, nucleic acid, and polyphosphate, often synthesizing special granules for their storage (17). Other bacteria become metabolically dormant, an active process that is covered elsewhere in this volume. Lastly, pelagic wanderers may have oligotrophic capability and use the available exogenous nutrients in modulated metabolic activity. There are not always clear-cut demarcations between strategies, and species may employ combinations of them (31). Some of the metabolically modulated cells have properties that uniquely define them (Table 2) and have been aptly termed growth precursor cells (GPCs) (20). Because this cell type is not

reproductive, they have also been labeled viable but not culturable (12), a phrase that has clinical implications and carries an appropriate epidemiological warning in the case of pathogens in the marine environment. When nutrient concentrations permit, GPCs become reproductive cells (Table 2).

Vibrio is an example of one genus that adapts to both oligotrophic and copiotrophic nutrient regimens, including a rugose form, contributing to biofilm formation (43). As also discussed elsewhere in this volume, *Vibrio's* presentation in nutrient-rich animal hosts is very different from that in the open water where it forms oligotrophic ultracells (32) and/or becomes a GPC (20). This process is externally regulated, as are 2-40 adaptations, discussed below. *Vibrio* sp. do not program an obligate GPC stage into their life cycles. It is a noncompulsory form, believed to be induced as an environmental sensory response. A genus of bacteria that obligately form GPC as part of their developmental cycle is *Hyphomonas*.

Hyphomonas (Prosthecate, Budding, Marine Bacteria)

Hyphomonas species are marine procaryotes that bud at the distal tip of a prosthecum (40, 41) and grow heterotrophically, using proteins and amino acids (25). This genus is widely distributed in the oceans (40, 65) and is important in the nutritional chain of several types of habitats, particularly in the ability to adapt to

TABLE 2 Properties of nutritionally adapted cell types

Property	Cell type		
	Growth-precursor	Reproductive	Transition phase
Replication	No	Yes	No
Strategy	k	R	S
Energy charge	Low	High	Low
Protein synthesis	Little	Yes	Yes
Niche	Planktonic	Adherent	Newly hostile
DNA replication	No	Yes	Yes

stressful conditions, including low nutrient concentrations (44).

Hyphomonas species have been isolated from several different hydrothermal vent basins (26), from the deep sea, and from surface waters (38). Some species form rosettes (i.e., mother cells stick to one another with prosthecea pointing outward in a floral pattern), suggesting a spatially localized capsular adhesin (structure that adheres the bacterium to other organisms or to surfaces, in this case nonspecifically). Some *Hyphomonas* species (e.g., *H. jannaschiana*) are facultative barophiles (16), growing more rapidly at 300 atm (1 atm = 101.29 kPa) than at 1 atm. They have a maximum growth temperature of 70°C at 200 atm. Perhaps most importantly, *Hyphomonas* spp. are ubiquitous colonizers of underwater surfaces (33, 60).

Marine Bacterium 2-40 and ICPs

There is another type of nutrient limitation to be considered, aside from paucity. In some cases, potential nutrients are copious but not readily utilizable. Some species of microorganisms specialize in the degradation of recalcitrant compounds to derive energy and/or carbon from them (recycle them). Examples include inorganic compounds such as atmospheric nitrogen and, in the case of carbon, insoluble complex polysaccharides (ICPs).

It is not a trivial matter to degrade ICPs, for they pose several challenges (71). Due to insolubility and complexation with other compounds, the bonds are not always accessible. There are also different types of bonds, which require bringing a number of different enzymes to bear (8). *Clostridium thermocellum* solves the degradation of cellulose (6) by synthesizing structures (cellulosomes) that arrange degradative enzymes in a surface array (4) together with substrate-binding proteins (see review by Béguin and Lemaire [7]). Thus, direct contact with the substrate is established to take advantage of momentary solubilization of parts of the molecule, and a number of different enzymes are optimally arrayed for an ordered attack. Cellulosome synthesis represents a

large commitment of the cell's resources, since many structures are synthesized, each with >26 different proteins. Therefore, it would not be surprising to find the commitment to their synthesis to be highly regulated.

We have recently obtained evidence that this strategy may not be limited to terrestrial bacteria. Periphytic marine/estuarine bacterium strain 2-40 (2-40) was isolated growing on salt marsh grass, *Spartina alterniflora*, from a salt marsh near the Chesapeake Bay. It is a strictly aerobic, gram-negative, pleomorphic, rod-shaped bacterium. The organism has an average size of 0.5 μm wide by 1.5 to 3.0 μm long when utilizing monosaccharide carbon sources. It is motile by a single polar flagellum, has a G+C content of 45.66 mol%, and utilizes carbohydrates for growth. Like many estuarine bacteria, it can tolerate a wide variety of temperatures (5–40°C), pH, and salinity (2–10% sea salts) (2). Cells synthesize a black melanin pigment during late exponential-stationary phases of growth (28) and may become elongated or even filamentous (70).

Although it has been suggested that it be assigned to the genus *Alteromonas* on the basis of its phenotypic characteristics (2), its fatty acid and membrane protein profile along with its 16S RNA analysis suggests that it probably represents a new marine genus. In addition to synthesizing proteases, lipases, and tyrosinases (28), 2-40 can degrade to monosaccharides over 13 insoluble ICPs from plants, animals, and microorganisms, including agar, alginate, cellulose, carrageenan, chitin, glucan, laminarin, pectin, pullulan, starch, and xylan (68). The degradation of at least three of these correlate (69) with formation of cellulosome-like structures (5).

Bacteria that degrade any ICP are important in nature as participants in the carbon cycle. To cite only one example, billions of tons of chitin, composed of repeating β-1,4-linked N-acetyl-D-glucosamine (NAG) residues are deposited each year into the environment by insects, fungi, and crustaceans (1). Thus, it is the most abundant aminopolysaccharide in nature and second to cellulose in total ICP abundance. The configuration of chitin influences its accessibility to chitinase and thereby its degradation, colloidal chitin being more readily attacked and crystalline chitin being less susceptible (23).

There are three major configurations of chitin. The most abundant form (e.g., in invertebrate exoskeletons) is α-chitin, which is also the most stable form, since the NAG chains run antiparallel with extensive hydrogen bonding. The second form is β-chitin, in which the NAG chains are aligned in parallel sheets. The third configuration, γ-chitin (similar to peptidoglycan), is a mix of parallel and antiparallel sheets of NAG chains. Thus, chitin is recalcitrant to degradation due to insolubility, configuration, and bonding. It can also be cross-linked to proteins, glucans, or organic salts, adding to its recalcitrance (57). Even so, because of the abundance of chitin, hundreds of eucaryotic and procaryotic species can degrade it. Only one, however, 2-40, has been suggested, so far, to use the cellulosome strategy to do so. (It is speculated that many other species of bacteria also employ the ordered enzyme-array strategy but have not yet been identified.)

LIFE CYCLE AND MORPHOGENESIS OF HYPHOMONAS

Hyphomonas

Hyphomonas, like other prosthecate, budding bacteria, has a biphasic life cycle (Fig. 1) (58). The progeny (bud), the swarm cell, is motile by means of a single flagellum. It can chemotactically sense favorable areas such as nutrient-rich surfaces sometimes nearby; but it also has the capability to form distant colonies, because as a GPC (Table 2), it is well adapted to survive in the pelagic zone. Among other attributes, it has a low metabolic rate (21), has polyhydroxybutyrate storage reserves, and is microspherical (0.4 mm diameter). Thus, *Hyphomonas* obligately shed GPC progeny suited to survive the pelagic zone.

On the other hand, the prosthecate reproductive stage is morphologically and physio-logically equipped to establish, maintain, and survive in marine biofilms (13). The prosthecate form is larger than the swarm cell (the main body being a prolate spheroid 1 to 2 μm long, with a prosthecum 1 to 2 μm long and 0.2 μm wide). An amino acid-rich surface cues the swarm, GPCs, to differentiate into an adherent biofilm specialist (63) and to shift from the k-strategy to the R-strategy. Its energy charge increases (21), and it synthesizes a substantial number of new proteins (53, 54) and expresses new structures. Recently, we have extensively studied this transition and the temporality and spatiality of EPS expression in two species of *Hyphomonas*, MHS-3 from surface water and VP-6 from the Guaymas vent basin.

In MHS-3 (Fig. 1), as the prosthecum emerges from one pole, a comparatively extensive "holdfast" EPS is synthesized from the other (51) along with polar fimbriae (49). The EPS is expressed during the entire reproductive cell phase, while the fimbriae are transiently expressed (Fig. 1). The holdfast is involved in primary adhesion (termed *nonspecific adhesin* [50]) as well as in formation of the matrix of the biofilm. The holdfast was probed by immunoelectron microscopy, using monoclonal antibodies (MAbs) against *Hyphomonas* MHS-3 lipopolysaccharide (LPS) (49). These MAbs were used as a negative stain, based upon the premise that in short exposures to whole cells, the EPS would sterically hinder the approach of the MAb to its LPS target. In the case of strain MHS-3, the "holdfast" surrounds the entire mother cell but not the prosthecum (Fig. 2). The pelagic swarm cell does not synthesize holdfast. We also demonstrated this by semispecific EPS staining with gold-labeled *Bauhinia purpurea* lectin (49) and thin sections of polycationic ferritin-stained cells. Studies so far indicate that the onset of EPS deposition coincides precisely with the beginning of prosthecum outgrowth.

In the case of *Hyphomonas* VP-6, there is a significant variation on this theme (34, 35). There are two capsules. One is always present and surrounds the entire cell (Fig. 3). The

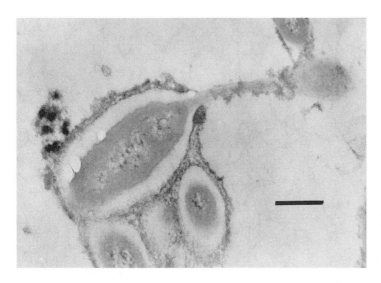

FIGURE 2 Thin section of polycationic ferritin-treated *Hyphomonas* MHS-3. Note the spatially defined capsule on the body of the prosthecate reproductive cell. Bar, 0.5 μm.

other is a temporally expressed, spatially defined, polar holdfast, present at the tip of the main body of the mother cell, opposite the prosthecum (Fig. 4). Both structures are adhesive. No fimbriae are synthesized.

A polar holdfast, capsular arrangement would allow the prosthecum to extend upward toward regions richer in nutrients and oxygen. Reproductive budding at the distal tip of the prosthecum allows the GPC progeny either to escape to the water column to establish a new community or to settle nearby to extend the existing community. Cells that remain trapped deep in the biofilm risk nutrient limitation, oxygen deprivation, and exposure to toxic substances. They become transition-phase cells (stationary-phase cells;

Table 2 and elsewhere in this volume). This "holdfast" survival strategy resembles that of another genus of procaryotes, *Caulobacter* (46). In *Caulobacter*, however, the polysaccharide is synthesized on the opposite pole (tip of the prosthecum), so that the reproductive cell body faces upward, with the prosthecum serving as the anchor (39).

To summarize, by virtue of its specialized physiology as well as morphology, the motile swarm cell is well adapted for survival in the oligotrophic water column, while the adherent, prosthecate, reproductive cell is suited to establish (3), maintain, and survive in marine biofilms. The respective types epitomize many of the properties set forth in Table 2. For example, the swarm cell has a low energy charge (21) and a high surface-to-volume ratio and does not synthesize detectable nucleic acid or protein (58). The reproductive cell has an R-strategy, and the shift from the k-strategy is temporal and requires the sensing of appropriate cues. This represents a good example of converging evolution with the oyster and other adherent marine invertebrates whose larval progeny are also obligately pelagic.

Some species of *Hyphomonas* may be even more even metabolically plastic, since they may also have autotrophic capability. We have demonstrated a functional Krebs cycle in *Hy-*

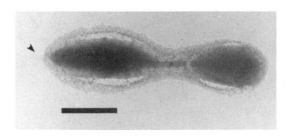

FIGURE 3 *Hyphomonas* VP-6 budding reproductive cell labeled with cationic ferritin. Arrow points to unlabeled holdfast. Bar, 1 μm.

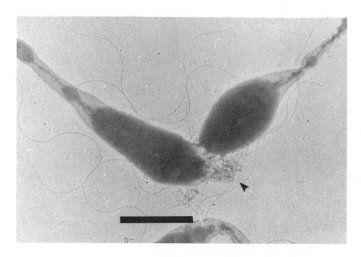

FIGURE 4 Two *Hyphomonas* VP-6 attached by fibrous holdfast. Cells were stained with uranyl acetate.

phomonas (19) and the synthesis of a protease (55) under heterotrophic environmental conditions; and the adherent reproductive stages, growing in microbial films, use protein and amino acids for energy. Autotrophically grown *Hyphomonas*, on the other hand, assimilate copious quantities of CO_2 (62). They grow with repeated transfers in water containing only salts, reduced sulfur, and 10% CO_2. There is no multiplication without sulfur and CO_2 (16). Such physiological plasticity confers unusual ability for primary surface colonization around the hydrothermal vent regions. Once a biofilm is established, *Hyphomonas* could switch to heterotrophic metabolism for rapid multiplication by using the accumulating organic material that may be sequestered by the growing biofilm (18, 66).

ICP-Degrading Bacterium 2-40

Unlike *Hyphomonas* development, 2-40 development does not follow a single obligate temporal sequence with two phases but actually two independent programs. The first is expressed when 2-40 utilizes simple sugars, especially glucose, and resembles the conventional morphogenic cell cycle described for other gram-negative rods such as *Escherichia* spp.; the alternate (and nonobligatory; i.e., facultative) phase is manifested when the bacterium must utilize ICPs for carbon and en-

ergy. Under these conditions, it expresses surface protuberances, which resemble the cellulosomes of *C. thermocellum*, when it is utilizing cellulose.

Both scanning and transmission electron microscopy reveal cell surface protuberances that correlate with the degradation of either agarose or chitin (Fig. 5) (61). Immunoelectron microscopy suggests that these structures contain agarase or chitinase (Fig. 6). Cells actively growing on ICPs may express hundreds of these structures, which we preliminarily term *degradosomes* (specifically, agarosome, chitinosomes, and alginosomes); 2-40 degradosome proteins cross-react (70) in Western blots with antisera against *C. thermocellum* cellulosome enzyme (52) or scaffolding protein (36).

When growing with ICPs, fine structure analysis reveals progressive changes in cell topology and morphogenesis during progression of cells to late stages of growth. These changes are consistent with the formation of ultramicrocells or GPCs (68). During starvation, 2-40 also forms membranous tubules (>20 μm long by 0.1 μm wide) putatively containing agarases or chitinases, structures that could be formed in response to local nutrient deprivation (68; unpublished data). *Hyphomonas* also forms them when growing in biofilms (48). These structures could protect and organize

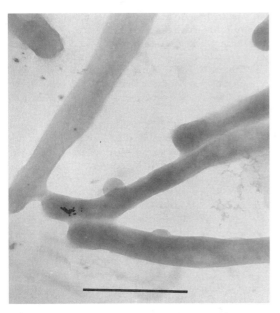

FIGURE 5 Fine structure of marine bacterium 2-40 grown with agarose as the sole carbon source. The nodes on the cell surface, viewed by transmission electron microscopy are degradosomes. Bar, 2 μm. Courtesy of L. Whitehead.

enzyme arrays for the degradation of more-distant, recalcitrant nutrient sources. Similar structures have recently been reported to be putatively involved in human (27) and fish

(45) pathogenesis, and it may be speculated that the same kinds of organized structures may be used to protect and optimize invasins.

UNANSWERED QUESTIONS

It has been relatively recently that bacteria have been discovered to be more developmentally complicated, interactively promiscuous, and structurally intricate than earlier notions of them as "bags of enzymes" would have us believe. Except for a small minority of the captive bacteria and an infinitesimal proportion of extant bacteria, understanding of their developmental capability remains descriptive, if it is known at all. Numerous ecological, genetic, and mechanistic questions remain compelling.

Does *Hyphomonas* swarm cell chemotaxis follow the two-component *Escherichia coli* model? How is this accomplished in a GPC? What is the mechanism of the coordinate regulation of the transition between GPC and reproductive cell? Is the *Caulobacter* model applicable? What cellular machinery participates in polar deposition of EPS? How does its chemistry make it a strong nonspecific adhesin?

In the case of 2-40, are different kinds of specialized degradosomes synthesized for each

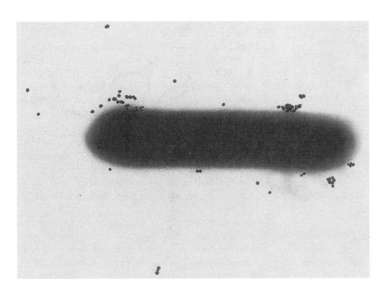

FIGURE 6 Immunolabeling of chitinosomes of marine bacterium 2-40. Cells were grown to middle logarithmic phase in chitin minimal medium before being exposed to colloidal gold-conjugated antichitinase antibody. Note the focus of label in chitinosomes that are not visible in this transmission electron micrograph. Courtesy of L. Whitehead.

of the 13 ICPs? What is the genetic organization for each enzyme system? Is there a single generic degradosome in which each enzyme system is packaged or are there specialized agarosomes, chitinosomes, etc., conserving only a part of the genetic machinery. What specifically cues the formation of ultracells? Are the degradative tubules representative of heretofore-undiscovered survival strategies? Are they involved in pathogenesis?

ACKNOWLEDGMENTS

S. Langille, E. Quintero, and L. Whitehead provided results that were incorporated into this paper. The research has been supported by grants from the Maryland Industrial Partnerships, NOAA/Maryland Sea Grant, and Oceanix Biosciences Corp.

REVIEWS AND KEY PAPERS

Béguin, P., and M. Lemaire. 1996. The cellulosome: an exocellular multiprotein complex specialized in cellulose degradation. *Crit. Rev. Biochem. Mol. Biol.* **31**:201–236.

Decho, A. W. 1990. Microbial exopolymer secretions in ocean environments: their role(s) in food webs and marine processes. *Oceanogr. Mar. Biol. Annu. Rev.* **28**:73–153.

Dow, C. S., R. Whittenbury, and N. G. Carr. 1983. The "shut down" or "growth precursor" cell—an adaptation for survival in a potentially hostile environment. *Symp. Soc. Gen. Microbiol.* **34**:187–247.

Harder, W., and L. Dijkhuizen. 1983. Physiological responses to nutrient limitation. *Annu. Rev. Microbiol.* **3**:1–23.

Kjelleberg, S., M. Hermansson, P. Marden, and G. Jones. 1987. The transient phase between growth and nongrowth of heterotrophic bacteria, with emphasis on the marine environment. *Annu. Rev. Microbiol.* **41**:25–49

Quintero, E. J., K. Busch, and R. M. Weiner. 1998. Spatial and temporal deposition of adhesive extracellular polysaccharide capsule and fimbriae by *Hyphomonas* MHS-3. *Appl. Environ. Microbiol.* **64**:1246–1255.

REFERENCES

1. Alexander, M. 1977. *Microbiology of Other Polysaccharides*, p. 188. John Wiley and Sons, Inc., New York.

2. Andrykovitch, G., and I. Marx. 1988. Isolation of a new polysaccharide-digesting bacterium from a salt marsh. *Appl. Environ. Microbiol.* **54**:3–4.

3. Baier, R., A. Meyer, V. DePalma, R. King, and M. Fornalik. 1983. Surface microfouling during the induction period. *J. Heat Trans.* **105**:618–624.

4. Bayer, E. A., E. Setter, and R. Lamed. 1985. Organization and distribution of the cellulosome in *Clostridium thermocellum*. *J. Bacteriol.* **163**:552–559.

5. Bayer, M. 1990. Visualization of the bacterial polysaccharide capsule. *Curr. Top. Microbiol. Immunol.* **150**:129–157.

6. Béguin, P., and J.-P. Aubert. 1994. The biological degradation of cellulose. *FEMS Microbiol. Rev.* **13**:25–58.

7. Béguin, P., and M. Lemaire. 1996. The cellulosome: an exocellular multiprotein complex specialized in cellulose degradation. *Crit. Rev. Biochem. Mol. Biol.* **31**:201–236.

8. Belas, R., D. Barlett, and M. Silverman. 1988. Cloning and gene replacement mutagenesis of a *Pseudomonas atlantica* agarase gene. *Appl. Environ. Microbiol.* **54**:30–37.

9. Brown, C. M., D. C. Ellwood, and J. R. Hunter. 1977. Growth of bacteria at surfaces: influence of nutrient limitation. *FEMS Microbiol. Lett.* **1**:163–166.

10. Burkholder, J. E. Noga, C. Hobbs, H. Glasgow, Jr., and S. Smith. 1992. New "phantom" dinoflagellate is the causative agent of major estuarine fish kills. *Nature* **358**:407–410.

11. Christensen, B. E. 1989. The role of extracellular polysaccharides in biofilms. *J. Biotechnol.* **10**:181–202.

12. Colwell, R. R., and A. Huq. 1994. Vibrios in the environment: viable but nonculturable *Vibrio cholerae*, p. 117–133. *In* I. K. Wachsmuth, P. A. Blake, and Ø. Olsvik (ed.), *Vibrio cholerae and Cholera: Molecular to Global Perspectives*. Washington, D.C.

13. Corpe, W. A. 1973. Microfouling: the role of primary film forming bacteria, p. 598–609. *In* R. F. Ackjer, B. F. Brown, J. R. DePalma, and W. P. Iverson (ed.), *Proceedings of the Third International Congress on Marine Corrosion Fouling*. Northwestern University Press, Evanston, Ill.

14. Costerton, J. W., K. J. Cheng, G. G. Geesey, T. Ladd, J. Nickel, M. Dasgupta and T. Marrie. 1987. Bacterial biofilms in nature and disease. *Annu. Rev. Microbiol.* **41**:435–464

15. Costerton, J. W., G. G. Geesey and K. J. Cheng. 1978. How bacteria stick. *Sci. Am.* **120**:86–95.

16. Dagasan, L. 1985. *Hyphomonas* sp. modulate morphology, physiology and membrane protein composition in response to changing growth temperatures: focus on *H. jannaschiana*. Ph.D. thesis. University of Maryland, College Park.

17. **Dawes, E. A.** 1985. Starvation survival and energy reserves, p. 43–74. *In* J. Slater, R. Whittenbury and J. Wimpenny, (ed.) *Bacteria in Their Natural Environments*. Society for General Microbiology, London.

18. **Decho, A. W.** 1990. Microbial exopolymer secretions in ocean environments: their role(s) in food webs and marine processes. *Oceanogr. Mar. Biol. Annu. Rev.* **28:**73–153.

19. **Devine, R. A., and R. M. Weiner.** 1990. *Hyphomonas* species metabolize amino acids using Krebs cycle enzymes. *Microbios* **62:**137–153.

20. **Dow, C. S., R. Whittenbury, and N. G. Carr.** 1983. The "shut down" or "growth precursor" cell—an adaptation for survival in a potentially hostile environment. *Symp. Soc. Gen. Microbiol.* **34:**187–247.

21. **Emala, M. A., and R. M. Weiner.** 1983. Modulation of adenylate energy charge during the swarmer cycle of *Hyphomicrobium neptunium*. *J. Bacteriol.* **153:**1558–1561.

22. **Gauthier J., and G. Vasta.** 1993. Continuous culture of the Eastern oyster parasite, *Perkinsus marinus*. *J. Invertebr. Pathol.* **62:**321–323.

23. **Gooday, G. W.** 1990. The ecology of chitin degradation. *Adv. Microb. Ecol.* **11:**387–430.

24. **Harder, W., and L. Dijkhuizen.** 1983. Physiological responses to nutrient limitation. *Annu. Rev. Microbiol.* **3:**1–23.

25. **Havenner, J., B. McCardell, and R. Weiner.** 1979. Development of defined, minimal and complete media for the growth of *Hyphomicrobium neptunium*. *Appl. Environ. Microbiol.* **38:**18–23.

26. **Jannasch, H. W., and C. O. Wirsen.** 1981. Morphological survey of microbial mats near deep sea hydrothermal vents. *Appl. Environ. Microbiol.* **41:**528–538.

27. **Kadurugamuwa, J. L., and T. J. Beveridge.** 1995. Virulence factors are released from *Pseudomonas aeruginosa* in association with membrane vesicles during normal growth and exposure to gentamicin: a novel mechanism of enzyme secretion. *J. Bacteriol.* **177:**3998–4008.

28. **Kelley, S. K., V. E. Coyne, D. D. Sledjeski, W. C. Fuqua, and R. M. Weiner.** 1990. Identification of a tyrosinase from a periphytic marine bacterium. *FEMS Microbiol. Lett.* **67:**275–280.

29. **Kennish, M. J.** 1989. *Practical Handbook of Marine Science*, Section 2: Chemical oceanography, p. 49–88. CRC Press, Inc., Boca Raton, Fla.

30. **Kjelleberg, S., and M. Hermansson.** 1984. Starvation-induced effects on bacterial surface characteristics. *Appl. Environ. Microbiol.* **48:**497–503.

31. **Kjelleberg, S., M. Hermansson, P. Marden, and G. Jones.** 1987. The transient phase between growth and nongrowth of heterotrophic bacteria, with emphasis on the marine environment. *Annu. Rev. Microbiol.* **41:**25–49.

32. **Kjelleberg, S., B. A. Humphrey, and K. C. Marshall.** 1982. Effect of interfaces on small, starved marine bacteria. *Appl. Environ. Microbiol.* **43:**1166–1172.

33. **Labare, M. L., R. M. Weiner, S. Coon, S. Mathias, and M. Walch.** 1997. Biofilms sequester tributyl tin from Chesapeake Bay waters to concentrations that block oyster development. *Appl. Environ. Microbiol.* **63:**4107–4110.

34. **Langille, S. L.** 1996. Capsular and holdfast extracellular polymeric substances of *Hyphomonas* strain VP-6 mediate adhesion to solid substrata. Ph.D. dissertation. University of Maryland, College Park.

35. **Langille, S. L., and R. M. Weiner.** 1998. Spatial and temporal deposition of *Hyphomonas* VP-6 capsules. *Appl. Environ. Microbiol.* **64:**2906–2913.

36. **Leibovitz, E., H. Ohayon, P. Gounon, and P. Béguin.** 1997. Characterization and subcellular localization of the *Clostridium thermocellum* scaffolding dockerin binding protein SdbA. *J. Bacteriol.* **179:**2519–2523.

37. **Marshall, K. C.** 1992. Biofilms: an overview of bacterial adhesion, activity, and control at surfaces. ASM News. **58:**202–207.

38. **Melick, M., K. Guthrie, R. Gherna and R. Weiner.** The addition of three new species to the genus *Hyphomonas:* molecular taxonomy reveals a heterogeneous taxon. In preparation.

39. **Merker, R., and J. Smit.** 1988. Characterization of the adhesive holdfast of marine and freshwater caulobacters. *Appl. Environ. Microbiol.* **54:**2078–2085.

40. **Moore, R. L.** 1981. The biology of *Hyphomicrobium* and other prosthecate, budding bacteria. *Annu. Rev. Microbiol.* **35:**567–594.

41. **Moore, R. L., and R. M. Weiner.** 1989. Genus *Hyphomonas*, p. 1904–1910. *In* J. T. Staley, M. P. Bryant, N. Pfenning, J. G. Holt, (ed.) *Bergey's Manual of Systematic Bacteriology*, vol. 3. The Williams & Wilkins Co., Baltimore.

42. **Moore, R. L., R. M. Weiner, and R. Gebers.** 1984. Genus *Hyphomonas* Pongratz 1957 nom. rev. emend. and *Hyphomonas polymorpha* Pongratz 1957 nom. rev. emend., and *Hyphomonas neptunium* (Leifson, 1964) comb. nov. emend. (*Hyphomicrobium neptunium*). *Int. J. Syst. Bacteriol.* **34:**71–73.

43. **Morris, J. G., Jr., J. Johnson, E. Rice, C. Tacket, G. Losonsky, M. Stein, and J. Nataro.** 1993. *Vibrio cholerae* can assume a rugose survival form which resists chlorination but retains virulence for humans, p. 177–182. Abstr.

29th Joint Conf. on Cholera and Related Diarrheal Diseases. NIH, Bethesda, Md.

44. **Nikitin, D. I., G. Y. Vishnewetskaya, K. M. Chumakov, and I. V. Zlatkin.** 1990. Evolutionary relationship of some stalked and budding bacteria (genera *Caulobacter*, "*Hyphobacter*," *Hyphomonas*, and *Hyphomicrobium*) as studied by the new integral taxonomic method. *Arch. Microbiol.* **153:**123–128.

45. **Noonan, B., and T. J. Trust.** 1995. Molecular characterization of an *Aeromonas salmonicida* mutant with altered surface morphology and increases systemic virulence. *Mol. Microbiol.* **15:**65–75.

46. **Poindexter, J.** 1981. The caulobacters: ubiquitous, unusual bacteria. *Microbiol. Rev.* **45:**155–170.

47. **Poindexter, J.** 1984. Physiological and morphological adaptations: role of prostheca development in oligotrophic aquatic bacteria, p. 33–40. *In* M. J. Klug and C. A. Reddy (ed.), *Current Perspectives in Microbial Ecology.* American Society for Microbiology, Washington, D.C.

48. **Quintero, E.** 1994. Characterization of adhesion and biofilm formation by the marine procaryote MHS-3. Ph.D. dissertation. University of Maryland, College Park.

49. **Quintero, E., K. Busch, and R. Weiner.** 1998. Spatial and temporal deposition of adhesive extracellular polysaccharide capsule and fimbriae by *Hyphomonas* MHS-3. *Appl. Environ. Microbiol.* **64:**1246–1255.

50. **Quintero, E. and R. Weiner.** 1995. Evidence for the adhesive function of the exopolysaccharide of *Hyphomonas* MHS-3 in its attachment to surfaces. *Appl. Environ. Microbiol.* **61:**1897–1903.

51. **Quintero, E., and R. Weiner.** 1995. Physical and chemical characterization of the polysaccharide capsule of the marine bacterium, *Hyphomonas* MHS-3. *J. Ind. Microbiol.* **15:**347–351.

52. **Salamitou, S., O. Raynaud, M. Lamaire, M. Coughlan, P. Beguin, and J.-P. Aubert.** 1994. Recognition specificity of the duplicated segments present in *Clostridium thermocellum* endoglucanase CelD and in the cellulosome-integrating protein CipA. *J. Bacteriol.* **176:**2822–2827.

53. **Shen, N., L. Dagasan, D. Sledjeski, and R. M. Weiner.** 1989. Major outer membrane proteins unique to reproductive cells of *Hyphomonas jannaschiana. J. Bacteriol.* **171:**2226–2228.

54. **Shen, N., and R. Weiner.** Isolation and characterization of proteins with S-layer properties from the prothescate bacteria, *Hyphomonas jannaschiana. Microbios* **93:**7–16.

55. **Shi, J., V. Coyne, and R. Weiner.** 1997. Identification of an alkaline metalloprotease produced by the hydrothermal vent bacterium *Hyphomonas jannaschianna* VP3. *Microbios* **91:**15–26.

56. **Sutherland, I. W.** 1983. Microbial exopolysaccharides—their role in microbial adhesion in aqueous systems. *Crit. Rev. Microbiol.* **10:**173–219.

57. **Svitil, A. L., S. M. Ní Chadhain, J. A. Moore, and D. L. Kirchman.** 1997. Chitin degradation proteins produced by the marine bacterium *Vibrio harveyi* growing on different forms of chitin. *Appl. Environ. Microbiol.* **63:**408–413.

58. **Wali, T. M., G. R. Hudson, D. A. Danald, and R. M. Weiner.** 1980. Timing of swarmer cell cycle morphogenesis and macromolecular synthesis by *Hyphomicrobium neptunium* in synchronous culture. *J. Bacteriol.* **144:**406–412.

59. **Wardell, J. N., C. M. Brown, and B. Flannigan.** 1983. Microbes and surfaces, p. 351–378. *In* J. H. Slater, R. Whittenbury, and J. W. T. Wimpenny (ed.), *Microbes in Their Natural Environments.* Cambridge Univ. Press, London.

60. **Weidner, S., W. Arnold, and A. Puhler.** 1996. Diversity of uncultured microorganisms associated with the seagrass *Halophila tipulacea* estimated by restriction fragment length polymorphism analysis of PCR-amplified 16S rRNA genes. *Appl. Environ. Microbiol.* **62:**766–771.

61. **Weiner, R., D. Chakravorty, and L. Whitehead.** 1998. The architecture of degradative complex polysaccharide enzyme arrays in a marine bacterium has implications for bioremediation, p. 171–176. *In* Y. LeGal and H. O. Halvorson (ed.), *New Developments in Marine Biotechnology.* Plenum Press, New York.

62. **Weiner, R., L. Dagasan, and J. Tuttle.** Evidence for chemolithotrophic metabolism in *Hyphomonas.* Manuscript in preparation.

63. **Weiner, R., L. Dagasan, and J. Tuttle.** 1997. Function of bacterial (*Hyphomonas*) capsular exopolymers in biofouling, p. 373–386. *In* N. Saxena (ed.), *Recent Advances in Marine Science and Technology, 96.* University of Hawaii Press, Honolulu.

64. **Weiner, R., D. Sledjeski, E. Quintero, S. Coon, and M. Walch.** 1993. Periphytic bacteria cue oyster larvae to set on fertile benthic biofilms, p. 217–220. *In* R. Guerrero and C. Pedros Alio, (ed.) *Proceedings of the 6th International Symposium on Microbiological Ecology.* Spanish Society for Microbiology, Barcelona.

65. **Weiner, R. M., R. A. Devine, D. M. Powell, L. Dagasan, and R. L. Moore.** 1985. *Hyphomonas oceanitis* sp. nov., *Hyphomonas hirschiana* sp. nov., and *Hyphomonas jannaschiana* sp. nov. *Int. J. Syst. Bacteriol.* **35:**237–243.

66. **Weiner, R. M., S. Langille, and E. Quintero.** 1995. Structure function and immunochemistry of bacterial capsular exopolysaccharides. *J. Ind. Microbiol.* **15:**339–346.

67. **Weiner, R. M., M. Walch, M. P. Labare, D. B. Bonar, and R. R. Colwell.** 1989. Effect of biofilms of the marine bacterium *Alteromonas colwelliana* on set of the oysters *Crassostrea gigas* (Thunberg) and *C. virginica* (Gmelin). *J. Shellfish Res.* **8:**117–123.

68. **Whitehead, L.** 1997. Complex polysaccharide degrading enzyme arrays synthesized by a marine bacterium. Ph.D. dissertation. University of Maryland, College Park.

69. **Whitehead, L., G. Andrykovitch, V. Chandoke, V. Smith, S. Stosz, and R. Weiner.** 1995. Membrane structures in a marine bacterium are synthesized coincidentally with insoluble biopolymer degradation, p. 572. Abstr. 95th Annu. Meet. Am. Soc. Microbiol. 1995. American Society for Microbiology, Washington, D.C.

70. **Whitehead, L., and R. Weiner.** Cell surface structures on a marine bacterium involved in the degradation of agarose and chitin. In preparation.

71. **Whitehead, L. A., S. K. Stosz, and R. M. Weiner.** 1996. Degradation of recalcitrant insoluble polysaccharides by a marine bacterium. Abstr. 96th Annu. Meet. Am. Soc. Microbiol. 1996. American Society for Microbiology, Washington, D.C.

72. **Zobell, C. E.** 1943. The effect of solid surfaces upon bacterial activity. *J. Bacteriol.* **46:**39–56.

SURVIVAL STRATEGIES IN THE STATIONARY PHASE

A. Matin, M. Baetens, S. Pandža, C. H. Park,
and S. Waggoner

3

At the end of the exponential phase, microbial cultures enter a phase of decelerating growth, followed by the stationary phase, in which no net growth occurs. The end of the exponential growth phase can result from several factors: for example, accumulation in the medium of toxic metabolites or changes in some physical factor such as temperature, redox potential, pH, etc. The decelerating and stationary phases that are the focal point of this review are those that result from exhaustion from the medium of an essential growth nutrient.

This situation—partial or complete starvation for an essential nutrient—is of direct ecological relevance, since in most natural environments, microorganisms are subjected to this stress. From time to time, a large influx of food may lead to rapid growth of the resident flora; but such episodes are few and far between, so that the general microbial experience in nature is one of semi- or total famine, which is relieved only occasionally by brief periods of plenitude. This can be inferred from the nutrient concentration in natural environments as well as the estimated in situ microbial growth rates.

The amount of dissolved organic matter in oceans is ca. 0.8 mg of carbon per liter, much of which is not biodegradable; in a freshwater lake, the concentration of individual carbon substrates was found to be 6 to 10 μg/liter (74), and in an estuary, microbial growth rate appeared to be close to zero (16). Most aquifers contain less than 1 mg of dissolved organic matter per liter, with only traces in the solid material (30). Soil too is a hostile environment in which the organic matter varies from 0.8 to 2%. Of this, 50 to 80% is humus (107), which is a recalcitrant molecule with a half-life of 250 to 5,000 years (39). The remaining components are plant residues (viz., sugars, organic and amino acids, etc.), which get used up rapidly. The estimated generation times of bacteria in nature can be in hundreds of days (16).

Whether the pathogens experience a similar dearth of nutrients inside their hosts is less well studied. Their in vivo growth rates are often much lower than their genetic potential for maximal growth (34a, 67). While stresses other than nutrient scarcity undoubtedly have a role in this phenomenon, several considerations implicate nutrient limitation as well.

A. Matin, M. Baetens, S. Pandža, C. H. Park, and S. Wag-goner, Department of Microbiology and Immunology, Stanford University School of Medicine, Sherman Fairchild Science Building, Stanford, CA 94305.

Microbial Ecology and Infectious Disease, Edited by Eugene Rosenberg
©1999 American Society for Microbiology, Washington, D.C.

The host mobilizes high-affinity substrate-capturing ligands that most likely impose starvation on the invading microbe; even when abundant nutrients are available, rapid growth of the pathogen would result in quickly outstripping the food supply, and as discussed below, the gene expression pattern inside the host is consistent with the presence of nutritional and other stress.

Within the constraints of its genotype, a bacterium can express a wide spectrum of characteristics depending on the environmental conditions. Given the importance of starvation in bacterial life, it is therefore important to examine the bacterial phenotype under starvation conditions. A paradox of studies on bacterial regulation and physiology, however, is that major emphasis has been on bacteria grown in lavish environments. But bacteria experiencing nutrient dearth have begun to receive considerable attention, and it has become clear that they possess a unique phenotype, resulting from unique global gene regulatory mechanisms. This regulation and its physiological consequences are the subjects of this chapter. Only non-sporeforming bacteria are considered.

STARVATION PHENOTYPE

The morphological changes exhibited by non-sporeformers upon starvation are less impressive than is the case with sporeformers. These changes include fragmentation, giving rise to smaller and round cells; protoplast shrinkage, which enlarges the periplasmic space; and nucleoid condensation (Fig. 1).

This simplicity masks a more complex underlying molecular realignment, however. Some 50 to 80 "starvation" proteins are induced, depending on the missing nutrient (34, 38). Many of these are unique to the starvation state, while others are also synthesized during growth but show increased levels in this phase. With respect to the time of synthesis following the onset of starvation, the starvation proteins in *Escherichia coli* fall into four categories that may form a dependent series (77), i.e., inhibition of the induction of

one class can interfere with that of the subsequent classes. The time needed for the completion of the synthesis of various classes of proteins (the "differentiation" period) depends on the bacterium and the starvation conditions. This period is longer, for example, in *Pseudomonas putida* than in *E. coli*; and in the latter organism, it can last from 2 to 4 h, depending on the nature of nutrient limitation (e.g., carbon vs. nitrogen) and the nature of the preceding growth conditions (e.g., glucose vs. succinate medium). Interestingly, the temporal class of a given starvation protein remains unaltered under the different starvation conditions (32, 94).

In the differentiation period, synthesis of most of the growth-related proteins ceases. Within a short time after the onset of starvation, some 50% of such proteins stop synthesis, and only 20 to 30% continue to be synthesized at the end of the differentiation period (94).

This differentiation accompanies fundamental physiological changes. There is a marked amplification of the cell's scavenging capacity for the missing nutrient, attained both through induction of high-affinity uptake and metabolic enzymes as well as acquisition of the capacity to utilize diverse sources for the needed nutrient. Concurrently, there is a progressive increase in the resistance of the bacterium not only to starvation itself but also to a variety of other stresses, viz., heat, cold, hyperosmosis, pH extremes, Cl_2 and ClO_2, and possibly also irradiation and organic solvents (35, 45–47, 57, 95, 104). Maximal resistance is attained by the end of the differentiation period. That these phenotypic traits result from new protein synthesis is shown by the fact that protein synthesis inhibition in the early phases of starvation prevents their development.

REGULATION OF THE STARVATION RESPONSE

Starvation, particularly that for the carbon and energy source, is a more encompassing stress than many other deleterious situations. The diminished redox and energetic status of the

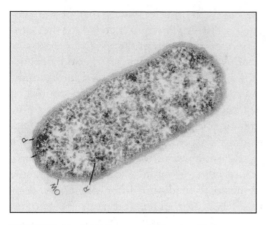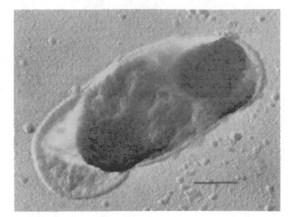

FIGURE 1 A 72 h-starved *E. coli* cell vs. an exponential-phase cell (from reference 86).

cell has several deleterious consequences. Dealing with oxygen radicals becomes more difficult, thus producing an oxidative stress. H^+ and other ionic flux through the electron transport chain, the ATPase, antiporters, and symporters are undermined, compromising cytoplasmic pH homeostasis and generating pH stress. The same holds for the reactions required to concentrate ions and solutes into the cells to maintain the turgor pressure, producing osmotic stress. This debilitated state makes the cellular repair mechanisms of paramount importance, but many of these themselves require energy and reducing power. This necessitates induction of more-efficient and/or higher levels of repair enzymes and chaperones to prevent damage to essential cell constituents. In the differentiation phase, a rapid turnover of cell constituents is necessary to provide the raw material for the synthesis of starvation proteins and other macromolecules. This necessitates discriminatory mechanisms to select for degradation only the nonessential constituents. Discretion is required also in selecting the source(s) for long-term energy generation, and control is needed to keep endogenous metabolism at a low level (9). Starvation thus confronts the cell with multiple stresses, and the ability to survive it better requires superior capacity to resist the constituent stresses. That is probably why starvation resistance accompanies cross-protection against stresses in general.

The fact that temporal classes exist, that starvation induces many of the same genes that are induced in response to other stresses, and that only a subset of other stress-regulon genes is affected indicate that the regulation of the starvation response is complex. Indeed, several sigma factors plus ancillary elements are involved in this regulation. The major starvation sigma factor is σ^S, which has been studied intensively, as discussed in the next section. In this section we discuss the role of other sigma factors in the starvation response.

The "vegetative" sigma factor, σ^{70}, which plays a major role in gene transcription during rapid exponential growth, continues to be important in the starvation response of *E. coli*. Its levels do not change in the stationary phase, at least up to 2 h after starvation begins (48). A major factor that shifts the $E\sigma^{70}$-regulated gene expression from growth to starvation related is the increase in cellular cyclic AMP (cAMP) levels. Approximately two-thirds of the carbon starvation genes, termed the *cst* genes, require cAMP for increased expression during starvation. For the induction of several of these genes, increased cellular cAMP is not only a necessary but also a sufficient condition (63), but for others the regulation is more complex (62).

Most of the *cst* genes appear to be concerned with enhancing the cell's capacity to scavenge the carbon substrates and thus escape starvation, although there are probably some exceptions. One *cst* gene that has been characterized in some detail, *cstA*, appears to be concerned with peptide utilization, a source of nutrient likely to be available in the gut; the induction of this gene illustrates the fact that when one substrate for a nutrient is depleted, *E. coli* prepares to utilize alternate sources likely to be available in its environment (96). The *cst* gene induction is not required for the development of resistance under carbon starvation, since Δ*cya E. coli* strains are completely normal in developing starvation and other attendant resistances. Such strains do not show increased synthesis of the Cst proteins during starvation but induce only a subset of starvation proteins. These non-cAMP-dependent proteins, which consist of ca. one-third of the total starvation proteins, are termed the Pex proteins (products of the *pex* genes). While induction of many *cst* genes is confined to carbon starvation, that of the *pex* genes occurs in response to other individual nutrients as well. Moreover, these genes are also induced by a variety of other stresses. It was therefore suggested that it is the *pex* gene induction that is primarily responsible for the general resistance of the starved cells (34, 63); subsequent studies have supported this premise, as a starvation-associated protective role has been demonstrated for the Pex proteins DnaK, GroEL, HtpG (44), PexA (OtsBA) (38, 49a) and PexB (DpS) (2, 59). The induction of many of the *pex* genes involves secondary sigma factors. However, *cstC* has a protective role under nitrogen starvation conditions (24).

Other species of RNA polymerase that have a role in the starvation response are Eσ^{32}, Eσ^{54}, and possibly also Eσ^E. σ^{32}, which has been studied primarily in the context of the heat shock response in *E. coli*, is also a starvation sigma factor in this bacterium. Its levels increase during carbon starvation and the *rpoH* (the gene that codes for σ^{32}) null

mutants are impaired in starvation survival. They fail to induce at least three Pex (heat shock) proteins upon starvation (namely, DnaK, GroEL and HtpG), and their survival impairment in starvation appears to be due to a lack of sufficient levels of these proteins (44). As discussed below, these proteins have a general protective role. Using a *dnaK* null mutant, Rockabrand et al. (87) reported a role for DnaK in starvation-induced cellular general resistance, but it is unclear how much of this effect is directly due to DnaK deficiency, rather than to the reduced σ^S levels that this deficiency also causes during starvation (88). The mechanism by which σ^{32} levels increase during starvation is not known. The *rpoH* promoter region contains a cAMP-binding site, but there is no evidence that this site has a role in this phenomenon (113).

Eσ^{54}, which is a product of the *rpoN* gene, controls a carbon starvation-survival gene in *P. putida* (50). σ^{54} has been studied primarily in the context of its control of nitrogen metabolism. Its involvement in the carbon-starvation response is of interest for reasons that include the facts that the gene that it controls codes for a G protein (50), and the *rpoN* operon encodes additional genes that may constitute a sensory pathway in carbon starvation (65, 84).

Eσ^E has not been examined for a role in regulating the starvation response. This sigma factor is induced by the accumulation of misfolded proteins in the periplasmic space (91) and may be concerned with their repair. It is likely that misfolded protein content of the enlarged periplasm (Fig. 1) increases in starvation, and thus σ^E could well be a starvation protein.

ROLE OF σ^S

A mutation in the *rpoS* gene results in the cell's inability to induce over 30 proteins during starvation, which include several Pex, as well as heat- and osmotic-shock proteins (68). The mutation also compromises survival under carbon, nitrogen, or oxygen starvation as well as starvation-mediated cross-protection to heat, oxidative, and osmotic stresses (52, 68). The stress sensitivity of the *rpoS* mutants is not confined to the stationary phase, as they show enhanced sensitivity also in exponential phase (38).

Regulation of σ^S Levels

TRANSCRIPTION, TRANSLATION, AND STABILITY

In *E. coli*, σ^S levels increase severalfold as cultures enter the decelerating phase of growth because of carbon starvation. Chemostat studies showed that the increase in the levels of this sigma factor bears a direct relationship to the progression of this phase and is complete before the onset of the stationary phase.

To determine the basis of this increase, Zgurskaya et al. (114) directly quantified the rates of *rpoS* gene transcription and *rpoS* mRNA translation in different growth phases. These rates were calculated by measuring mRNA and σ^S levels and their half-lives. The *rpoS* transcription rate as well as the *rpoS* mRNA translational efficiency decreased as the culture progressed through the decelerating phase; eventually, the translational efficiency dropped by ca. 50%. As a result, the σ^S synthesis rate declined from ca. 55 in the exponential to 13 pmol per mg of protein per minute in the stationary phase. Thus, the increase in σ^S concentration in the stationary-phase cultures occurs despite a large decrease in its synthesis. Parallel measurements showed that the stability of the sigma protein increased progressively in the decelerating phase 7- to 16-fold, resulting in the overall net increase in the sigma levels (Fig. 2). That the σ^S stability increases in the stationary phase had been reported earlier (53, 112).

The instability of σ^S in the exponential phase specifically requires the presence of the ClpXP protease (97). This protease is a member of multimeric ATP-dependent proteases and consists of two subunits. The ClpP protein by itself has only a weak peptidase activity; but in combination with a chaperone with ATPase activity (ClpA, ClpC, ClpX, and pos-

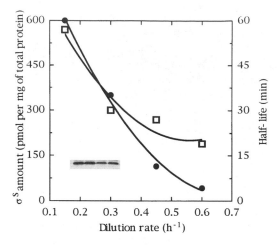

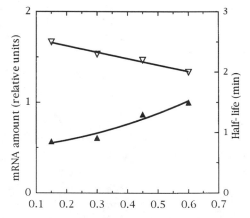

FIGURE 2 The σ^S levels (pmol/mg protein; □) and half-lives (min; ●) of *E. coli* grown in a chemostat under glucose limitation at various dilution rates (from reference 115).

sibly ClpB), it becomes a protease with a certain degree of specificity. This specificity resides in the chaperone part, which presents various protein substrates to the protease (33, 90).

E. coli mutants devoid of either *clpP* or *clpX* showed high levels of σ^S in the exponential phase, and half-life determinations in vivo revealed that in the absence of either of these proteins, the sigma factor was highly stable regardless of the growth phase. The absence of other proteases, viz., Lon or ClpAP, did not affect σ^S levels. Since the ClpXP protease levels did not decrease in stationary-phase cells, it appears that σ^S becomes resistant to this protease in this phase (97). The mechanism of this resistance is unknown. A role for DnaK has been reported in that DnaK deficiency reduced σ^S levels in the stationary phase by destabilizing it in this phase (88). C. H. Park and A. Matin (unpublished) have found that σ^S coprecipitates with certain proteins only in the exponential phase; this association may produce a conformation in which the sigma protein is susceptible to proteolysis. In fact, association of σ^{32} with certain chaperones (DnaK, DnaJ, and GrpE) in nonstressed cells is believed to be the reason for its sensitivity to a variety of proteases such as Lon, FtsH (HflB), and ClpQY (HslVU). In heat-stressed cells, the chaperones dissociate from the sigma factor, as they have a higher affinity for the denatured proteins that accumulate under these conditions; the resulting conformational change in the sigma protein apparently makes it refractory to proteolysis (89, 113).

Whatever proteins may be concerned with altering σ^S stability, they do not seem to include most of the housekeeping E. coli chaperones (other than DnaK, as discussed above), since mutants deficient in GroEL, DnaJ, GrpE, or CbpA were not affected in their σ^S levels in any growth phase (97).

Studies with σ^S protein-containing internal deletions provided strong evidence that the 173- to 188-amino acid stretch of this protein might be at least a part of the target site for the ClpXP protease, since its deletion rendered the sigma factor highly stable in a ClpXP-proficient background, regardless of the growth phase (97). This site approximates the region of the sigma factor that interacts with the −10 sequence of the promoter. A recent computer-assisted database analysis concluded that all proteins that interact with ClpX possess the LDA/L motif on or near a predicted α-helix; this motif is present in σ^S. Furthermore, the substrates for the ClpXP protease may possess an additional sequence, which varies from protein to protein (108). If so, the 173- to 188-amino acid stretch of σ^S could be the second binding site for ClpX.

While σ^{32} is a target for many proteases, σ^S sensitivity appears to be confined only to ClpXP protease. The high degree of stability that the sigma factor attains in the absence of this protease (97) renders the possible involvement of other proteases unlikely.

POSSIBLE REASONS FOR DIFFERENT CONCLUSIONS OF DIRECT MEASUREMENTS VS. FUSION RESULTS
Until the more direct studies of Zgurskaya et al. (114), the consensus view had been that the increase in σ^S levels in E. coli during starvation was a cumulative result of increased protein stability, increased rpoS mRNA translational efficiency, and increased rpoS transcription. The involvement of the latter two mechanisms was inferred from the use of transcriptional and translational fusions, as well as from methionine incorporation in the case of translational efficiency. It is relevant to consider why the conclusions of these approaches differed from those of the more direct measurements.

The rpoS-lacZ transcriptional fusions show an approximately two-fold induction in the stationary phase. The rpoS gene has a complex regulatory region consisting of three promoters, one of which lies within the coding sequence of the upstream (nlpD) gene (38). A possible explanation for the difference in the results obtained with the fusions and in the direct measurements is that the hybrid rpoS-lacZ mRNA forms secondary structures that are influenced by the growth phase. This is consistent with the finding that transcriptional fusions with different lengths of the rpoS coding region inserted between the regulatory region of the rpoS gene and the lacZ coding region exhibit different degrees of induction in the stationary phase (68).

As already stated, two lines of evidence indicated increased rpoS translational efficiency in the stationary phase. We first consider the intriguing behavior of the various translational fusions to this gene that suggested this possibility. The β-galactosidase induction pattern of these fusions during transition between different growth phases mimicked the actual change in the σ^S levels (as quantified by Western analysis) only if they contained a stretch of the *rpoS* coding region beyond 515 nucleotides (nt) (53, 68a, 75). Fusions lacking this stretch showed nearly fully induced levels already in the exponential phase. Computer-assisted sequence analysis suggested a region of complementarity between the translational start site of the rpoS mRNA and its coding sequences beyond 551 nt (68a).

It was therefore proposed that the *rpoS* mRNA stretch beyond 551 nt may constitute an "antisense element," (53) that caused the mRNA to bend upon itself, masking translational initiation sites and thereby inhibiting translation (Fig. 3A). This situation prevailed, according to this postulate, in the exponential-phase cells. But upon entry into the stationary phase, the secondary structure relaxed, leading to a more efficient translation of the mRNA. Synthesis or activation of some protein factor(s) in the stationary phase could be the reason for the relaxation of the mRNA secondary structure (68a). A similar mechanism is thought to contribute to the increased σ^{32} levels during heat shock, although the nature of the factor(s) accounting for the messenger losing its secondary structure in the stressed cells is not yet established (113).

However, the target region thought to account for σ^S sensitivity to the ClpXP protease in the exponential phase (173- to 188-amino acid stretch) (97) is encoded by 519 to 564 nt of the *rpoS* mRNA, i.e., encompassing the region where the antisense element for translational control is supposed to reside. Thus, the fusion results could, with equal justification, be interpreted as indicating either translational control, or posttranslational control. As discussed, the former interpretation invokes formation of mRNA secondary structure in the *rpoS-lacZ* hybrid mRNA (containing the antisense element) in the exponential phase, thereby hampering translation and accounting for the observed low levels of β-galactosidase. But if translation was in fact not hampered, the result in such fusions would be production of RpoS-LacZ hybrid proteins containing the

target region for the ClpXP protease. The end result would still be low β-galactosidase levels in such fusions in exponential phase but for a different reason, namely, the ClpXP-mediated degradation of the hybrid protein (Fig. 3B). In view of the more direct studies indicating a more efficient translation of *rpoS* mRNA in exponential phase than in stationary phase, it is reasonable to conclude that the fusion results are due to posttranslational regulation (114).

The second line of evidence indicating increased translational efficiency of *rpoS* mRNA in the stationary phase consisted of increased incorporation of labeled methionine in σ^S in this phase (53). But, as discussed elsewhere (114), this is more likely to reflect concurrent increase in the σ^S protein stability under these conditions.

While increased σ^S stability alone accounts for increased levels of the sigma factor under the above starvation conditions in *E. coli*, it remains possible, of course, that transcription and translational regulation have a role in σ^S control in other situations and/or organisms. In *Pseudomonas aeruginosa*, for example, an *rpoS-lacZ* transcriptional fusion shows a much greater induction (five-fold) upon entry into the stationary phase (27), raising the likelihood for control at the transcriptional level. Similarly, several mechanisms of translational control could play a role in specific situations. One example is the protein HF-I, which probably relaxes helical regions around the mRNA ribosomal binding site (11), thereby promoting translation. Involvement of HF-I in σ^S synthesis has been demonstrated, but there is, as yet, no evidence either that this protein has a specific role in *rpoS* mRNA translation or that it acts differentially in controlling this translation in exponential and stationary phase cells. On the contrary, strains lacking HF-I are deficient in σ^S synthesis in both these growth phases, and this protein also affects expression of other genes (71, 72). While these findings suggest that HF-I may be a more general translation factor, under some conditions it may be specifically involved in σ^S synthesis (73). A specific role in σ^S translational regulation for two small un-

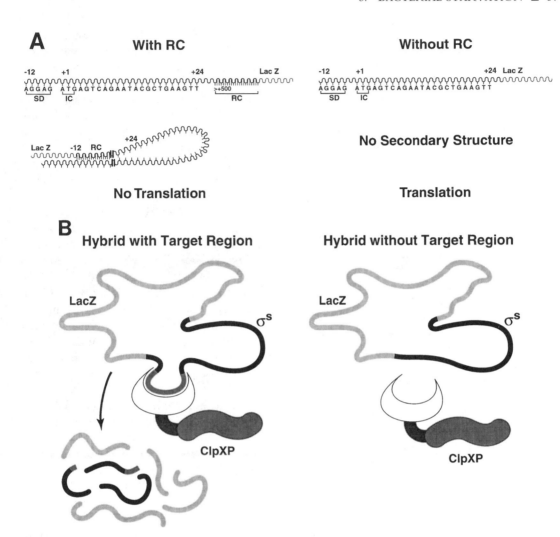

FIGURE 3 Two different mechanisms of low β-galactosidase production in exponential phase by *E. coli* translational fusions. (A) Possession of the "antisense element" by the *rpoS-lacZ* hybrid mRNA leading to secondary structure formation, and prevention of translation. (B) Possession of the ClpXP target site by the RpoS-LacZ hybrid protein leading to its degradation by the protease. See text for further details. RC, region of complementarity.

translated RNAs has been proposed, namely, those encoded by the *dsrA* (98) and *oxyS* (3) genes, with the former stimulating translation at low temperatures, and the latter possibly inhibiting it under oxidative stress.

OTHER REGULATORS

The histonelike protein H-NS may also lower *rpoS* translational efficiency and σ^S half-life in exponential-phase cells (6, 112). H-NS synthesis increases in the stationary phase, which

should result in further decreases in σ^S translation and stability (18, 105) instead of what actually occurs. Mutants deficient in UDP-glucose also lose the ability to down regulate σ^S levels in exponential phase, evidently through posttranscriptional regulation (38). The stringent response regulator, ppGpp, is required for the synthesis of σ^S at the onset of starvation. However, ppGpp^O mutants synthesize normal levels of the sigma factor upon longer starvation (28), indicating a role for this molecule mainly in proper timing of σ^S synthesis in starvation. A ppGpp^O strain exhibited higher levels of *rpoS* mRNA, arising entirely from an increase in stability of the mRNA and not from any effect on *rpoS* (114). How ppGpp affects the course of σ^S induction during starvation remains unclear; it may involve interaction of ppGpp with the conserved region of σ^{70} (40).

SENSING STARVATION

Two groups independently reported the existence of a protein termed SprE (85) or RssB (70) in *E. coli*, which is homologous to the response-regulator component of the classical two-component system of environmental sensing. SprE contains a unique carboxy-terminal output domain. Mutants in the *sprE* gene show undiminished levels of σ^S in exponential phase, and the overproduction of SprE decreases σ^S levels, but only in a ClpXP-proficient background (85). Thus, SprE may, in conjunction with a sensor protein, communicate the starvation signal through its output domain to the ClpXP protease, controlling its activity and regulating σ^S levels. That the σ^S half-life markedly increased in the *sprE* mutants is consistent with this possibility (70, 85).

Recent studies (115) make it doubtful, however, that RssB/SprE acts directly on the protease. Instead, it may affect σ^S. Thus, modulation of RssB/SprE levels altered σ^S stability without influencing that of the λO protein, which is also a substrate for the ClpXP protease. In a *clpP* mutant, large amounts of σ^S accumulated, regardless of whether SprE was present or not; but the σ^S that accumulated in the absence of SprE was severalfold more active in inducing transcriptional fusions to σ^S-dependent genes. This may be because SprE interacted with σ^S in the same approximate region with which the sigma factor binds to the promoter, i.e., the ca. 173- to 188-amino acid stretch (see above).

σ^S-Dependent Promoters

A consensus sequence for σ^S-dependent promoters has proved elusive. A probable reason is that σ^S and σ^{70} resemble each other closely, and subtle factors may determine whether a gene is transcribed by one or the other. Another reason is that it is frequently not known if a putatively σ^S-controlled promoter is in fact directly dependent on it for transcription. Several genes in vitro are transcribed by both sigma factor holoenzymes, although there are exceptions in which transcription depends exclusively on either of the holoenzyme species (75). As it is difficult to reproduce precisely, in vitro, the flux of conditions inside a cell experiencing different kinds of stresses, it would be rash to conclude that the absence of selectivity indicated by the in vitro results is physiologically wholly relevant. Indeed, there is evidence that the cellular ionic composition (which can vary significantly under different environmental conditions) influences whether a gene is transcribed by Eσ^S or Eσ^{70} (19). Furthermore, the core RNA polymerase appears to undergo subtle changes during starvation (79).

Nevertheless, some generalizations about the nature of the promoter recognized by Eσ^S have emerged. It appears that the -10 consensus sequence for such promoters is CTATACT (21). This sequence, it is evident, bears a close resemblance to the -10 region recognized by Eσ^{70}-regulated promoters. No -35 consensus sequence for Eσ^S promoters is apparent, but an AT-rich sequence is present at this approximate site in most such promoters. The curved DNA that such a sequence produces is probably important in the recognition of a promoter by Eσ^S. Eσ^S competes with H-NS that too binds to curved AT-rich DNA sequences. The *csgA* gene (which encodes the curlin subunit protein) has a curved DNA regulatory region and is repressed by H-NS. This repression is antagonized by increased σ^S levels (78). Similarly, the H-NS repression of the *luxR1* and *luxC* genes, which also possess a curved regulatory region, is overcome by σ^S (106).

The AT-rich region does not entirely preclude the possibility that no characteristic -35 nucleotides exist for Eσ^S promoters. In several such promoters, conserved cytosines at positions −35 and/or −34 are often followed by a guanine at position −33. The importance of this configuration is shown by the fact that conversion of the −35/34 CC to TT in the $E\sigma^S$ osmY promoter changes it into a promoter recognized exclusively by $E\sigma^{70}$; similarly, altering an $E\sigma^{70}$ promoter (proU) to replace TT with CC in similar positions produces the opposite result (109).

To assess the relative roles of −10 and −35 regions of different promoters in $E\sigma^S$ recognition, Tanaka et al. (101) constructed various chimeras of E. coli σ^S and σ^{70} promoters and tested them in vitro for transcription by the two polymerase holoenzymes. The −10 region and upstream sequences, beginning at position −17, proved crucial for σ^S promoter specificity. Any change in the −10 hexamer (TATAAT) produced decreased promoter strength, the requirement being more stringent for $E\sigma^{70}$ than for $E\sigma^S$ (101). That the σ^{70} −10 hexamer was recognized by $E\sigma^S$ was shown in vivo by Wise et al. (109), using transcriptional fusion assays. Furthermore, random mutagenesis of the σ^S-dependent fic promoter confirmed that the −10 hexamer was crucial for recognition by $E\sigma^S$. All mutations that resulted in defective transcription were confined to the −10 region (41).

While the overlap in the specificity of the two sigma holoenzymes may be exaggerated by the in vitro results, it may, on the other hand, be a means by which the cell achieves flexibility in transcribing a given gene under different conditions. For genes controlled by other "alternate" sigma factors in E. coli, this end is attained by the possession of multiple promoters in the regulatory region. This is the case, for example, for the heat shock genes, which contain generally both the σ^{32}- and σ^{70}-recognized promoters. The similarity of σ^S and σ^{70} promoters may achieve the same end with greater economy. σ^S promoters could thus have evolved on purpose as inherently weak promoters that can be recognized either by $E\sigma^S$ or $E\sigma^{70}$, or both, depending on the cellular conditions, viz., the relative concentration of the two RNA polymerase holoenzymes, minor changes in the core RNA polymerase, the cytoplasmic ionic composition, and the presence of specific ancillary factors. An example of the last mentioned is provided by pexB (dps) gene regulation. Increased expression of this gene under carbon starvation or osmotic stress depends on σ^S. However, even though the same transcriptional start site continues to be used, its expression becomes independent of this sigma factor under oxidative stress (59). Under the latter conditions, the increased expression is mediated by σ^{70} and the integration host factor instead. Expression during exponential growth requires another ancillary factor, OxyR (2). A further example is the gene katG that codes for hydroperoxidase I. This gene is transcribed by $E\sigma^S$, but in the presence of OxyR, it can be transcribed also by $E\sigma^{70}$. The csi gene can similarly be transcribed by either $E\sigma^S$ or $E\sigma^{70}$, but here the condition for transcription by the latter is the presence of cAMP/CRP (62). The promiscuity of $E\sigma^S$ promoters apparently exists also in other bacteria. Thus, the P_m promoter in P. putida is transcribed by $E\sigma^{70}$ in the exponential phase and by $E\sigma^S$ in the stationary phase (61).

PHYSIOLOGICAL ROLE OF STARVATION PROTEINS

With respect to their role, the starvation proteins fall into several categories: escape from starvation; endogenous metabolism; global regulation; and protection and repair. The starvation proteins concerned with escape from starvation were reviewed recently by one of us (65) and are not considered further.

Endogenous Metabolism

Only minimal information is available about these proteins. Recently, Fraley et al. (24) found that the starvation protein CstC is a close homologue of the E. coli N-α-acetylornithine-δ-aminotranferase enzyme, encoded by the argD gene. The growth and starvation phenotype of a cstC mutant suggested that whereas ArgD is involved in amino acid biosynthesis, CstC may be involved in carrying out a similar step in amino acid catabolism. Schneider et al. (92a) independently reported that *cstC* (which they refer to as *astC*) is the first gene in a five-gene operon (*astCADBE*) that codes for the AST pathway of amino acid catabolism. Thus, the CstC protein may have a role in endogenous metabolism of the starving *E. coli* cells. The upstream region of the *astCADBE* operon contains regulatory sites for several sigma and ancillary factors, suggesting careful and complex regulation of amino acid breakdown during starvation (24), in which σ^S and σ^{54} may compete with each other. Pyruvate oxidase and phosphoenolpyruvate carboxykinase are other proteins in this category that are induced by starvation. They may have a role in energy generation and/or biosynthesis in the starving cell.

Global Regulators

Two examples of these proteins, σ^S and σ^{32}, have already been considered. In addition, the σ^S-controlled proteins, PexB (DpS), AppY, and BolA, have global roles. Removal or overproduction of PexB influences the synthesis of several proteins, including the Pex proteins (2, 59). The PexB regulon may be concerned with oxidative resistance of starved cells (2). Both the AppY and BolA proteins possess a helix-turn-helix motif typical of many DNA-binding proteins (1, 5). AppY induction links the starvation response to that of *cyxAB* and *hyaABCDEF* genes (4, 10), which are part of the anaerobiosis regulon. A protein controlled by BolA is DacC (12; D-alanine carboxypeptidase), which, by increasing the peptidoglycan cross-linkage, accounts, at least in part, for the increased strength of the cell wall of starved cells.

Protective and Repair Proteins

KatG and KatE (hydroperoxidase I and II, respectively) destroy H_2O_2, XthA (exonuclease III) is probably more adept at DNA repair under starvation conditions and, as discussed above, PexB (DpS) may control other proteins

concerned with oxidative protection and DNA repair (38). Another DNA-repair starvation protein is AidB, which may be concerned with reversing DNA methylation (51). The pilin porin PapC probably has a role in heat and osmotic resistance of the starved cells, as do the proteins encoded by the *ecp-htrE* operon. Furthermore, the *otsBA* (*pexA*) operon-encoded proteins, by stimulating trehalose biosynthesis in starved cells, increase the membrane strength of these cells (38). In addition, a large number of starvation proteins is involved in protein protection and repair.

REPAIR OF CONFORMATIONAL DAMAGE

These proteins constitute a large and diverse class (37). The eukaryotic counterpart of DnaK (Hsp70) for example, is encoded by 9 different genes in humans, and 14 in yeast. Many of these homologs cannot function interchangeably (43). These proteins play an indispensable role in normal cell physiology, such as binding to nascent polypeptides to ensure proper folding, protein transport, and disassembly of clathrin-coated vesicles (22). Indeed, according to recent work, a defect in chaperone function may be the basis of prion formation; prions are associated with serious diseases such as scrapie and Creutzfeldt-Jakob disease (58). In yeast, the psi+ factor, which causes an abnormal translational termination frequency, is thought to be a prionlike form of the normal protein Sup35. Overproduction of the chaperone, Hsp104, can revert psi+ to the normal Sup35 protein (103).

Chaperones can either minimize damage or outright protect proteins from denaturation during stresses. Thus, stress-denatured firefly luciferase can be reactivated in *E. coli* cells only when functional DnaK, DnaJ, and GrpE proteins are present during the inactivation period (93). A similar phenomenon relates to DnaK and transgenic human growth hormone (HGH) overproduction in *E. coli*. The inclusion body formation representing denatured HGH could be mitigated only if DnaK was overproduced before HGH production (7). In eukaryotic cells, Hsp70, in conjunction with Hsp90 and Hsp25, prevents heat-induced protein denaturation (25). In addition, there is evidence that chaperones can renature proteins denatured by stress. Thus, DnaK can solubilize aggregates of several heat-denatured proteins in vitro (29) and so can Hsp104 in yeast (83).

It is not known how chaperones protect proteins from stress damage; but the repair of stress-damaged proteins is probably an extension of their normal function of bringing about correct folding of substrate proteins (82). Based on the in vitro conversion of unfolded luciferase into active enzyme (100), Hartl (36) proposed the following mechanism. DnaJ interacts with the unfolded polypeptide and presents it to the DnaK-ATP complex (81). ATP hydrolysis follows, resulting in a ternary complex between the substrate, DnaJ, and DnaK-ADP. The nucleotide-exchange factor, GrpE, releases ADP from DnaK, resulting in the release of DnaJ. DnaK now binds ATP, which triggers the release of the substrate protein, thus completing the cycle. Besides DnaJ, a close analog of this protein, CbpA, is induced in starvation in a σ^S-dependent manner (111), suggesting that initiation of the DnaK repair cycle may be particularly important in starvation. Another chaperone system, GroEL/ES, has also been extensively studied (8, 110) and is likely to be involved in protection and renaturation of stress-damaged proteins.

REPAIR OF COVALENT DAMAGE

Proline peptide bonds can exist in either the normal *trans* configuration or the *cis* form (23), the latter interfering with protein folding or refolding (49). Peptidyl-prolyl-*cis-trans* isomerases (PPIases) able to catalyze proline isomerization have been identified in many organisms (92), nine in *E. coli* alone (42). One PPIase is the protein SurA, which was originally identified because mutants in *surA* were compromised in starvation survival (102). The role of SurA in normal physiology is to bring about proper folding of periplasmic and outer membrane proteins (55, 91), and its induction

in the stationary phase probably indicates that denatured periplasmic proteins most likely accumulate under these conditions.

The ability to accelerate refolding of denatured proteins has been demonstrated in vitro for PpiA and PpiB (17). These enzymes are not heat inducible; whether starvation or other stresses induce them is not known. Regardless, the fact that they interact with HtpG in their repair function connects them with the stress response.

L-Isoaspartyl protein carboxyl methyltransferase, the product of the *pcm* gene in *E. coli*, deals with covalent repair of the isoaspartate residue, which is the "abnormal" form of asparaginyl residues. This enzyme can catalyze a reaction that leads eventually to the conversion of isoaspartate to aspartate, thus removing the kink caused by isoaspartate and the barrier to correct protein folding. A *pcm* mutant of *E. coli* is impaired in starvation survival, presumably because of the inability to repair denatured proteins (26).

The enzymes involved in the recognition and repair of covalent damage would appear to be different from chaperones whose role is confined to conformational changes. However, inasmuch as the former perform the end-role of producing correct conformation, they act like chaperones. In addition, a chaperone, DnaJ, also possesses a protein-disulfide isomerase activity (99).

STARVATION/STRESS RESPONSE AND BACTERIAL PATHOGENESIS

This volume rightly emphasizes the relationship between studies on microbial ecology and their pathogenic process. This point is forcefully made by the results of starvation studies whose primary motivation was to understand nonpathogenic aspects of bacterial ecophysiology but whose results have proved to be relevant to bacterial pathogenesis.

We illustrate this point by focusing first on *Salmonella typhimurium*, a "model" organism for pathogenic studies. The pathogenic process of this bacterium is fraught with stresses (60). To establish an infection, this bacterium has to pass through the stomach, which has an average pH of ca. 1.5 over a 24-h period. Upon reaching the ileal mucosa it invades the gut-associated lymphoid tissue (GALT); a constituent of GALT are the Peyer's patches, and upon attaching to these, it is phagocytosed by the host macrophages. The phagocytosis, presumably meant to be a defensive move on the part of the host, is recruited by the bacterium to its own advantage, since it multiplies in the macrophages. Inside the macrophage, *S. typhimurium* encounters oxidative stress in the form of reactive oxygen intermediates and hypochlorite, acid stress since the pH of phagolysosomes is 4.5, and also, as discussed above, most likely nutritional stress.

Whether or not direct starvation is involved, many of the same physiological features uncovered as important in starvation survival play a role in its existence inside the macrophage. Thus, the σ^S-regulated stress response is crucial for this existence. The critical σ^S-regulated genes reside not only on the chromosome but also on a virulence plasmid. This plasmid contains the *spvR* and *spvABCD* operons (14). SpvR is a regulatory protein that, along with σ^S, modulates the expression of the *spvABCD* operon, whose products are essential for *S. typhimurium* mouse virulence; in addition, the expression of the *spvR* gene itself is controlled by σ^S. Consequently, the *spvABCD* operon is transcribed maximally in starving cells, which may be an indication that starvation is experienced by this bacterium inside the macrophages. Moreover, an *rpoS-lacZ* transcriptional fusion of *S. typhimurium* is induced when it is phagocytosed by macrophages; likewise, expression of the σ^S-dependent *katE* and *spvB* genes increases inside the macrophages and the epithelial cells (15). However, it remains possible that the signal for σ^S induction is only partially starvation, since it may be also short-chain fatty acids and *N*-butanoyl-L-homoserine lactone, the latter working in conjunction with the RhlR protein (54).

Several *rpoS* mutants of *S. typhimurium* are attenuated in virulence and can serve as an effective vaccine. Such mutants can invade

human embryonic intestinal epithelial cells and macrophages, but unlike the wild type, they cannot adhere to the Peyer's patches; these mutants also do not destroy the follicle-associated epithelium of the GALT (76).

Another starvation-phase, but σ^S-independent, gene with a role in the *S. typhimurium* pathogenic process is *slyA*. SlyA is a transcriptional regulator with sequence homology to other transcription factors including EmrR, MarR, PecS, and HprR, all of which are involved in the adaptation of bacteria to changing environmental conditions (69). The *slyA* mutant was more sensitive to hydrogen peroxide and to the products of the redox cycling compound paraquat; it was less virulent in mice and was compromised in survival in macrophages. A *slyA-lacZ* transcriptional fusion was markedly induced in stationary phase as well as inside the macrophages. Sodium dodecyl sulfate-polyacrylamide gel electrophoresis analysis showed that the *slyA* mutant produced fewer proteins during stationary phase, although it was not affected in exponential-phase protein-synthesis profile. During infection of macrophages, several proteins were absent in the *slyA* mutant, indicating that SlyA affects *S. typhimurium* gene expression once inside the macrophage (13). HtrA, another stress protein that has been implicated in the pathogenesis of *S. typhimurium*, is a serine protease that degrades misfolded periplasmic proteins; *htrA* mutants are impaired in their ability to replicate in macrophages. HtrA protein is important also in the pathogenesis of *Brucella abortus*. While the loss of this protein does not affect the ability of this bacterium to replicate in macrophages, survival is reduced 10-fold. The *htrA* mutants of *S. typhimurium* and *Yersinia enterocolitica* can act as vaccines in mice (80).

Induction of several stress proteins has also been shown in *Mycobacterium tuberculosis* (56) and *Listeria monocytogenes* (34a) during their existence in macrophages. In the latter bacterium, loss of a stress/starvation protein, ClpC, markedly impairs replicative ability in macrophages. Intravenous infection of mice with the *clpC* mutant was not lethal, as opposed to wild-type infection. The growth rate of the *clpC* mutant, although similar to that of the wild type in the early stages of infection, was restricted in late stages (90). In *Haemophilus influenzae*, mutants in the *sodA* gene (which encodes type b superoxide dismutase) are defective in establishing sustained colonization of the rat nasopharynx (20). In *P. aeruginosa*, the σ^E (AlgU)-mucoidy phenotype is associated with the capacity to establish a chronic colonization of the respiratory tract of cystic fibrosis patients (31); σ^E is a stress sigma factor.

UNRESOLVED QUESTIONS/ FUTURE RESEARCH

Studies on the molecular biology and physiology of bacteria in decelerating and stationary growth phases are very much in a state of infancy, and there are several aspects that will continue to incite interest and yield fruitful information. The questions that stand out from the ongoing studies reviewed above include σ^S regulation. What links this regulation to the environmental signals? What protein(s) communicates with SprE/RssB, or other equivalent protein(s), and what leads to σ^S becoming resistant to the ClpXP protease under stress conditions? Exploration of these questions will impinge on the larger issue of what determines the specific nature of σ^S sensitivity to the ClpXP protease. The basis of proteolytic specificity, about which little is known, is of fundamental importance in cell biology. Another aspect worthy of investigation within the context of σ^S is the basis of the seeming promiscuity of the promoters it transcribes.

The molecular biological studies to elucidate the regulation of gene expression in starving cells can have practical payoff. In in situ bioremediation, for example, dissociation of expression of the desired degradative activity from the need for rapid growth is highly desirable. This objective has been achieved by the use of starvation promoters, but there is need for improvement (64, 66).

We need to understand better how the cell becomes more resistant in the starved state, which means more thorough elucidation of the biochemical role of the starvation/stress proteins. This understanding can provide radically new ways for controlling microbes, both when their survival is undesirable (e.g., disease), and when it is (e.g., released engineered organisms to achieve beneficial changes in the environment). Related to this line of investigation is our need to understand in more precise terms what physiological traits bacteria need to initiate their pathogenic process and what precise role stress proteins have in this process. New approaches to control bacterial disease are urgently needed, given the alarming increase in bacterial resistance to our current arsenal of antibiotics and other antimicrobials.

ACKNOWLEDGMENTS

Recent work reported from this laboratory was supported by NSF, EPA, and DOE grant numbers DCB-9207101, DE-FG03-93ER61684, and R823390, respectively. We thank Sara White for excellent secretarial help.

REVIEWS AND KEY PAPERS

Chen, C.-Y., L. Eckmann, S. J. Libby, F. C. Fang, S. Okamoto, M. F. Kagnoff, J. Fierer, and D. G. Guiney. 1996. Expression of *Salmonella typhimurium rpoS* and *rpoS*-dependent genes in the intracellular environment of eukaryotic cells. *Infect. Immun.* **64:**4739–4743.

Ding, Q., S. Kusano, M. Villarejo, and A. Ishihama. 1995. Promoter selectivity control of *Escherichia coli* RNA polymerase by ionic strength: differential recognition of osmoregulated promoters by $E\sigma^D$ and $E\sigma^S$ holoenzymes. *Mol. Microbiol.* **16:**649–656.

Fink, A. L. 1998. Preface, p. iii–iv. *In* A. Fink and Y. Goto (ed.), *Molecular Chaperones in the Life Cycle of Proteins: Structure, Function and Mode of Action.* Marcel Dekker, Inc. New York.

Hengge-Aronis, R. 1996. Regulation of gene expression during entry into stationary phase, p. 1497–1512. *In* F. C. Neidhardt, R. Curtiss III, J. L. Ingraham, E. C. C. Lin, K. B. Low, Jr., B. Magasanik, W. S. Reznikoff, M. Riley, M. Schaechter, and H. E. Umbarger (ed.), *Escherichia coli and Salmonella typhimurium: Cellular and Molecular Biology.* American Society for Microbiology, Washington, D.C.

Matin, A. 1996. Role of alternate sigma factors in starvation protein synthesis—novel mechanisms of catabolite repression. *Res. Microbiol.* **147:**494–504.

Muffler, A., D. D. Traulsen, D. Fischer, R. Lange, and R. Hengge-Aronis. 1997. The RNA-binding protein HF-I plays a global regulatory role which is largely, but not exclusively, due to its role in expression of the sigma S subunit of RNA polymerase in *Escherichia coli. J. Bacteriol.* **179:**297–300.

Zgurskaya, H., M. Keyhan, and A. Matin. 1997. The σ^S level in starving *Escherichia coli* cells increases solely as a result of its increased stability, despite decreased synthesis. *Mol. Microbiol.* **24:**643–651.

REFERENCES

1. Aldea, M., C. Hernandez-Chico, A. G. De La Campa, S. R. Kushner, and M. Vicente. 1989. Identification, cloning, and expression of *bolA*, an *ftsZ*-dependent morphogene of *Escherichia coli. J. Bacteriol.* **170:**5169–5176.

2. Altuvia, S., M. Almiron, G. Huisman, R. Kolter, and G. Storz. 1994. The *dps* promoter is activated by OxyR during growth and IHF and sigma-S in stationary phase. *Mol. Microbiol.* **13:**265–272.

3. Altuvia, S., D. Weinstein-Fischer, A. Zhang, L. Postow, and G. Storz. 1997. A small, stable RNA induced by oxidative stress: role as a pleiotropic regulator and antimutator. *Cell* **90:**43–53.

4. Atlung, T., and L. Brondsted. 1994. Role of the transcriptional activator AppY in regulation of the *cyx appA* operon of *Escherichia coli* by anaerobiosis, phosphate starvation, and growth phase. *J. Bacteriol.* **171:**5414–5422.

5. Atlung, T., A. Nielsen, and F. G. Hansen. 1989. Isolation, characterization, and nucleotide sequence of *appY*, a regulatory gene for growth-phase-dependent gene expression. *J. Bacteriol.* **171:**1683–1691.

6. Barth, M., C. Marschall, A. Muffler, D. Fischer, and R. Hengge-Aronis. 1995. Role for the histone-like protein H-NS in growth phase-dependent and osmotic regulation of σ^S and many σ^S-dependent genes in *Escherichia coli. J. Bacteriol.* **177:**3455–3464.

7. Blum, P., M. Velligan, N. Lin, and A. Matin. 1992. DnaK-mediated alterations in human growth hormone protein inclusion bodies. *Biotechnology* **10:**301–304.

8. Boisvert, D. C., J. Wang, Z. Otwinowski, A. L. Horwich, and P. B. Sigler. 1996. The 2.4 Å crystal structure of the bacterial chaperonin GroEL complexed with ATPγS. *Nature Struct. Biol.* **3:**170–177.

9. Boylen, C., and J. C. Ensign. 1970. Intracellular substrates for endogenous metabolism during long-term starvation of rod and spherical cells of *Arthrobacter crystallopoites. J. Bacteriol.* **103:**578–587.

10. Brondsted, L., and T. Atlung. 1994. Anaerobic regulation of the hydrogenase I (*hya*) operon of *Escherichia coli. J. Bacteriol.* **176:**5423–5428.

11. Brown, L., and T. Elliott. 1996. Efficient translation of the RpoS sigma factor in *Salmonella typhimurium* requires host factor I, an RNA-binding protein encoded by the *hfq* gene. *J. Bacteriol.* **178:**3763–3770.

12. Buchanan, C. E., and O. Sowell. 1982. Synthesis of penicillin-binding protein 6 by stationary phase *Escherichia coli. J. Bacteriol.* **114:**1068–1073.

13. Buchmeier, N., S. Bossie, C.-Y. Chen, F. C. Fang, D. G. Guiney, and S. J. Libby. 1997. SlyA, a transcriptional regulator of *Salmonella typhimurium*, is required for resistance to oxidative stress and is expressed in the intracellular environment of macrophages. *Infect. Immun.* **65:**3725–3730.

14. Chen, C.-Y., N. A. Buchmeier, S. Libby, F. C. Fang, M. Krause, and D. G. Guiney. 1995. Central regulatory role for the RpoS sigma factor in expression of *Salmonella dublin* plasmid virulence genes. *J. Bacteriol.* **177:**5303–5309.

15. Chen, C.-Y., L. Eckmann, S. J. Libby, F. C. Fang, S. Okamoto, M. F. Kagnoff, J. Fierer, and D. G. Guiney. 1996. Expression of *Salmonella typhimurium rpoS* and *rpoS*-dependent genes in the intracellular environment of eukaryotic cells. *Infect. Immun.* **64:**4739–4743.

16. Coffin, R., and J. Sharp. 1987. Microbial trophodynamics in the Delaware Estuary. *Mar. Ecol. Progr. Ser.* **41:**253–266.

17. Compton, L. A., J. M. Davis, J. R. MacDonald, and H. P. Bächinger. 1992. Structural and functional characterization of *Escherichia coli* peptidyl-prolyl *cis-trans* isomerases. *Eur. J. Biochem.* **206:**927–934.

18. Dersch, P., K. Schmidt, and E. Bremer. 1993. Synthesis of the *Escherichia coli* K-12 nucleoid-associated DNA-binding protein H-NS is subjected to growth-phase control and autoregulation. *Mol. Microbiol.* **8:**875–889.

19. Ding, Q., S. Kusano, M. Villarejo, and A. Ishihama. 1995. Promoter selectivity control of *Escherichia coli* RNA polymerase by ionic strength: differential recognition of osmoregulated promoters by $E\sigma^D$ and $E\sigma^S$ holoenzymes. *Mol. Microbiol.* **16:**649–656.

20. D'Mello, R. A., P. R. Langford, and J. S. Kroll. 1997. Role of bacterial Mn-cofactored superoxide dismutase in oxidative stress responses, nasopharyngeal colonization, and sustained bacteremia caused by *Haemophilus influenzae* type b. *Infect. Immun.* **65:**2700–2706.

21. **Espinosa-Urgel, M., and A. Tormo.** 1993. σ^S-Dependent promoters in *Escherichia coli* are located in DNA regions with intrinsic curvature. *Nucleic Acids Res.* **20:**3667–3670.

22. **Fink, A. L.** 1998. Preface, p. iii–iv. *In* A. Fink and Y. Goto (ed.), *Molecular Chaperones in the Life Cycle of Proteins: Structure, Function and Mode of Action.* Marcel Dekker, Inc. New York.

23. **Fisher, G., J. Heins, and A. Barth.** 1983. The conformation around the peptide bond between the P1- and P-2 positions is important for catalytic activity of some proline-specific proteases. *Biochim. Biophys. Acta* **742:**452–462.

24. **Fraley, C., J. H. Kim, M. P. McCann, and A. C. Matin.** 1998. The *Escherichia coli* starvation gene, *cstC*, is regulated by cAMP, RpoS and RpoN and is involved in amino acid catabolism. *J. Bacteriol.* **180:**4287–4290.

25. **Freeman, B. C., and R. I. Morimoto.** 1996. The human cytosolic molecular chaperones hsp90, hsp70 (hsc70) and hdj-1 have distinct roles in recognition of a non-native protein and protein folding. *EMBO J.* **12:**2969–2979.

26. **Fu, J. C., L. Ding, and S. Clarke.** 1991. Purification, gene cloning, and sequence analysis of an L-isoaspartyl protein carboxyl methyltransferase from *Escherichia coli. J. Biol. Chem.* **266:** 14562–14572.

27. **Fujita, M., K. Tanaka, H. Takahashi, and A. Amemura.** 1994. Transcription of the principal sigma-factor genes, *rpoD* and *rpoS*, in *Pseudomonas aeruginosa* is controlled according to the growth phase. *Mol. Microbiol.* **13:**1071–1077.

28. **Gentry, D. R., V. J. Hernandez, L. H. Nguyen, D. B. Jensen, and M. Cashel.** 1993. Synthesis of the stationary-phase sigma factor σ^S is positively regulated by ppGpp. *J. Bacteriol.* **175:** 7982–7989.

29. **Georgopoulos, C., K. Liberek, M. Zylicz, and D. Ang.** 1994. Properties of the heat shock proteins of *Escherichia coli* and the autoregulation of the heat shock response, p. 209–249. *In* R. I. Morimoto, A. Tissieres, and C. Georgopoulos (ed.), *The Biology of Heat Shock Proteins and Molecular Chaperones.* Cold Spring Harbor Laboratory Press, Cold Spring Harbor, N.Y.

30. **Ghiorse, W. C., and J. J. Wilson.** 1988. Microbial ecology of the terrestrial subsurface. *Adv. Appl. Microbiol.* **33:**107–172.

31. **Gilligan, P. H.** 1991. Microbiology of airway disease in patients with cystic fibrosis. *Clin. Microbiol. Rev.* **4:**35–51.

32. **Givskov, M., L. Eberl, S. Moller, L. K. Poulsen, and S. Molin.** 1994. Responses to nutrient starvation in *Pseudomonas putida* KT2442: analysis of general cross-protection, cell shape, and macromolecular content. *J. Bacteriol.* **176:**7–14.

33. **Gottesman, S.** 1996. Proteases and their targets in *Escherichia coli. Annu. Rev. Genet.* **30:**465–506.

34. **Groat, R. G., J. Schultz, E. Zychlinsky, A. Bockman, and A. Matin.** 1986. Starvation proteins in *Escherichia coli:* kinetics of synthesis and role in starvation survival. *J. Bacteriol.* **168:**486–493.

34a. **Hanawa, T., T. Yamamoto, and S. Kamiya.** 1995. *Listeria monocytogenes* can grow in macrophages without the aid of proteins induced by environmental stress. *Infect. Immun.* **63:**4595–4599.

35. **Harakeh, M. S., J. Berg, J. C. Hoff, and A. Matin.** 1985. Susceptibility of chemostat-grown *Yersinia enterocolitica* and *Klebsiella pneumoniae* to chlorine dioxide. *Appl. Environ. Microbiol.* **49:**69–72.

36. **Hartl, F. U.** 1996. Molecular chaperones in cellular protein folding. *Nature* **381:**571–580.

37. **Hendrick, J. P., and F. U. Hartl.** 1993. Molecular chaperone functions of heat-shock proteins. *Annu. Rev. Biochem.* **62:**349–384.

38. **Hengge-Aronis, R.** 1996. Regulation of gene expression during entry into stationary phase, p. 1497–1512. *In* F. C. Neidhardt, R. Curtiss III, J. L. Ingraham, E. C. C. Lin, K. B. Low, Jr., B. Magasanik, W. S. Reznikoff, M. Riley, M. Schaechter, and H. E. Umbarger (ed.), *Escherichia coli and Salmonella Typhimurium: Cellular and Molecular Biology.* American Society for Microbiology, Washington, D.C.

39. **Henis, Y.** 1987. Survival and dormancy in microorganisms, p. 1–108. *In* Y. Henis (ed.), *Survival and Dormancy in Microorganisms.* John Wiley & Sons, Inc., New York.

40. **Hernandez, V. J., and M. Cashel.** 1995. Changes in conserved region 3 of *Escherichia coli* σ^{70} mediated ppGpp-dependent functions *in vivo. J. Mol. Biol.* **252:**536–549.

41. **Hiratsu, K., H. Shinagawa., and K. Makino.** 1995. Mode of promoter recognition by the *Escherichia coli* RNA polymerase holoenzyme containing the σ^S subunit: identification of the recognition sequence of the *fic* promoter. *Mol. Microbiol.* **18:**841–850.

42. **Hottenrott, S., T. Schumann, A. Plückthun, G. Fischer, and J.-U. Rahfeld.** 1997. The *Escherichia coli* SlyD is a metal ion–regulated peptidyl-prolyl cis-trans-isomerase. *J. Biol. Chem.* **272:** 15697–15701.

43. **James, P., C. Pfund, and E. A. Craig.** 1997. Functional specificity among Hsp70 molecular chaperones. *Science* **275:**387–389.

44. **Jenkins, D., E. Auger, and A. Matin.** 1991. Role of RpoH, a heat shock regulator protein,

in *Escherichia coli* carbon starvation protein synthesis and survival. *J. Bacteriol.* **173**:1992–1996.

45. **Jenkins, D. E., S. Chaisson, and A. Matin.** 1990. Starvation-induced cross protection against osmotic challenge in *Escherichia coli*. *J. Bacteriol.* **172**:2779–2781.

46. **Jenkins, D. E., J. E. Schultz, and A. Matin.** 1988. Starvation-induced cross protection against heat or H_2O_2 peroxide challenge in *Escherichia coli*. *J. Bacteriol.* **170**:3910–3914.

47. **Jeon, T.-J., and K.-J. Lee.** 1998. Synthesis and requirement of *Escherichia coli* heat shock proteins GroEL and DnaK for survival under phenol stress conditions. *J. Microbiol.* **36**:26–33.

48. **Jishage, M., A. Iwata, S. Ueda, and A. Ishihama.** 1996. Regulation of RNA polymerase sigma subunit synthesis in *Escherichia coli*: intracellular levels of four species of sigma subunits under various growth conditions. *J. Bacteriol.* **178**:5447–5451.

49. **Kern, G., D. Kern, F. X. Schmid, and G. Fischer.** 1994. Reassessment of the putative chaperone function of prolyl-cis/trans-isomerases. *FEBS Lett.* **348**:145–148.

49a.**Kim, J. H., E. Auger, R. Solly, and A. Matin.** 1993. *E. coli* starvation genes: cloning and analysis of *pexA*, abstr. I-52. Abstr. Annu. Meet. Am. Soc. Microbiol. 1993.

50. **Kim, Y., L. S. Watrud, and A. Matin.** 1995. A carbon starvation survival gene of *Pseudomonas putida* is regulated by σ^{54}. *J. Bacteriol.* **177**:1850–1859.

51. **Landini, P., L. Hajec, and M. R. Volkert.** 1994. Structure and transcriptional regulation of the *Escherichia coli* adaptive response gene *aidB*. *J. Bacteriol.* **176**:6583–6589.

52. **Lange, R., and R. Hengge-Aronis.** 1991. Identification of a central regulator of stationary-phase gene expression in *Escherichia coli*. *Mol. Microbiol.* **5**:49–59.

53. **Lange, R., and R. Hengge-Aronis.** 1994. The cellular concentration of the σ^S subunit of RNA polymerase in *Escherichia coli* is controlled at the levels of transcription, translation, and protein stability. *Genes Dev.* **8**:1600–1612.

54. **Latifi, A., M. Foglino, K. Tanaka, P. Williams, and A. Lazdunski.** 1996. A hierarchical quorum-sensing cascade in *Pseudomonas aeruginosa* links the transcriptional activators LasR and RhlR (VsmR) to expression of the stationary-phase sigma factor RpoS. *Mol. Microbiol.* **21**:1137–1146.

55. **Lazar, S. W., and R. Kolter.** 1996. SurA assists the folding of *E. coli* outer membrane proteins. *J. Bacteriol.* **178**:1770–1773.

56. **Lee, B-Y, and M. A. Horwitz.** 1995. Identification of macrophage and stress-induced proteins of *Mycobacterium tuberculosis*. *J. Clin. Invest.* **96**:245–249.

57. **Lee, I. S., J. Lin, H. K. Hall, B. Bearson, and J. W. Foster.** 1995. The stationary phase sigma factor σ^S (RpoS) is required for a sustained acid tolerance response in virulent *Salmonella typhimurium*. *Mol. Microbiol.* **17**:155–167.

58. **Liautard, J. P.** 1991. Are prions misfolded molecular chaperones? *FEBS Lett.* **294**:155–157.

59. **Lomovskaya, O., J. P. Kidwell, and A. Matin.** 1994. Characterization of the σ^{38}-dependent expression of a core *Escherichia coli* starvation gene, *pexB*. *J. Bacteriol.* **176**:3928–3935.

60. **Mackaness, G. B.** 1962. Cellular resistance to infection. *J. Exp. Med.* **116**:381–406.

61. **Marques, S., M. T. Gallegos, and J. L. Ramos.** 1995. Role of σ^S in transcription from the positively controlled P_m promoter of the TOL plasmid of *Pseudomonas putida*. *Mol. Microbiol.* **18**:851–857.

62. **Marschall, C., and R. Hengge-Aronis.** 1995. Regulatory characteristics and promoter analysis of *csiE*, a stationary phase-inducible gene under the control of σ^S and the cAMP-CRP complex in *Escherichia coli*. *Mol. Microbiol.* **18**:175–184.

63. **Matin, A.** 1991. The molecular basis of carbon-starvation-induced general resistance in *Escherichia coli*. *Mol. Microbiol.* **5**:3–10.

64. **Matin, A.** 1994. Starvation promoters of *Escherichia coli:* their function, regulation and use in bioprocessing and bioremediation. Recombinant DNA Technology II. *Ann. NY Acad. Sci.* **722**:277–291.

65. **Matin, A.** 1996. Role of alternate sigma factors in starvation protein synthesis—novel mechanisms of catabolite repression. *Res. Microbiol.* **147**:494–504.

66. **Matin, A., C. D. Little, C. D. Fraley, and M. Keyhan.** 1995. Use of starvation promoters to limit growth and selectively express trichloroethylene and phenol transformation activity in recombinant *Escherichia coli*. *Appl. Environ. Microbiol.* **61**:3323–3328.

67. **Maw, J., and G. G. Meynell.** 1968. The true division and death rates of *Salmonella typhimurium* in the mouse spleen determined with superinfecting phage P22. *Br. J. Exp. Pathol.* **49**:597–613.

68. **McCann, M., J. Kidwell, and A. Matin.** 1991. The putative σ factor KatF has a central role in Pex protein synthesis and development of starvation-mediated general resistance in *Escherichia coli*. *J. Bacteriol.* **173**:4188–4194.

68a.**McCann, M., C. Fraley, and A. Matin.** 1993. The putative σ factor KatF is regulated posttranscriptionally during carbon starvation. *J. Bacteriol.* **175**:2143–2149.

69. **Miller, P. F., and M. C. Sulavik.** 1996. Overlaps and parallels in the regulation of intrinsic multiple-antibiotic resistance in *Escherichia coli. Mol. Microbiol.* **21**:441–448.

70. **Muffler, A., D. Fischer, S. Altuvia, G. Storz, and R. Hengge-Aronis.** 1996. The response regulator RssB controls stability of the σ^S subunit of RNA polymerase in *Escherichia coli. EMBO J.* **15**:1333–1339.

71. **Muffler, A., D. Fischer, and R. Hengge-Aronis.** 1996. The RNA-binding protein HF-I, known as a host factor for phage $Q\beta$ RNA replication, is essential for *rpoS* translation in *Escherichia coli. Genes Dev.* **10**:1143–1151.

72. **Muffler, A., D. D. Traulsen, D. Fischer, R. Lange, and R. Hengge-Aronis.** 1997. The RNA-binding protein HF-I plays a global regulatory role which is largely, but not exclusively, due to its role in expression of the sigma S subunit of RNA polymerase in *Escherichia coli. J. Bacteriol.* **179**:297–300.

73. **Muffler, A., D. D. Traulsen, R. Lange, and R. Hengge-Aronis.** 1996. Posttranscriptional osmotic regulation of the σ^S subunit of RNA polymerase in *Escherichia coli. J. Bacteriol.* **178**:1607–1613.

74. **Munster, U., and R. J. Chrost.** 1990. Advanced biochemical and molecular approaches to aquatic microbial ecology, p. 8–46. *In* J. Overbeck and R. J. Chrost (ed.), *Brock/Springer Series in Contemporary Biosciences*. Springer-Verlag, New York.

75. **Nguyen, L. H., D. B. Jensen, N. E. Thompson, D. R. Gentry, and R. R. Burgess.** 1993. In vitro functional characterization of overproduced *Escherichia coli katF/rpoS* gene product. *Biochemistry* **32**:11112–11117.

76. **Nickerson C. A., and R. Curtiss III.** 1997. Role of sigma factor RpoS in initial stages of *Salmonella typhimurium* infection. *Infect. Immun.* **65**:1814–1823.

77. **Nystrom, T., K. Flardh, and S. Kjellberg.** 1990. Response to multiple nutrient starvation in marine *Vibrio* sp. strain CCUG 15956. *J. Bacteriol.* **172**:7085–7097.

78. **Olsen, A., A. Arnqvist, M. Hammar, S. Sukupolvi, and S. Normark.** 1993. The *rpoS* sigma factor relieves H-NS-mediated transcriptional repression of *csgA*, the subunit gene of fibronectin-binding curli in *Escherichia coli. Mol. Microbiol.* **7**:523–536.

79. **Ozaki, M., A. Wada, N. Fujita, and A. Ishihama.** 1991. Growth phase-dependent modification of RNA polymerase in *Escherichia coli. Mol. Gen. Genet.* **230**:17–23.

80. **Pallen, M. J., and B. W. Wren.** 1997. The HtrA family of serine proteases. *Mol. Microbiol.* **26**:209–221.

81. **Palleros, D. R., K. L. Reid, L. Shi, W. J. Welch, and A. L. Fink.** 1993. ATP-induced protein-Hsp70 complex dissociation requires K^+ but not ATP hydrolysis. *Nature* **365**:664–666.

82. **Palleros, D. R., W. J. Welch, and A. L. Fink.** 1991. Interaction of hsp70 with unfolded proteins: effects of temperature and nucleotides on the kinetics of binding. *Proc. Natl. Acad. Sci. USA* **88**:5719–5723.

83. **Parsell, D. A., A. S. Kowal, M. A. Singer, and S. Lindquist.** 1994. Protein disaggregation mediated by heat shock protein Hsp104. *Nature* **372**:475–478.

84. **Powell, B. S., D. L. Court, T. Inada, and Y. Nakamura.** 1995. Novel proteins of the phosphotransferase system encoded within the *rpoN* operon of *Escherichia coli. J. Biol. Chem.* **270**:4822–4839.

85. **Pratt, L., and T. Silhavy.** 1996. The response regulator SprE controls the stability of RpoS. *Proc. Natl. Acad. Sci. USA* **93**:2488–2492.

86. **Reeve, C. A., P. S. Amy, and A. Matin.** 1984. Role of protein synthesis in the survival of carbon-starved *Escherichia coli* K-12. *J. Bacteriol.* **160**:1041–1046.

87. **Rockabrand, D., T. Arthur, G. Korinek, K. Livers, and P. Blum.** 1995. An essential role for the *Escherichia coli* DnaK protein in starvation-induced thermotolerance, H_2O_2 resistance, and reductive division. *J. Bacteriol.* **177**:3695–3703.

88. **Rockabrand, D., K. Livers, T. Austin, R. Kaiser, D. Jensen, R. Burgess, and P. Blum.** 1998. Roles of DnaK and RpoS in starvation-induced thermotolerance of *Escherichia coli. J. Bacteriol.* **180**:846–854.

89. **Rohrwild, M., O. Coux, H.-C. Huang, R. P. Moerschell, S. J. Yoo, J. H. Seol, C. H. Chung, and A. L. Goldberg.** 1996. HslV-HslU: a novel ATP-dependent protease complex in *Escherichia coli* related to the eukaryotic proteasome. *Proc. Natl. Acad. Sci. USA* **93**:5808–5813.

90. **Rouquette, C., M-T. Ripio, E. Pellegrini, J.-M. Tascon, J.-A. Vazquez-Boland, P. Berche.** 1996. Identification of a ClpC ATPase required for stress tolerance and in vivo survival of *Listeria monocytogenes. Mol. Microbiol.* **21**:977–987.

91. **Rouvière, P. E., and C. A. Gross.** 1996. SurA, a periplasmic protein with peptidyl-prolyl isomerase activity, participates in the assembly of outer membrane porins. *Genes Dev.* **10**:3170–3182.

92. **Schmid, F. X., L. M. Mayr, M. Mücke, and E. R. Schönbrunner.** 1993. Prolyl isomerases:

role in protein folding. *Adv. Protein Chem.* **44:** 25–66.

92a. **Schneider, B. L., A. K. Kiupakis, and L. J. Reitzer.** 1998. Arginine catabolism and the arginine succinyltransferase pathway in *Escherichia coli. J. Bacteriol.* **180:**4278–4286.

93. **Schroeder, H., T. Langer, F. U. Hartl, and B. Bukau.** 1993. DnaK, DnaJ and GrpE form a cellular chaperone machinery capable of repairing heat-induced protein damage. *EMBO J.* **12:**4137–4144.

94. **Schultz, J. E., G. I. Latter, and A. Matin.** 1988. Differential regulation by cyclic AMP of starvation protein synthesis in *Escherichia coli. J. Bacteriol.* **170:**3903–3909.

95. **Schultz, J. E., and A. Matin.** 1987. Regulation of carbon starvation genes in *Escherichia coli. In* Homeostatic mechanisms in microorganisms. *FEMS Symp.* **44:**50–60.

96. **Schultz, J. E., and A. Matin.** 1991. Molecular and functional characterization of a carbon starvation gene of *Escherichia coli. J. Mol. Biol.* **218:**129–140.

97. **Schweder, T., K. Lee, O. Lomovskaya, and A. Matin.** 1996. Regulation of *Escherichia coli* starvation sigma factor (σ^S) by ClpXP protease. *J. Bacteriol.* **178:**470–476.

98. **Sledjeski, D. D., and S. Gottesman.** 1995. A small RNA acts as an antisilencer of the H-NA-silenced *rcsA* gene of *Escherichia coli. Proc. Natl. Acad. Sci. USA* **92:**2003–2007.

99. **Song, J. L., and C. C. Wang.** 1995. Chaperone-like activity of protein disulfide-isomerase in the refolding of rhodanese. *Eur. J. Biochem.* **231:**312–316.

100. **Szabo, A., T. Langer, H. Schroeder, J. Flanagan, B. Bukau, and F. U. Hartl.** 1994. The ATP hydrolysis-dependent reaction cycle of the *Escherichia coli* Hsp70 system DnaK, DnaJ, and GrpE. *Proc. Natl. Acad. Sci. USA* **91:**10345–10349.

101. **Tanaka, K., S. Kusano, N. Fujita, A. Ishihama, and H. Takahashi.** 1995. Promoter determinants for *Escherichia coli* RNA polymerase holoenzyme containing σ^{38} (the *rpoS* gene product). *Nucleic Acids Res.* **23:**827–834.

102. **Tormo, A., M. Almiron, and R. Kolter.** 1990. *surA*, an *Escherichia coli* gene essential for survival in stationary phase. *J. Bacteriol.* **172:** 4339–4347.

103. **Tuite, M. F., and S. L. Lindquist.** 1996. Maintenance and inheritance of yeast prions. *Trends Genet.* **12:**467–471.

104. **Tuveson, R. W.** 1981. The interaction of a gene (*nur*) controlling near-UV-sensitivity and the *polA1* gene in strains of *E. coli* K12. *Photochem. Photobiol.* **33:**919–923.

105. **Ueguchi, C., Kakeda, M., and Mizuno, T.** 1993. Autoregulatory expression of the *Escherichia coli hns* gene encoding a nucleoid protein: H-NS functions as a repressor of its own transcription. *Mol. Gen. Genet.* **236:**171–178.

106. **Ulitzur, S., A. Matin, C. Fraley, and E. Meighen.** 1997. H-NS protein represses transcription of the lux systems of *Vibrio fischeri* and other luminous bacteria cloned into *Escherichia coli. Curr. Microbiol.* **35:**336–342.

107. **Waksman, S. A.** 1927. *Principles of Soil Microbiology.* The Williams and Wilkins Co., Baltimore.

108. **Wawrzynow, A., B. Banecki, and M. Zylicz.** 1996. The Clp ATPases define a novel class of molecular chaperones. *Mol. Microbiol.* **21:** 895–899.

109. **Wise, A., R. Brems, V. Ramakrishnan, and M. Villarejo.** 1996. Sequences in the -35 region of *Escherichia coli rpoS*-dependent genes promote transcription by $E\sigma^S$. *J. Bacteriol.* **178:** 2785–2793.

110. **Xu, Z., A. L. Horwich, and P. B. Sigler.** 1997. The crystal structure of the asymmetric GroEL-GroES-(ADP)$_7$ chaperonin complex. *Nature* **388:**741–750.

111. **Yamashino, T., M. Kakeda, C. Ueguchi, and T. Mizuno.** 1994. An analogue of the DnaJ molecular chaperone whose expression is controlled by σ^S during the stationary phase and phosphate starvation in *Escherichia coli. Mol. Microbiol.* **13:**475–483.

112. **Yamashino, T., C. Ueguchi, and T. Mizuno.** 1995. Quantitative control of the stationary phase specific sigma factor, σ^S, in *Escherichia coli*: involvement of the nucleoid protein HNS. *EMBO J.* **14:**594–602.

113. **Yura, T., H. Nagai, and H. Mori.** 1993. Regulation of heat-shock response in bacteria. *Annu. Rev. Microbiol.* **47:**321–350.

114. **Zgurskaya, H., M. Keyhan, and A. Matin.** 1997. The σ^S level in starving *Escherichia coli* cells increases solely as a result of its increased stability, despite decreased synthesis. *Mol. Microbiol.* **24:**643–651.

115. **Zhou, Y., and S. Gottesman.** 1998. Regulation of proteolysis of the stationary-phase sigma factor RpoS. *J. Bacteriol.* **180:**1154–1158.

ADHESION AND INVASION MECHANISMS

INTRODUCTION

Emanuel Hanski

Adherence of bacteria to host cells is an essential step leading to development of an infection. This is particularly important in areas such as the mouth, small intestine, and bladder where mucosal surfaces are washed by fluids. In these areas, only bacteria that can adhere to mucosal surfaces will be able to stay and occupy a specific niche. Even in relatively stagnant areas such as the colon and vaginal tract, bacteria must have a way of attaching themselves firmly to host cells to establish an infection. Most studies on adhesion by bacterial pathogens have focused on the binding of a single bacterium to receptors on the host cell surface. However, bacteria can also form dense, multiorganism layers on surfaces (biofilms), in which the first layer of the bacteria are attached to this basal layer usually by a polysaccharide matrix. Biofilms are of unquestioned importance for the survival of bacteria in many environmental settings. This is particularly important in hospital-acquired infections in patients with indwelling devices such as urinary or venous catheters or implants such artificial heart valves or voice prostheses.

Biofilms are more resistant to antibiotics than are free-living bacteria and are partially protected from phagocytes. Thus, the formation of biofilm on an implant has adverse consequences for the patient.

Once adherence has occurred, the bacteria may replicate at this site or move deeper into host tissues before significant replication occurs. Damage to the host may occur at any point in this process, because of either products of synthesis such as bacterial toxins or the harmful effects of normal defense mechanisms. Thus, usually two potential fates await a bacterial pathogen. One is extracellular colonization, and the other is internalization of various cells that include professional phagocytes and nonphagocytes, such as epithelial and endothelial cells. Entry of bacteria to the latter type of cells involves induction of changes in the host cell cytoskeleton that finally result in forcing engulfment of the bacteria by these cells. Within host cells, the bacteria usually escape from the phagocytic vesicle into the cell cytoplasm. There are many advantages to be gained in the host cytoplasm, including an abundance of nutrients, protection from antibodies and complement, and partial protection from some antibiotics.

Secreted or surface-exposed bacterial proteins have long been known to play central

Emanuel Hanski, Clinical Microbiology, Hadassah Medical School, Hebrew University, Ein Karem, Jerusalem 91120, Israel.

roles in bacterial–host interactions. In the past 7 years, the highly conserved multicomponent type III secretion system has been found in many gram-negative bacteria that cause disease in animals and plants. This secretion system is responsible for transporting (injecting) effector molecules directly from bacterial cytoplasm to the host cytoplasm across three membranes, two of the bacterial pathogen and one of the host cell. Within the host, these effector proteins act as bacterial toxins, modifying specific host functions. Thus bacterial adherence may, in addition to the consequence described above, also facilitate the delivery of specific virulence factor into the host cells.

In this section, Jack London discusses formation of dental plaque. Bacteria that make up over 80% of this material coexist in an extremely complex arrangement. There may be as many as 200 species in one site that can be categorized as primary or secondary colonizers. The intricate bacteria–bacteria and bacteria–host cell interactions determine formation and maintenance of oral biofilms. Likewise, Henk J. Busscher and coworkers discuss formation of a biofilm on indwelling voice prostheses. They show that active probiotic bacteria such as thermophilic streptococci reduce initial adherence of *Candida* strains to silicone rubber.

Ilan Tsarfati and colleagues describe the changes occurring in the organization of the epithelial cell cytoskeleton upon entry of *Streptococcus pyogenes* and *Candida albicans*. Ilan Rosenshine and Yuan Fang discuss the virulence of enteropathogenic *Escherichia coli* (EPEC). They demonstrate that the expression of several virulence factors is regulated by conditions such as temperature, growth phase, and pH. These factors encode components of the type III protein secretion system, through which affector proteins are translocated into the host cell. Anthrax toxin, produced by the bacterium *Bacillus anthracis*, is composed of three proteins: protective antigen (PA), edema factor (EF), and lethal factor (LF). PA binds to specific cell surface receptors, and upon proteolytic activation to a 63-kDa fragment, forms membrane channels that mediate entry of EF and LF. John Collier and colleagues discuss the structure of the PA channel formed in lipid bilayers.

FROM DENTAL PLAQUE TO ORAL BIOFILM: A MOLECULAR ODYSSEY

Jack London

4

A 17th-century report detailing the morphological variation of microorganisms found in material removed from between the teeth is most likely the first description of a biofilm to be published in the scientific literature (20). The full extent of the morphological and genetic diversity found among the oral microbiota was not appreciated until they were carefully enumerated in contemporary taxonomic surveys (69, 70, 78, 79). Ecological studies described the temporal population changes within plaque communities and established that these deposits were dynamic, evolving biofilm (82). Following oral prophylaxis, teeth are coated with gram-positive oral streptococci and actinomyces within a matter of hours. After several days, a population of gram-negative bacteria appear, and if the deposit is not disturbed by physical intervention, the gram-negative population will become dominant, resulting in soft tissue inflammation. The subsequent demonstration of specific bacteria-to-host (29, 34, 84) and bacteria-to-bacteria attachments added yet another level of complexity to oral colonization and biofilm formation (35). This chapter examines the makeup of the oral flora, the physical and biochemical properties of the interactions, and current ideas about the nature of oral biofilms.

ORAL MICROFLORA

The oral cavity plays host to a large assortment of unicellular prokaryotic and various eukaryotic microorganisms including yeast and amoeboid forms. Current estimates suggest that subgingival or periodontal plaque contains 20 genera of bacteria representing over 200 species (69, 70, 78, 79); the total number of taxa found in the mount is significantly larger, about 450. Even before the nature of bacteria-to-host or bacteria-to-bacteria interactions was understood, it was clear that bacterial plaque was composed of large numbers of diverse bacteria that varied with the age of the deposited material. A cleaned tooth is colonized almost immediately by indigenous strains of *Streptococcus oralis*, *Streptococcus mitis*, *Streptococcus sanguis*, and *Streptococcus gordonii*; competing for space on the tooth surface are *Actinomyces* spp., *Haemophilus* spp., and *Viellonella* spp. Within 12 h, a 24-mm^2 area of enamel can be colonized with 10^7 CFU of bacteria (72). An accretion of gram-negative anaerobic bacteria follows, with accumulation of noxious meta-

Jack London, National Institute of Dental Research, National Institutes of Health, Bethesda, MD 20892.

Microbial Ecology and Infectious Disease, Edited by Eugene Rosenberg
©1999 American Society for Microbiology, Washington, D.C.

bolic products and cytotoxic cell components. These set up inflammatory responses that destroy epithelial tissue to produce a pocket beneath the gingival margin (28). The developing pocket usually contains a larger consortium of genera including *Streptococcus, Gamella, Propionibacterium, Actinomyces, Lactobacillus, Peptostreptococcus, Eubacterium, Bifidobacterium, Fusobacterium, Porphyromonas, Prevotella, Capnocytophaga, Bacteroides, Dialister, Actinobacillus, Veillonella, Wolinella, Eikenella, Haemophilus,* and *Treponema* (69, 70). The periodontal plaque deposit is also home to members of the *Archaeae.* The archeons are represented by methane producers belonging to the genus *Methanobrevibacterium* (48) and a group of as yet unidentified sulfate-reducing bacteria (40, 83). The appearance of archeons and the diversification seen among other types of prokaryotes can be attributed to an expanding and varied food chain within the developing pocket.

GLYCOCALYXES, TROPISMS, AND SPECIFIC INTERACTIONS

It has become axiomatic that oral lactic acid bacteria are causative agents of carious enamel lesions by virtue of their ability to produce organic acids from sugar fermentation. *Streptococcus mutans* had been identified as a potential caries-producing pathogen earlier in this century (13). Koch's postulates were fulfilled some 40 years later with the demonstration of its pathogenic potential and transmissibility in animal models (23). However, it was not until isolates of *S. mutans* were characterized biochemically that a rationale for the deposition of these bacteria on a tooth surface emerged. When grown in the presence of sucrose, the streptococcus synthesized an adherent polysaccharide matrix capable of trapping bacteria (30). At the time, the accumulation of bacteria in plaque was still considered to be a random process, and specificity of accretion was not an issue. The polysaccharide matrix also was thought to concentrate metabolically produced acids near the tooth surface, which accelerated the dissolution of enamel.

Concomitant with the *S. mutans* studies, a number of reports established that certain oral microorganisms were readily isolated from specific areas of the oral cavity. For example, *Streptococcus salivarius* was found on the tongue and in saliva but less frequently on teeth (84), *Bacteroides* species were plentiful in or below the gingival crevice (34), *S. mutans* exhibited an affinity for enamel surfaces as did strains of *S. mitis* and *S. sanguis* (84). These and other studies suggested that oral bacteria exhibit tropisms or predilections for particular niches within the mouth.

Both avenues of research, tissue specificity and adherence, established a framework for the next testable hypothesis, namely, that plaque was an organized biofilm. It was demonstrated that commercially available dextrans, similar to the glucans produced by *S. mutans*, caused the aggregation of *S. mutans* cells (31), producing an "ersatz" plaque ex vitro. Subsequently, saliva and extracts of plaque were shown to contain substances that could aggregate a number of oral bacteria (36). High-molecular-weight mucins were one of the salivary components implicated in the aggregation process. Later research showed that streptococci belonging to the *S. mutans* group synthesized surface-binding proteins specific for glucans; the binding proteins anchor the bacteria to the adherent polysaccharide (44, 65).

In addition to mucins, other salivary constituents adhere to teeth, forming a pellicle coating. These polysaccharides and proteins act as receptor molecules for oral bacteria. As the pure components of the saliva became available, they were tested in solution or adsorbed to solid supports that mimicked the tooth surface, e.g., hydroxyapatite particles or enamel chips (12, 42). Salivary proteins including the family of proline-rich proteins (PRP), α-amylase, and statherin have been shown to serve as bacterial receptors on such supports. Initially, radiolabeled *Streptococcus* sp. and *Actinomyces naeslundii* were shown to bind to acidic PRPs (32, 33); the list presently includes *Eikenella corrodens, Actinomyces israelii, S.*

mutans, *Streptococcus uberis*, *Fusobacterium nucleatum* and *Porphyromonas gingivalis* (2, 47). Libraries of synthetic peptides derived from the sequence analyses of the acid PRPs aided in identifying those segments of the molecule that serve as receptor sites (2, 3, 47). Both *P. gingivalis* and *F. nucleatum* can bind to statherin (6, 29), and various streptococci attach to α-amylase–coated substrates (5, 41, 76). The paradigm describing primary colonization is grounded in pellicle-bacteria interactions.

Concomitant with the early saliva studies, another set of important observations established that genetically unrelated oral bacteria were capable of independently aggregating with one another (35). These findings led to formulation of a model for secondary colonization model in which these "aggregating factors" permitted early colonizers to serve as scaffolds for other oral bacteria. The interaction, mediated by a receptor molecule on one cell type and an adhesive molecule on the partner, is generally referred to as coaggregation (56, 57, 61) but is also known as coadhesion or cohesion. A number of these studies included preliminary assessments to determine which partner bore surface receptor molecules and which synthesized the complementary adhesive molecules. Most, but not all, of the receptor molecules appeared to be heat stable polysaccharides, while many of the heat-labile adhesive molecules were postulated to be proteins (52, 57). Both assumptions proved to be generally valid. The assays, in their simplest form, involve mixing suspensions of two bacterial species and looking for macroscopic clumping; results can be estimated visually or quantified by use of radiolabeled bacteria or spectrophotometric assays (52, 57). From the large body of work that now exists in the literature, it can be concluded that coaggregation is the norm rather than the exception among oral bacteria. This trait is a hallmark of the oral econiche.

ADHESINS: SPECIFICITY AND PROPERTIES

The paradigm that defined adhesive proteins, adhesins, was significantly altered just over a decade ago when mutational studies revealed that *Escherichia coli* mannose-specific adhesin activity was independent of the type 1 pilin gene expression (81). Previous work had suggested or assumed that adhesin activity resided within the pilin subunit. This report provided the first evidence that an adhesin could be an independently synthesized, fimbria-associated protein. The report stimulated a number of new investigations and changed the course of ongoing adhesin studies. Since then, many laboratories have demonstrated by one means or another that adhesins are accessory proteins associated with pili, cell walls, or outer membranes of both pathogenic and saprophytic bacteria (61, 63).

The extensive cataloging of oral bacteria-to-bacteria interactions identified numerous opportunities to explore the nature of adhesins, especially adhesive proteins found on secondary colonizers. Adhesins that recognize one or more sugars in a complementary polysaccharide receptor have been designated lectinlike proteins (7, 9, 11). A second category of adhesins functions via protein-protein interactions (1, 8, 17). The number of lectin adhesins that have been partially or fully purified is relatively small because often they are synthesized in comparatively small numbers (80, 87) or their physical properties make purification difficult (61, 62).

Several approaches have been employed to identify and characterize bacterial adhesins. For lectinlike adhesins, those mono- or disaccharides that best inhibit a specific pairwise coaggregation can be coupled to an appropriate support to fabricate an affinity column. The affinity matrix is then combined with cell surface preparations containing adhesin and eluted with the appropriate sugar (51). Low yields and nonspecifically adhering proteins tend to minimize the value of this approach. An indirect procedure entails generating coaggregation-negative mutants by conventional mutagenesis or by enriching for naturally occurring mutant populations. The latter was accomplished by repetitive rounds of coaggregation in which addition of fresh receptor-bearing partner cells were used to remove a diminishing number of wild-type adhesin-bearing cells (52). This technique yields readily detectable, phenotypically stable, adhesin-negative clones. An electrophoretic comparison of wild-type and mutant cell surface proteins is used to identify the missing or altered putative adhesin protein(s) in the mutant preparation.

In a modification of this procedure, rabbit polyclonal antisera were prepared against wild-type cells bearing the adhesin. Inhibition of coaggregation by the antiserum was interpreted to mean that the serum contained adhesin-specific antibodies. Aliquots of antiserum were repeatedly absorbed with mutant cell suspensions to enrich for the adhesin-specific antibodies (45). An adsorbed antiserum that retained the ability to inhibit coaggregation was used in immunoblot analyses to detect the adhesin in wild-type cell surface preparations (45). A more labor-intensive approach involved the preparation of one or more libraries of adhesin-specific monoclonal antibodies (MAbs). Like polyclonal antisera, such libraries are easily screened by monitoring inhibition of coaggregation.

CASE STUDIES IN THE IDENTIFICATION, ISOLATION, AND CHARACTERIZATION OF ADHESINS

Prevotella loescheii

With few exceptions, one of the most confounding problems with studies of oral bacteria has been the lack of genetic information, chromosomal mapping, and easily applicable recombinant DNA technologies. For this reason, two libraries of mouse MAbs were prepared against the surface proteins of *P. loescheii* (86). The expectation was that the hydridomas would produce blocking antibodies specific for the adhesins mediating coaggregation of *P. loescheii* with its two partners *S. oralis* 34 (a galactoside-inhibitable reaction) and *A. israelii* PK14 (a sugar-insensitive reaction). Incubating ascites fluid from the respective hybridoma clones with prevotellae cells prior to addition

of the partner cells revealed that a number of different clones produced blocking antibodies (86). Purified antibodies or Fab fragments proved to be potent inhibitors of the cell-cell interactions. Electrophoretograms of *P. loescheii* cell-surface preparations treated with the set of radiolabeled MAbs that blocked coaggregation with the streptococcal partner clearly identified a monomeric protein with an estimated molecular mass of 75 kDa (85). MAbs that inhibited coaggregation between the prevotellae and actinomyces reacted with a 43-kDa polypeptide (85). The topological location of these respective adhesins was pinpointed by treating *P. loescheii* cells with MAb-coated gold particles and examining the cells with transmission electron microscopy. The coated gold particles associated only with the distal ends of the fimbriae (87). The same sets of MAbs were radiolabeled with I^{125} and were used in quantitative binding experiments to estimate the total number of adhesins on the surface of the cells; the study yielded values of roughly 200 actinomyces-specific adhesins and 400 streptococcus-specific adhesins per cell (87).

The binding analyses also indicated that the affinities (K_a) of some of the MAbs were relatively high, suggesting that antibodies conjugated to an appropriate matrix might selectively remove adhesins from *P. loescheii* surface preparations (87). Individual trials with streptococcal adhesin-specific antibody affinity columns yielded up to 200 μg of adhesin protein per 10 g of cells (wet weight) of an electrophoretically homogeneous protein. The protein was shown to be composed of six identical 75-kDa subunits; the pI of the native material was 8.0 (62). When dissociated from the affinity matrix, the lectinlike adhesin retained its ability to bind to streptococcal cells and prevent coaggregation with *P. loescheii* cells, confirming that the protein was indeed an adhesin (62). The purified adhesin also adhered to a variety of neuraminidase-treated red blood cells, causing them to agglutinate. *S. oralis* 34 participates in a number of galactoside-inhibitable coaggregations, including strains of *Actinomyces naeslundii*, *Veillonella* sp., and other streptococci. The adhesin was capable of blocking all of these interactions (London, unpublished data). Preliminary experiments suggested that all of these bacteria recognized a common or related carbohydrate receptor.

N-terminal amino acid analysis of the purified adhesin yielded the sequence of the initial 28 residues (62). Degenerate DNA probes were derived by reverse translation of sequence data employing codon usage from another bacteroides species (66). These were used to identify the lectinlike adhesin gene in a GEM-11 bacteriophage library of *P. loescheii* cDNA. The DNA fragment was cloned into pGEM7Zf(+) and then transformed in a strain of *E. coli*. DNA sequencing identified a putative 22-amino-acid signal sequence followed by all but 1 of 28 amino acids predicted from N-terminal sequencing. Unexpectedly, the next 3 nucleotides encoded a termination codon, UAA, followed by a stretch of 27 nucleotides, another ochre terminator and large open reading frame. Repeated sequencing of this region with other vectors and constructs indicated that the UAA codons did not result from sequencing errors. Another second round of adhesin sequencing identified the first 31 residues and resolved the impasse. The segment of 27 nucleotides located between the pair of UAA terminators separated the codons for amino acids 28 and 29 (asparagine and valine) of the mature protein. These nucleotides were not being translated. Analysis of the region following the first termination codon and computer-derived conformational models showed that the essential structural elements needed for ribosomal "hopping," a rare phenomenon in which a portion of message is not translated, are present (67). The archtypical hop occurs within the bacteriophage T4 topoisomerase gene where a segment of 60 nucleotides is not translated (89). Where a reading gap occurs in other systems, a second polypeptide can be generated from the same gene (67); that does not seem to be the case with the *P. loescheii* adhesin. Thus, the function of the hop in a constituitively expressed gene remains ambiguous.

Capnocytophaga Species

The oral gram-negative gliding bacteria that belong to the genus *Capnocytophaga* possess lectin-type adhesins that recognize receptors containing methyl sugars or amino sugars. *Capnocytophaga ochracea* interacts with *S. oralis* ATCC55229 (formerly *S. sanguis* H1), *A. naeslundii* PK984, and *A. israelii* PK16 via two distinguishable sugar-inhibitable interactions (88). Coaggregation with the first two mentioned partners is inhibited by L-rhamnose or D-fucose, while interaction with *A. israelii* requires both a methyl sugar and N-acetylneuraminic acid. *Capnocytophaga gingivalis* coaggregates with *A. israelii* PK16 via an aminogalactoside- or neuraminlactose-inhibitable coaggregation (45, 46).

In contrast to *P. loescheii*, capnocytophagae adhesins appear to be incorporated into their outer membranes (45, 80). Membrane preparations purified by sucrose density gradient centrifugation retain the ability to aggregate the various partner cells (45). Rabbit polyclonal antisera prepared against intact cells of the respective *Capnocytophaga* sp. and adsorbed with mutants of the appropriate coaggregation-negative phenotype detected putative 150-kDa adhesins in wild-type membrane preparations on immunoblots (45, 80). The antisera also inhibited the appropriate coaggregations at relatively low IgG concentrations. Monoclonal antibodies selected for their ability to inhibit coaggregation did not effectively remove adhesins from surfactant-dissociated membrane preparations (80). However, radiolabeled MAbs were useful for estimating the number of adhesin molecules per cell; like *P. loescheii*, each cell bore between 200 and 300 adhesin molecules (80).

Much of the research on adhesins of oral bacteria has used procedures like those cited here. Immunological methodologies, the acquisition of naturally occurring or genetically generated mutants, or a combination of the two approaches have been employed to build a case for the existence of adhesins. Adhesin preparations that retain any binding activity appear to be comparatively rare.

Streptococcus Species Adhesins

As a group, the oral streptococci exhibit a high degree of evolutionary sophistication. Members of this group make up a substantial proportion of the primary colonizers by virtue of their affinity for various salivary pellicle proteins. Some have adhesins for soft tissue, and some have evolved proteins that permit both intergeneric and intrageneric cell-to-cell interactions; intrageneric coaggregation only occurs among a few groups of oral bacteria (56, 57). Initial descriptions of nonlectin adhesins on *S. sanguis* 12, *S. parasanguis* FW213, and *S. gordonii* PK488 suggested that they were very different entities (21, 27, 53). The first two were fimbria-associated adhesins that mediated binding to saliva-coated hydroxyapatite particles, while the third participated in coaggregation with an actinomyces. When the three adhesin genes *ssaB*, *fimA*, and *scaA*, respectively, were sequenced, they were found to be least 80% identical and possess a putative 19-amino-acid signal sequence, and all were lipoproteins (22, 26, 54). The *scaA* gene product was subsequently shown to possess Mn^{2+} transporter activity (55), and it is not clear whether scaA is bifunctional or whether a mutation within *scaA* altered expression of the adhesin activity. Whether FimA or Ssab are also Mn^{2+} transport proteins is unresolved, as is the precise nature of their respective saliva-coated hydroxyapatite receptors.

S. gordonii DL1 adheres to *Candida albicans* via a complex series of interactions. Inactivation of genes that encode the large cell wall-associated proteins CshA and CshB partially inhibits *S. gordonii* DL1 from adhering to the yeast cells (43). Further, inactivation of the genes encoding the surface proteins SspA and SspB increases the effect twofold and nearly obliterates adherence. The interaction between these various streptococcal proteins, a cell wall polysaccharide, and components on the yeast cell remains to be elucidated. In-activating the genes for either CshA or CshB produced a second set of major phenotypic changes in strain DL1; the CshA-negative mutant lost its ability to participate in galactoside-sensitive coaggregations with *A. naeslundii* ATCC 12104 and PK606 (68). The sugar-insensitive interactions between *S. gordonii* DL1 and *A. naeslundii* T14V, *A. naeslundii* WVU627, *S. oralis* C104, and *S. oralis* 34 were lost when both CshA and B were not expressed. Antibodies prepared against the N-terminal region of recombinant CshA also inhibited coaggregation between DL1 and *A. naeslundii* T14V and PK606. It appeared, therefore, that CshA acts as a putative multifunctional adhesin (44, 68).

Actinomyces Species

A. naeslundii T14V fimbriae became a prototypic model for the study of these structures on oral bacteria. Two types of antigenically distinguishable, but genotypically similar, fimbriae were isolated and identified (10, 92, 93). Type 1 fimbriae participated in the attachment of *A. naeslundii* strains to saliva-coated hydroxyapatite; the nonlectin adhesive activity was shown to be specific for acidic PRPs in the salivary fluid. Type 2 fimbriae mediated coaggregation with *S. oralis* 34 and other similar streptococci via a lectinlike protein specific for galactoside receptors. Cloning, sequencing, and expression of type 1 and 2 genes and immunological characterization of the recombinant products established that the adhesive properties attributed to the fimbriae were not contained within the peptide structure itself. Like other examples in the literature, the adhesin appears to be a minor constituent that is firmly associated with the macromolecular structure. Gold particles coated with PRP antibodies were used to visualize the positions of the adhesive proteins on type 1 fimbriae; electron micrographs showed that the particles were sparsely associated with the peripheral portions of the type 1 fimbriae (60).

Porphyromonas gingivalis

Following its identification as a potential oral pathogen, the surface constituents of *P. gingi-*

valis were scrutinized to uncover factors that might contribute to its virulence. Strains of this gram-negative bacterium coaggregate with various oral bacteria including *F. nucleatum, Treponema denticola, A. naeslundii, S. oralis,* and *S. gordonii* (37, 38, 59, 77, 91) and attach to a number of supports. Adhesive peptides associated with fimbriae and extracellular proteases have received much attention over the past decade. *P. gingivalis* fimbriae were isolated and characterized, and the information gained was used to clone and sequence its subunit (fimbrillin) gene (19, 94). As cited earlier, *P. gingivalis* attaches to surfaces coated with acidic PRPs and statherin. Through the use of synthetic peptides that mimic various domains of the fimbrillin subunit, it was shown that the carboxyl terminus of the fimbrillin monomer (residues 266–288 and 318–337) was responsible for binding to PRPs (2, 47). The peptide with the sequence PQGPPQ was the most effective inhibitor in the binding assay. Coincidentally, nearly overlapping regions of the carboxyl terminus of the recombinant fimbrillin (residues 266–286, 293–306, and 307–326) were the most effective inhibitors in the statherin binding assays (3). In both instances, effective binding seems to require multiple sites on the fimbrillin molecule.

Cloning of the *P. gingivalis* cysteine protease genes is beginning to clarify some of the earlier confusion about the numbers, types, and specificities of these enzymes and their associated adhesins. The gene *prpR1*, found in *P. gingivalis* W50, encodes a polypeptide consisting of four distinct domains, pro, alpha, beta, and gamma (8, 17, 75). The polypeptide is processed to a heterodimeric form of alpha and beta subunits, the former contains the arginine-specific catalytic site, while the beta region possesses adhesin/hemagglutinin activity. The complex appears to bind to erythrocytes in a protein-protein interaction, and subsequent lysis of the eukaryotic cell presumably supplies the bacterium with a source of heme. There are several homologous beta-type loci in the *P. gingivalis* genome, one of these was cloned and sequenced; because of

similarities to the TonB-linked receptors, it was designated *tla* (TonB-linked adhesin). Insertional inactivation of *tla* in the *P. gingivalis* W50 wild type rendered the mutant unable to grow at low concentrations of heme (1).

Other Adhesins

The preceding section by no means constitutes a complete recapitulation of the adhesin literature for oral bacteria; the examples cited here serve to emphasize their functional diversity and the approaches used to identify and characterize these proteins. Relying heavily or solely on mutagenesis as a means of uncovering adhesins carries with it certain pitfalls. Some surface proteins serve as scaffolding for other constituents such as adhesins or are important in organizing the topology of the cell surface, and mutations that alter or delete these polypeptides can result in an adhesin-negative phenotype. In recognition of such possibilities, terms such as "adhesin-relevant" or "adhesin-related" are used to describe the gene product that affects adhesin function.

LIFE IN THE ORAL BIOFILM

What is truly unique about the bacteria in oral biofilms is the specificity with which they attach to surfaces and to each other. Almost all of the oral strains examined to date possess the ability to adhere to either soft tissue, hard tissue, or neighboring bacteria already anchored to some substratum (57, 63). To date, only sporadic reports mentioning coaggregation among intestinal bacteria, rumen bacteria, or naturally occurring zooglea can be found in the literature. Oral bacteria that possess multiple adhesins can serve as a bridge in biofilms between two unrelated forms; e.g., *P. loescheii* links *S. oralis* 34 to *A. israelii* PK14 (62). Strains of *F. nucleatum, S. sanguis,* or *S. oralis* appear to act as central mooring points by virtue of their multiple surface adhesin/receptor molecules that enable them to partner with a variety of genotypically distinct oral bacteria (57, 77, 90). The composition, specificities, and immunological aspects of polysaccharide receptor molecules found on the surfaces of oral bacteria have been reviewed recently (7, 11).

The structure and function of aquatic biofilms and the advantages accruing to members of such communities have received a great deal of attention lately (15, 16). Some of these exist as elaborate "mushroomlike" structures with channels that facilitate gas exchange and make nutrients available to resident bacteria (15). In addition to providing a hospitable environment, these edifices also protect the consortium from certain antibacterial agents and, presumably, predation. Supragingival plaque deposits on oral hard tissues also exhibit some degree of structure (e.g., aggregates and columnar microcolonies [49], but nothing quite so intricate as the "mushrooms"). Periodontal biofilms exhibit even less structure, and the bacteria are very densely packed. However, the absence of complex, readily discernible structures seems to have little effect on plaque vitality. Most of the bacteria present in a fresh sample of periodontal plaque can be recovered upon cultivation (69, 70), and vigorous swimming, gliding, and pulsating motility is observed among constituent members (49). Photomicrography showed that large clusters of anchored spirochetes are among the most active in these deposits; conceivably, their "in phase" undulation in mature plaque deposits may create a turbulence that mimics the convective channel currents of "mushrooms."

Attempts to use model systems to reproduce conditions in oral biofilms have yielded intriguing preliminary data. A mixture of nine species of oral bacteria was introduced into an anaerobically maintained chemostat containing a complex medium. Under these conditions, *F. nucleatum*, *P. gingivalis*, and *Veillonella dispar* predominated, while *A. naeslundii*, *S. gordonii*, *S. oralis*, *S. mutans*, *Lactobacillus casei*, and the aerobe *Neisseria subflava* were found in lower numbers (4, 50). When the population achieved steady-state conditions, it was used to inoculate an aerobically maintained constant-depth film fermentor housing multiple biofilm supports. The presence of air would presumably simulate conditions in the mouth and provide a means of assessing the effect of oxygen on the mixed population. Analyses of early biofilms formed under aerobic conditions showed a marked decrease in the viable numbers of the three anaerobes (to roughly 0.1% of the original population), while the primary colonizers, *N. subflava*, *S. oralis*, and *S. gordonii*, rapidly achieved dominance. However, in less than 100 h, the fusobacteria and veillonellae recovered and quickly repopulated the biofilm. Within 200 h, *P. gingivalis* became the most populous microbe in the biofilm. The fact that the aerobes and facultative aerobes quickly restored anaerobic conditions by depleting the oxygen supply in the culture is not remarkable; the survival and recovery of the anaerobes, especially *P. gingivalis*, during the transition period was unexpected. Whether survival of the anaerobes was simply due to oxygen scavenging or whether specific metabolic events such as production of antioxidants by other members of the biofilm flora supported repopulation of the anaerobes was not reported. With the appropriate aggregation-negative mutants, it may be possible to determine if cell-to-cell contact between small numbers of aerotolerant and oxygen-sensitive microbes is sufficient to protect the latter against the effects of oxygen.

The intuitive experiments demonstrating tissue tropisms, adherence to host tissues, and coaggregation have culminated in searches for more-sophisticated interactions that occur within the plaque biofilm. Communication within a biofilm can exist at several levels of complexity, beginning with simple exchanges such as cross-feeding of nutrients. A number of actual and possible examples of sharing have been discussed previously (39). More-complex signaling systems exist among bacteria, and some have been found in oral microbes or their close relatives. Among the enteric streptococci, pheromone-like peptides induce intraspecies mating events between strains that produce the peptides and partners that synthesize a specific receptor (14, 24). This system facilitates the transfer of conjugal plasmids. Another family of peptides, competence factors, activates a group of cell-surface and cytoplasmic proteins that permit certain streptococci to take up exogenous sources of DNA. This transformable state was first demonstrated in *Streptococcus pneumoniae* and has since been described for *S. gordonii*, *S. mutans*, and *Streptococcus crista* (64); a streptomycin-resistance gene is generally used as a marker to test the system. Since three of the four transformable streptococcal species are found in dental plaque, it seems likely that some form of genetic communication occurs in oral biofilms. How often the transfer of genetic material occurs between oral bacteria in a biofilm environment is the more relevant issue. The present state of knowledge should encourage DNA exchange experiments in either artificial or natural plaque deposits. A third class of signaling molecules, homoserine lactones and their analogs, permits select groups of gram-negative, aerobic bacteria to respond to population density. At appropriate concentrations, these small molecules act as transcriptional activators that trigger production of light-producing enzymes in certain commensal marine vibrios (25) or invasive enzymes in *Pseudomonas aeruginosa* (73, 74) and *Erwinia carotovora* (71). Similar molecules have been sought in culture fluids of oral gram-negative bacteria and plaque samples, without success (90). It may be that the oral bacteria have developed alternative or subtler means of communicating with one another, mechanisms that take advantage of the panoply of intimate cell-to-cell contacts that occur in the densely packed biofilms.

ACKNOWLEDGMENT

I thank Paul Kolenbrander and Henning Birkedal-Hansen for reading and commenting on the manuscript.

REVIEWS AND KEY PAPERS

Bradshaw, D. J., P. D. Marsh, G. K. Watson, and C. Allison. 1997. Oral anaerobes cannot survive oxygen stress without interacting with facultative/aerobic species as a microbial community. *Lett. Appl. Microbiol.* **25:**385–387.

Costerton, J. W., Z. Lewandowski, D. E. Caldwell, D. R. Korber, and H. M. Lappinscott. 1995. Microbial biofilms. *Annu. Rev. Microbiol.* **49:**711–745.

Costerton, J. W., Z. Lewandowski, D. Debeer, D. E. Caldwell, D. R. Korber, and G. James. 1994. Biofilms, the customized microniche. *J. Bacteriol.* **176:**2137–2142.

Fuqua, C., S. C. Winans, and E. P. Greenberg. 1996. Census and consensus in bacterial ecosystems: the LuxR-LuxI family of quorum-sensing transcriptional regulators. *Annu. Rev. Microbiol.* **50:**727–751.

Gibbons, R. J. 1996. Role of adhesion in microbial colonization of host tissues: a contribution of oral microbiology. *J. Dent. Res.* **75:**866–870.

Jenkinson, H. F., and R. J. Lamont. 1997. Streptococcal adhesion and colonization. *Crit. Rev. Oral Biol. Med.* **8:**175–200.

Kinniment, S. L., J. W. T. Wimpenny, D. Adams, and P. D. Marsh. 1996. Development of a steady-state oral microbial biofilm community using the constant-depth film fermenter. *Microbiology* **142:**631–638.

Kolenbrander, P. E., and J. London. 1992. Ecological significance of coaggregation in oral bacteria. *Adv. Microb. Ecol.* **12:**183–217.

London, J., and P. E. Kolenbrander. 1996. Coaggregation: enchancing colonization in a fluctuating environment, p. 249–279. *In* M. Fletcher, (ed.), *Molecular and Ecological Diversity of Bacterial Adhesion.* J. Wiley & Sons, Inc., New York.

REFERENCES

1. Aduse-Opoku, K., J. M. Slaney, M. Rangarajan, J. Muir, K. A. Young, and M. A. Curtis. 1997. The Tla protein of *Porphyromonas gingivalis* W50; a homolog of the RI protease precursor (PrpRI) is an outer membrane receptor required for growth on low levels of hemin. *J. Bacteriol.* **179:**4778–4788.

2. Amano, A., K. Kataoka, P. A. Raj, R. J. Genco, and S. Shizukuishi. 1996. Binding sites of salivary statherin for *Porphyromonas gingivalis* recombinant fimbrillin. *Infect. Immun.* **64:**4249–4254.

3. Amano, A., A. Sharma, J.-Y. Lee, H. T. Sojar, P. A. Raj, and R. J. Genco. 1996. Structural domains of *Porphyromonas gingivalis* recombinant fimbrillin that mediate binding to salivary proline-rich protein and statherin. *Infect. Immun.* **64:**1631–1637.

4. Bradshaw, D. J., P. D. Marsh, G. K. Watson, and C. Allison. 1997. Oral anaerobes cannot survive oxygen stress without interacting

with facultative/aerobic species as a microbial community. *Lett. Appl. Microbiol.* **25**:385–387.

5. **Brown, A. E., J. D. Rogers, and F. A. Scannapieco.** 1998. Homology of the amylase-binding protein A gene (abpA) of *Streptococcus gordonii* with genes from *Streptococcus mitis* and *Streptococcus sobrinus. J. Dent. Res.* **77**:134.

6. **Carlin A., P. Bratt, C. Stenudd, J. Olsson, N. Stromberg.** 1998. Agglutinin and acidic proline-rich protein receptor patterns may modulate bacterial adherence and colonization on tooth surfaces. *J. Dent. Res.* **77**:81–90.

7. **Cassels, F. J., C. V. Hughes, and J. L. Nauss.** 1995. Adhesin receptors of human oral bacteria and modeling of putative adhesin-binding domains. *J. Ind. Microbiol.* **15**:178–185.

8. **Ciborowski, P., M. Nishikata, R. D. Allen, and M. S. Lantz.** 1994. Purification and characterization of two forms of a high-molecular weight cysteine protease (porphypain) from *Porphyromonas gingivalis. J. Bacteriol.* **176**:4549–4557.

9. **Cisar, J. O., A. L. Sandberg, C. Abeygunawardana, G. P. Reddy, and C. A. Bush.** 1995. Lectin recognition of host-like saccharide motifs in streptococcal cell wall polysaccharides. *Glycobiology* **5**:655–662.

10. **Cisar, J. O., A. L. Sandberg, and S. E. Mergenhagen.** 1984. The function and distribution of different fimbriae on strains of *Actinomyces viscosus* and *Actinomyces naeslundii. J. Dent. Res.* **63**:393–396.

11. **Cisar, J. O., A. L. Sandberg, G. P. Reddy, C. Abeygunawardana, and C. A. Bush.** 1997. Structural and antigenic types of cell wall polysaccharides from viridans group streptococci with receptors for oral actinomyces and streptococcal lectins. *Infect. Immun.* **65**:5035–5041.

12. **Clark, W. B., L. L. Bammann, and R. J. Gibbons.** 1978. Comparative estimates of bacterial affinities and adsorption sites on hydroxyapatite surfaces. *Infect. Immun.* **19**:846–853.

13. **Clarke, J. K.** 1924. On the bacterial factor in the aetiology of dental caries. *Br. J. Exp. Pathol.* **5**:141–146.

14. **Clewell, D. B.** 1993. Bacterial sex pheromone-induced plasmid transfer. *Cell* **73**:9–12.

15. **Costerton, J. W., Z. Lewandowski, D. E. Caldwell, D. R, Korber, and H. M. Lappin-scott.** 1995. Microbial biofilms. *Annu. Rev. Microbiol.* **49**:711–745.

16. **Costerton, J. W., Z. Lewandowski, D. Debeer, D. E. Caldwell, D. R. Korber, and G. James.** 1994. Biofilms, the customized microniche. *J. Bacteriol.* **176**:2137–2142.

17. **Curtis, M. A.** 1997. Analysis of the protease and adhesin domains of the PrpRI of *Porphyromonas gingivalis. J. Periodont. Res.* **32**:133–139.

18. **Cui, Y., A. Chaterjee, Y. Lui, C. K. Dumenyo, and A. K. Chaterjee.** 1995. Identification of a global repressor gene, *RMSA*, of *Erwinia cavotoavora* subsp. *carotovora* that controls extracellular enzymes, N-(3-oxohexanoyl)-L-homoserine lactone, and pathogenicity in soft-rotting *Erwinia* spp. *J. Bacteriol.* **177**:5108–5115.

19. **Dickinson, D. P., M. A. Kubiniec, F. Yoshimura, and R. J. Genco.** 1988. Molecular cloning and sequencing of the gene encoding the fimbrial subunit protein of *Bacteroides gingivalis. J. Bacteriol.* **170**:1658–1665.

20. **Dobell, C.** 1932. *Antony van Leeuwenhoek and His "Little Animals,"* p. 238–255. Harcourt, Brace and Co., New York.

21. **Fachon-Kalweit, S., B. Elder, and P. Fives-Taylor.** 1985. Antibodies that bind to fimbriae block adhesion of *Streptococcus sanguis* to saliva coated hydroxyapatite. *Infect. Immun.* **48**:617–624.

22. **Fenno, J. C., D. J. LeBlanc, and P. Fives-Taylor.** 1989. Nucleotide sequence analysis of a type 1 fimbrial gene of *Streptococcus sanguis* FW213. *Infect. Immun.* **57**:3527–3533.

23. **Fitzgerald, R. J., and P. H. Keyes.** 1960. Demonstration of the etiologic role of streptococci in experimental caries in the hamster. *J. Am. Dent. Assoc.* **61**:9–31.

24. **Fujimoto, S., M. Bastos, K. Tanimoto, F. An, K. Wu, and D. B. Clewell.** 1997. The pAD1 sex pheromone response in *Enterococcus faecalis. Adv. Exp. Med. Biol.* **418**:1037–1040

25. **Fuqua, C., S. C. Winans, and E. P. Greenberg.** 1996. Census and consensus in bacterial ecosystems: the LuxR-LuxI family of quorum-sensing transcriptional regulators. *Annu. Rev. Microbiol.* **50**:727–751.

26. **Ganeshkumar, N., P. M. Hannam, P. E. Kolenbrander, and B. C. McBride.** 1991. Nucleotide sequence of a gene coding for a saliva-binding protein (SsaB) from *Streptococcus sanguis* 12 and possible role of the protein in coaggregation with actinomyces. *Infect. Immun.* **59**:1093–1099.

27. **Ganeshkumar, N., M. Song, and B. C. McBride.** 1988. Cloning of a *Streptococcus sanguis* adhesin which mediates binding to saliva-coated hydroxyapatite. *Infect. Immun.* **56**:1150–1157.

28. **Genco, R. J., and J. Slots.** 1984. Host responses in periodontal disease. *J. Dent. Res.* **63**:441–451.

29. **Gibbons, R. J.** 1996. Role of adhesion in microbial colonization of host tissues: a contribution of oral microbiology. *J. Dent. Res.* **75:**866–870.

30. **Gibbons R. J., and S. B. Banghart.** 1967. Synthesis of extracellular dextran by cariogenic bacteria and its presence in human dental plaque. *Arch. Oral Biol.* **12:**11–23.

31. **Gibbons, R. J., and R. J. Fitzgerald.** 1969. Dextran-induced agglutination of *Streptococcus mutans*, and its potential role in the formation of microbial dental plaques. *J. Bacteriol.* **98:**341–346.

32. **Gibbons, R. J., and D. I. Hay.** 1988. Human salivary acidic protein-rich proteins and statherin promote the attachment of *Actinomyces viscosus* LY7 to apatitic surfaces. *Infect. Immun.* **56:**439–445.

33. **Gibbons, R. J., and D. I. Hay.** 1989. Adsorbed salivary acidic proline-rich proteins contribute to the adhesion of *Streptococcus mutans* JBP to apatitic surfaces. *J. Dent. Res.* **68:**1303–1307.

34. **Gibbons, R. J., B. Kapsimalis, and S. S. Socransky.** 1964. The source of salivary bacteria. *Arch. Oral Biol.* **9:**101–103.

35. **Gibbons, R. J., and M. Nygaard.** 1970. Interbacterial aggregation of plaque bacteria. *Arch. Oral Biol.* **15:**1397–1400.

36. **Gibbons, R. J., and D. M. Spinell.** 1970. Salivary-induced aggregation of plaque bacteria, p. 207–215. *In* McHugh, W. D. (ed.), *Symposium on Dental Plaque.* Livingstone, Edinburgh.

37. **Goulborne, P. A., and R. P. Ellen.** 1991. Evidence that *Porphyromonas* (*Bacteroides*) *gingivalis* fimbriae function in adhesion to *Actinomyces viscosus. J. Bacteriol.* **173:**5266–5274.

38. **Grenier, D.** 1992. Demonstration of a bimodal coaggregation reaction between *Porphyromonas gingivalis* and *Treponema denticola. Oral Microbiol. Immunol.* **7:**280–284.

39. **Grenier, D., and D. Mayrand.** 1986. Nutritional relationships between oral bacteria. *Infect. Immun.* **60:**616–620.

40. **Grimm, W. D., J. S. van der Hoeven, and C. W. A. van den Kiebom.** 1997. Colonization of barrier membranes for periodontal regeneration by sulfate-reducing bacteria. *J. Dent. Res.* **76:**802.

41. **Gwynn, J. P., and C. W. I. Douglas.** 1994. Comparison of amylase-binding proteins in oral streptococci. *FEMS Microbiol. Lett.* **124:**373–379.

42. **Hillman, J. D., J. van Houte, and R. J. Gibbons.** 1970. Sorption of bacteria to human enamel powder. *Arch. Oral Microbiol.* **15:**899–903.

43. **Holmes, A. R., R. McNab, and H. F. Jenkinson.** 1996. *Candida albicans* binding to the oral bacterium *Streptococcus gordonii* involves multiple adhesin-receptor interactions. *Infect. Immun.* **64:**4680–4685.

44. **Jenkinson, H. F., and R. J. Lamont.** 1997. Streptococcal adhesion and colonization. *Crit. Rev. Oral Biol. Med.* **8:**175–200.

45. **Kagermeier, A., and J. London.** 1986. Identification and preliminary characterization of a lectinlike protein from *Capnocytophaga gingivalis* (emended). *Infect. Immun.* **51:**490–494.

46. **Kagermeier, A., J. London, and P. E. Kolenbrander.** 1984. Evidence for the participation of N-acetylated amino sugars in the coaggregation between *Capnocytophaga* species strain DR2001 and *Actinomyces israelii* PK16. *Infect. Immun.* **44:**299–305.

47. **Kataoka, K., A. Amano, M. Kuboniwa, H. Horie, H. Nagata, and S. Shizukuishi.** 1997. Active sites of salivary-rich protein for binding to *Porphyromonas gingivalis* fimbriae. *Infect. Immun.* **65:**3159–3164.

48. **Kemp, C. W., N. A. Curtis, S. S. Robrish, and W. H. Bowen.** 1983. Biogenesis of methane in primate dental plaque. *FEBS Lett.* **155:**61–64.

49. **Keyes, P. H., and T. E. Rams.** 1983. A rationale for management of periodontal diseases: rapid identification of microbial 'therapeutic targets' with phase-contrast microscopy. *J. Am. Dent. Assoc.* **106:**803–812.

50. **Kinniment, S. L., J. W. T. Wimpenny, D. Adams, and P. D. Marsh.** 1996. Development of a steady-state oral microbial biofilm community using the constant-depth film fermenter. *Microbiology* **142:**631–638.

51. **Klier, C. M., P. E. Kolenbrander, A. G. Roble, M. L. Marco, S. Cross, and P. S. Handley.** 1997. Identification of a 95 kDa putative adhesin from *Actinomyces* serovar WVA963 strain PK1259 that is distinct from type 2 fimbrial subunits. *Microbiology* **143:**835–846.

52. **Kolenbrander, P. E.** 1982. Isolation and characterization of coaggregation-defective mutants of *Actinomyces viscosus, Actinomyces naeslundii* and *Streptococcus sanguis. Infect. Immun.* **37:**1200–1208.

53. **Kolenbrander, P. E., and R. N. Andersen.** 1990. Characterization of *Streptococcus gordonii* (*S. sanguis*) PK488 adhesin-mediated coaggregation with *Actinomyces naeslundii* PK606. *Infect. Immun.* **58:**3064–3072.

54. **Kolenbrander, P. E., and R. N. Andersen.** 1994. Nucleotide sequence of the *Streptococcus gordonii* PK488 coaggregation adhesin gene, *scaA*, and ATP binding cassette. *Infect. Immun.* **62:**4469–4480.

55. **Kolenbrander, P. E., R. N. Andersen, R. A. Baker, and H. F. Jenkinson.** 1998. The adhesion-associated *sca* operon in *Streptococcus gordonii* encodes an inducible high-affinity ABC transporter for Mn^{2+} uptake. *J. Bacteriol.* **180:** 290–295.

56. **Kolenbrander, P. E., R. N. Andersen, and L. V. H. Moore.** 1990. Intrageneric coaggregation among strains of human oral bacteria: potential role in primary colonization of the tooth surface. *Appl. Environ. Microbiol.* **56:**3890–3894.

57. **Kolenbrander, P. E., and J. London.** 1992. Ecological significance of coaggregation in oral bacteria. *Adv. Microb. Ecol.* **12:**183–217.

59. **Lamont, R. J., C. A. Bevin, S. Gil, R. E. Perrson, and B. Rosan.** 1993. Involvement of *Porphyromonas gingivalis* fimbriae in adherence to *Streptococcus gordonii*. *Oral Microbiol. Immunol.* **8:** 272–276.

60. **Leung, K.-P., W. E. Fischlschweiger, D. I. Hay, and W. B. Clark.** 1990. Binding of colloidal gold-labeled salivary proline-rich proteins to *Actinomyces viscosus* type 1 fimbriae. *Infect. Immun.* **58:**1986–1991.

61. **London, J.** 1991. Bacterial adhesins. *Annu. Rep. Med. Chem.* **26:**239–247.

62. **London, J., and J. Allen.** 1990. Purification and characterization of a *Bacteroides loescheii* adhesin that interacts with prokaryotic and eucaryotic cells. *J. Bacteriol.* **172:**2527–2534.

63. **London, J., and P. E. Kolenbrander.** 1996. Coaggregation: enhancing colonization in a fluctuating environment, p. 249–279. *In* M. Fletcher (ed.), *Molecular and Ecological Diversity of Bacterial Adhesion.* J. Wiley & Sons, Inc., New York.

64. **Lunsford, R. D.** 1998. Streptococcal transformation: essential features and applications of a natural gene exchange system. *Plasmid* **39:**10–20.

65. **Ma, Y. S., M. O. Lassiter, J. A. Banas, M. Y. Galperin, K. G. Taylor, and R. J. Doyle.** 1996. Multiple glucan-binding proteins of *Streptococcus sobrinus*. *J. Bacteriol.* **178:**1572–1577.

66. **Manch-Citron, J. N., J. Allen, M. J. Moos, and J. London.** 1992. The gene encoding a *Prevotella loescheii* lectin-like adhesin contains an interrupted sequence which causes a frameshift. *J. Bacteriol.* **174:**7328–7336.

67. **Manch-Citron, J. N., and J. London.** 1994. Expression of the *Prevotella loescheii* gene (*plaA*) is mediated by a programmed frameshifting hop. *J. Bacteriol.* **176:**1944–1948.

68. **McNab, R., A. R. Holmes, J. M. Clarke, G. W. Tannock and H. F. Jenkinson.** 1996. Cell surface polypeptide CshA mediates binding of *Streptococcus gordonii* to other oral bacteria and to immobilized fibronectin. *Infect. Immun.* **64:** 4202–4210.

69. **Moore, W. E. C., L. V. Holdeman, and E. P. Cato.** 1984. Variation in periodontal floras. *Infect. Immun.* **46:**720–726.

70. **Moore W. E. C., and L. H. Moore.** 1994. The bacteria of periodontal disease. *Periodontol. 2000* **5:**66–77.

71. **Mukherjee, A., Y. Y. Cui, Y. Liu, and A. K. Chaterjee.** 1997. Molecular characterization and expression of the *Erwinia carotovora hepN (Ecc)* gene, which encodes an elicitor of the hypersensitive reaction. *Mol. Plant Microbe Interact.* **10:** 462–471.

72. **Nyvad, B., and M. Kilian.** 1987. Microbiology of the early colonization of human enamel and root surfaces in vivo. *Scand. J. Dent. Res.* **95:**369–380.

73. **Pearson, J. P., L. Passador, B. H. Iglewski, and E. P. Greenberg.** A 2nd N-acetylhomoserine lactone signal produced by *Pseudomonas aerugenosa*. *Proc. Natl. Acad. Sci. USA* **92:**1490–1494.

74. **Pearson, J. P., E. C. Pesci, and B. H. Iglewski.** 1997. Roles of *Pseudomonas aeruginosa* las and rhl quorum-sensing systems in control of elastase and rhamnolipid biosynthesis genes. *J. Bacteriol.* **179:**5757–5767.

75. **Rangarajan, M., S. J. Smith, and M. A. Curtis.** 1997. Biochemical characterization of the argine-specific proteases of *Porphyromonas gingivalis* W50 suggests a common precursor. *Biochem. J.* **323:**701–709.

76. **Scannapieco, F. A., L. Solomon, and R. O. Wadenya.** 1994. Emergence in human dental plaque and host distribution of amylase-binding streptococci. *J. Dent. Res.* **73:**1627–1635.

77. **Shaniztki, B., D. Hurwitz, N. Smorodinsky, N. Ganeshkumar, and E. I. Weiss.** 1997. Identification of a *Fusobacterium nucleatum* PK1594 galactose-binding adhesin which mediates coaggregation with periodontopathic bacteria and hemagglutination. *Infect. Immun.* **65:**5231–5237.

78. **Socransky, S. S., and A. D. Haffajee.** 1994. Microbiology and immunology of periodontal disease. *Periodontol. 2000* **5:**7–168.

79. **Tanner, A. C. R., S. S. Socransky, and J. M. Goodman.** 1984. Microbiota of periodontal pockets losing crestal alveolar bone. *J. Periodont. Res.* **19:**279–291.

80. **Tempro, P., F. Cassels, R. Siraganian, A. Hand, and J. London.** 1989. Use of adhesin-specific monoclonal antibodies to identify and lo-

calize an adhesin on the surface of *Capnocytophaga gingivalis* DR2001. *Infect. Immun.* **57**:3418–3424.

81. **Uhlin, B., E. M. Norgren, M. Baga, and S. Normark.** 1985. Adhesin to human cells by *Escherichia coli* lacking the major subunit of a digalactoside-specific pilus adhesin. *Proc. Natl. Sci. Acad. USA* **82**:1800–1804.

82. **Theilade, E., W. H. Wright, S. B. Jensen, and H. Loe.** 1966. Experimental gingivitis in man. II. A longitudinal clinical and bacteriological investigation. *J. Periodont. Res.* **1**:1–13.

83. **van der Hoeven, J. S., and M. J. M. Schaeken.** 1997. Sulfate-reducing bacteria in the periodontal pocket. *J. Dent. Res.* **74**:587.

84. **van Houte, H., R. J. Gibbons, and S. B. Banghart.** 1970. Adherence as a determinant of the presence of *Streptococcus salivarius* and *Streptococcus sanguis* on the human tooth surface. *Arch. Oral Biol.* **15**:1025–1034.

85. **Weiss, E. I., J. London, P. E. Kolenbrander, and R. N. Andersen.** 1989. Fimbriae-associated adhesin of *Bacteroides loescheii* that recognizes receptors on prokaryotic and eucaryotic cells. *Infect. Immun.* **57**:2912–2913.

86. **Weiss, E. I., J. London, P. E. Kolenbrander, R. N. Andersen, C. Fischler, and R. Siraganian.** 1988. Characterization of monoclonal antibodies to fimbria-associated adhesins of *Bacteroides loescheii* PK1295. *Infect. Immun.* **56**:219–224.

87. **Weiss, E. I., J. London, P. E. Kolenbrander, A. R. Hand, and R. Siraganian.** 1988b. Localization and enumeration of fimbria-associated adhesins of *Bacteroides loescheii*. *J. Bacteriol.* **170**:1123–1128.

88. **Weiss, E. I., J. London, P. E. Kolenbrander, A. S. Kagermeier, and R. N. Andersen.** 1987. Characterization of lectinlike surface components on *Capnocytophaga ochracea* ATCC 33596 that mediate coaggregation with gram-positive oral bacteria. *Infect. Immun.* **55**:1198–1202.

89. **Weiss, R. B., W. M. Huang, and D. M. Dunn.** 1990. A nascent peptide is required for the ribosomal bypass of the coding gap in bacteriophage T4 gene *60*. Cell **62**:117–126.

90. **Whittaker, C. A., C. M. Klier, and P. E. Kolenbrander.** 1996. Mechanisms of adhesion by oral bacteria. *Annu. Rev. Microbiol.* **50**:513–552.

91. **Yao, E. S., S. P. Leu, A. Weinberg, and R. J. Lamont.** 1995. Adherence of *Treponema denticola* to *Porphyromonas gingivalis* and *Streptococcus crista*. *J. Dent. Res.* **74**:199.

92. **Yeung, M. K., and J. O. Cisar.** 1988. Cloning and nucleotide sequence of a gene for *Actinomyces naeslundii* WVU45 type 2 fimbriae. *J. Bacteriol.* **170**:3803–3809.

93. **Yeung, M. K., and J. O. Cisar.** 1990. Sequence homology between the subunits of immunologically and functionally distinct types of fimbriae of *Actinomyces* spp. *J. Bacteriol.* **172**:2462–2468.

94. **Yoshimura, F., K. Takahashi, Y. Nodasaka, and T. Suzuki.** 1984. Purification and characterization of a novel type of fimbriae from the oral anaerobe *Bacteroides gingivalis*. *J. Bacteriol.* **160**:949–957.

MICROBIAL INTERFERENCE IN THE COLONIZATION OF SILICONE RUBBER IMPLANT SURFACES IN THE OROPHARYNX: *STREPTOCOCCUS THERMOPHILUS* AGAINST A MIXED FUNGAL/ BACTERIAL BIOFILM

*Henk J. Busscher, Betsy van de Belt-Gritter, Minca Westerhof,
Ranny van Weissenbruch, Frans W. J. Albers,
and Henny C. van der Mei*

5

Patients after laryngectomy due to a malignant laryngeal tumor have to breathe through a tracheostoma and receive a voice prosthesis for speech rehabilitation. Voice prostheses are implanted as a shunt valve between the digestive tract and the trachea. By closing the tracheostoma with a finger, patients can direct an airflow through the valve into the oropharyngeal region where remaining muscular structures act as pseudo-vocal cords. The prolonged use of indwelling silicone rubber voice prostheses by laryngectomized patients is limited to 3 to 4 months on average (21). Thick biofilms consisting of a variety of oral and skin microorganisms, including streptococci, staphylococci, and yeasts, on the valve side of the prostheses, either cause leakage or increased airflow resistance (14, 17). Adhesion of yeasts is particularly troublesome, as they tend to grow into the silicone rubber (6, 17), as dem-

onstrated in Fig. 1, and thus avoid detachment by naturally occurring shear forces in the oropharyngeal cavity.

Attempts to increase the lifetime of indwelling voice prostheses are for this reason mainly aimed at reducing the adhesion of yeasts to the silicone rubber (15). There is anecdotal evidence among patients that consumption of buttermilk, which contains antimycotic-releasing *Lactococcus lactis* subspecies (1), prolongs the lifetime of indwelling voice prostheses. Recently, it has been suggested that consumption of 2 kg of Turkish yogurt per day effectively eliminates biofilm formation on indwelling voice prostheses. The mechanism by which this occurs has never been investigated, but it is hypothesized that the presence of *Streptococcus thermophilus* and *Lactobacillus bulgaricus*, two well-known probiotic bacterial strains (12, 20) in Turkish yogurt, may interfere with adhesion of yeasts to the silicone rubber. Lactobacilli have been long known for their capacity to interfere with the adhesion of uropathogens to epithelial cells (2, 18) and catheter materials (13), and the mechanisms of this interference have been demonstrated to include, among others, the release of proteinaceous biosurfactants (23).

Henk J. Busscher, Betsy van de Belt-Gritter, Minca Westerhof, and Henny C. van der Mei, Laboratory for Materia Technica, University of Groningen, Bloemsingel 10, 9712 KZ Groningen, The Netherlands.   *Ranny van Weissenbruch and Frans W. J. Albers*, Department of Otorhinolaryngology, University Hospital Groningen, Hanzeplein 1, 9713 EZ Groningen, The Netherlands.

Microbial Ecology and Infectious Disease, Edited by Eugene Rosenberg
©1999 American Society for Microbiology, Washington, D.C.

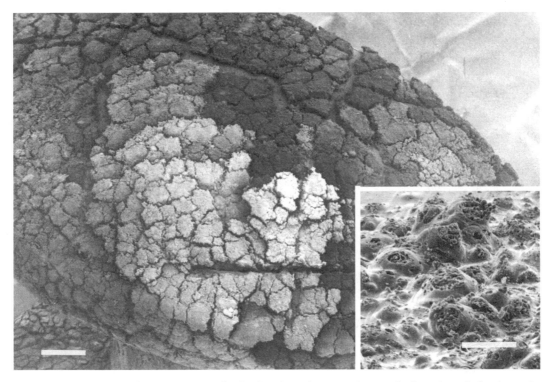

FIGURE 1 Scanning electron micrograph of a Groningen button voice prosthesis explanted after 4 months from a laryngectomized patient, showing heavy biofilm formation with ingrowth features (insert). Bar, 1 mm for the low-magnification micrograph and 10 μm for the insert.

Also *S. thermophilus* releases biosurfactants (8, 9) that are suggested to interfere with their own adhesion to substratum surfaces (4).

Recently (10), adhesion of yeasts (two *Candida albicans* and two *Candida tropicalis* strains isolated from naturally colonized voice prostheses) to silicone rubber was studied, with and without a salivary conditioning film in the absence and presence of adhering *S. thermophilus* B, a biosurfactant-releasing dairy isolate. A 1 to 4% coverage of the surface of silicone rubber substrata with adhering *S. thermophilus* B significantly reduced initial yeast adhesion, regardless of the presence of a salivary conditioning film. Mechanistically, this interference in yeast adhesion by *S. thermophilus* B was not due to geometrical effects, but to biosurfactant release by the adhering bacteria, because experiments with *S. thermophilus* B cells that had released their biosurfactants

prior to adhesion to silicone rubber and competition with yeasts did not show interference with initial yeast adhesion (see Table 1). Preadsorbing biosurfactants to silicone rubber prior to allowing yeasts to adhere was as effective against *C. albicans* GB 1/2 adhesion as covering 1 to 2% of the silicone rubber surface with adhering *S. thermophilus* B, but a preadsorbed biosurfactant layer was less effective against *C. tropicalis* GB 9/9.

The above approach to studying the effects of biosurfactant-releasing *S. thermophilus* B is a so-called reductionistic approach, in which the study is carried out with an emphasis on single strains, isolated from explanted voice prostheses. In vivo, the number of strains on voice prostheses is extremely large, and it is always doubtful whether any selection of strains made in a reductionistic approach will be representative of the complex microbial

TABLE 1 Adhesion of *Candida* strains to silicone rubber[a]

Yeast strain	Surface coverage (%) by *S. thermophilus* B	Relative initial cell deposition rate (%)		Relative cell number adhering at 4 h (%)	
		b[−b]	b[+]	b[−]	b[+]
C. albicans GB 1/2	1	113	60	121	67
	4	123	15	78	32
	Biosurfactants only	N.A.[c]	69	N.A.	77
C. tropicalis GB 9/9	1	125	64	96	89
	4	107	51	118	43
	Biosurfactants only	N.A.	103	N.A.	124

[a] Yeast strains were tested in competition with adhering *S. thermophilus* B and to silicone rubber with preadsorbed stationary-phase biosurfactants only. Results are expressed in percentages with respect to the control (0% coverage by *S. thermophilus* B). For details see Busscher et al. (10).

[b] b[−] variants of *S. thermophilus* B have released all their biosurfactants prior to being engaged in the experiments, while b[+] indicates the original biosurfactant-releasing strain.

[c] N.A., not applicable.

community colonizing voice prostheses. The reductionistic approach is opposed to a "teleological" approach, in which entire microbial communities are used for experiments without detailed isolation and identification of the strains and species involved in the microbial community used (19).

The aim of the present paper is to determine the effect of *S. thermophilus* B on the formation of oropharyngeal biofilms on silicone rubber voice prostheses in a modified Robbins device, using a teleological approach for the colonizing mixed fungal/bacterial biofilm.

VOICE PROSTHESES AND BIOFILM FORMATION IN THE MODIFIED ROBBINS DEVICE

"Low Resistance" Groningen button voice prostheses (kindly provided by Médin Instruments and Supplies, Groningen, The Netherlands) were placed in two transparent modified Robbins devices, shown schematically in Fig. 2. Each Robbins device was equipped with 10 Groningen button voice prostheses. The total cultivable microflora from an explanted Groningen button voice prosthesis, containing a variety of yeast and bacterial strains including *C. albicans*, *C. tropicalis* and streptococcal and staphylococcal strains, was cultured in a mixture of 30% brain

heart infusion broth (OXOID, Basingstoke, Great Britain) and 70% defined yeast medium [per liter: 7.5 g of glucose, 3.5 g of $(NH_4)_2SO_4$, 1.5 g of L-asparagine, 10 mg of L-histidine, 20 mg of DL-methionine, 20 mg of DL-tryptophan, 1 g of KH_2PO_4, 500 mg of $MgSO_4 \cdot 7 H_2O$, 500 mg of NaCl, 500 mg of $CaCl_2 \cdot 2 H_2O$, 100 mg of yeast extract, 500 μg of H_3BO_3, 400 μg of $ZnSO_4 \cdot 7 H_2O$, 120 μg of $Fe(III)Cl_3$, 200 μg of $Na_2MoO_4 \cdot 2 H_2O$, 100 μg of KI, 40 μg of $CuSO_4 \cdot 5 H_2O$] and used to inoculate the modified Robbins devices. Subsequently, a biofilm was allowed to grow on the voice prostheses for 3 days. On the fourth day, the devices were both flushed with phosphate-buffered saline, pH 7.0, to remove remnants of the growth medium.

In one Robbins device, serving as a control, 650 ml of phosphate buffer was then perfused, and the prostheses were left in the moist environment of the drained modified Robbins device. In the other Robbins device, a suspension of *S. thermophilus* B was perfused, after which it was left drained as well. To remove remnants of the streptococcal suspension, phosphate-buffered saline was perfused through the device prior to each succeeding perfusion. This perfusion scheme was repeated three times a day. At the end of the day, both Robbins devices were filled with growth medium for half an hour and left drained during

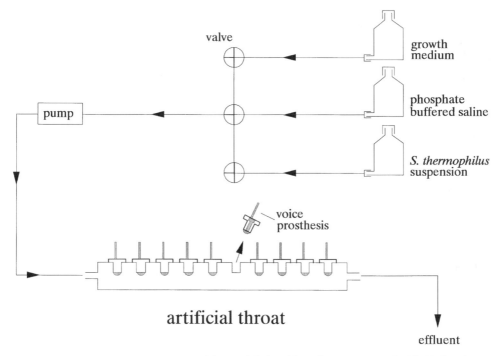

FIGURE 2 Schematic presentation of the modified Robbins device, equipped with 10 Groningen button voice prostheses.

the night. Phosphate-buffered saline was perfused through the devices first thing in the morning, prior to other perfusions.

Both experiments were continued for 9 days at room temperature, and the tracheal sides of the prostheses were left in ambient air without taking precautions to prevent infections from the air, similar to the situation with a stoma.

S. THERMOPHILUS
GROWTH CONDITIONS
S. thermophilus B, isolated from heat-exchanger plates in the downward section of a pasteurizer (3), was kindly provided by NIZO (Ede, The Netherlands) and additionally identified by us using the method of Bergey. Bacteria were stored in M17 broth (Oxoid, Basingstoke, England), supplemented with 1% sucrose, containing 7% (vol/vol) dimethyl sulfoxide at −60°C. For each, experiment subcultures (10 ml) were prepared by inoculating M17 broth, supplemented with 1% sucrose, with bacteria from a frozen stock (1% inoculum) and incubating overnight at 37°C. A second culture (200 ml) was incubated with 10 ml of an overnight subculture. After 16 h, cells were harvested by centrifugation at 4,000 $\times$ g, washed two times in water, and resuspended in water. To break bacterial chains, the bacterial suspension was sonicated for 30 s at 30 W (Vibra Cell model 375, Sonics and Materials Inc., Danbury, Conn.). Sonication was done intermittently while cooling in an ice-water bath. Finally, cells were suspended in water for perfusion of the modified Robbins device (see above). The cell concentration was fixed to a density of 3×10^8 cells/ml with the aid of a Bürker-Türk counting chamber.

EVALUATION OF BIOFILMS
After removal of the voice prostheses from the modified Robbins device, biofilm formation

on the valve sides of the prostheses was determined by electron microscopy and by plating the biofilms on agar. For scanning electron microscopy (SEM), samples removed from the Robbins device were flushed with 6.8% sucrose and 0.1 M cacodylate buffer (pH 7.4), fixed and stained in 2% glutardialdehyde and 0.2% ruthenium red in 0.1 M cacodylate buffer at 4°C, and flushed again. Postfixation and staining was carried out in 1% OsO_4 and 0.2% ruthenium red in cacodylate buffer by gently shaking for 3 h at room temperature. Buffer washes and dehydration involved the following rinsing procedures: 20 min in 6.8% sucrose in 0.1 M cacodylate buffer; 3 × 10 min bidistilled water; 20 min in (respectively) 30, 50, and 70% ethanol, and 4 × 30 min in 100% ethanol. After critical-point drying with CO_2 for 4 h, the specimens were mounted on SEM stubs and sputter-coated with gold/palladium (15 nm). SEM observations were made using the Jeol 6301, with different magnifications at 15 to 25 kV.

Microbial compositions of the biofilms were estimated after serial diluting by plating on brain heart infusion (for yeasts) and on blood agar plates (for bacteria) after removal of the biofilms by scraping and sonication. Agar plates were stored at 37°C under aerobic conditions for 4 days. Subsequently, the number of bacterial and fungal CFU per unit valve area (CFU/cm^2) was determined for each prosthesis.

OBSERVATIONS AND IMPLICATIONS

Figure 3 shows a representative SEM of a Groningen button voice prosthesis removed from the control Robbins device. Heavy biofilm formation can be observed extending over a major part of the valve, with clear ingrowth of microcolonies similar to that observed on explanted voice prostheses (compare Fig. 1). The comparison of the in vitro and in vivo biofilm features demonstrates the validity of the current use of the modified Robbins device to simulate oropharyngeal biofilms on voice prostheses.

Figure 4 compiles the number of bacteria and yeasts isolated from voice prostheses in the control Robbins device and from the voice prostheses exposed three times daily to a suspension of *S. thermophilus* B. Although *S. thermophilus* cells have never been isolated from these voice prostheses, it is clear that bacterial colonization is somewhat reduced, while colonization of the silicone rubber prostheses by yeasts is significantly below that in the control group. Figure 5 shows, however, that perfusing the Robbins device with thermophilic streptococci could not prevent ingrowth of isolated fungal microcolonies on isolated spots.

Since the first studies on probiotics by Metchnikoff, published in 1907, there has been a growing number of health claims based on the consumption of probiotics, including suppression of diarrhea, antitumor activity, stimulation of immunity, and relief of lactose intolerance. Unfortunately, the development of probiotics slowed down in the 1930s and 40s with the introduction of chemotherapy and penicillin (11). Now that the limits of antibiotics may almost be reached, interest in the use of probiotics for health benefits has renewed, and recently, a biotherapeutic effect of probiotic bacteria on candidiasis in immunodeficient mice was reported (24).

Formation of a biofilm can be divided into several sequential stages, commencing with the adsorption of conditioning film components (in the case of oropharyngeal biofilms these are salivary components), followed by initial microbial adhesion, anchoring of the adhering organisms, growth, and sometimes ingrowth of the adhering organisms (7, 22). A previous study (10) concentrated on the interference of biosurfactant-releasing thermophilic streptococci with initial adhesion of yeasts isolated from voice prostheses. Some of the results from this study are presented in Table 1 (10). These results suggest that these streptococci interfere with adhesion of yeasts not merely by a geometrical effect but that the release and subsequent adsorption of biosurfactants to the silicone rubber plays an essential role in preventing initial adhesion of yeasts. A

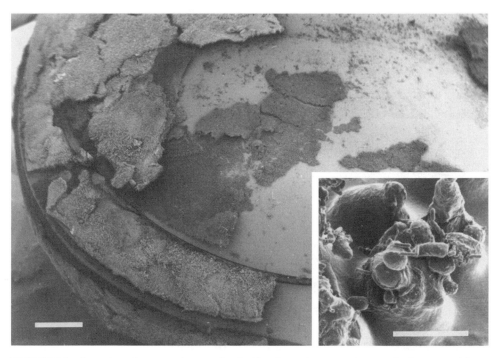

FIGURE 3 Scanning electron micrograph of a Groningen button voice prosthesis removed from the modified Robbins device in the control group after 7 days, showing heavy biofilm formation with ingrowth features (insert) similar to those observed in vivo (compare Fig. 1). Bar, 1 mm for the low-magnification micrograph and 50 μm for the insert.

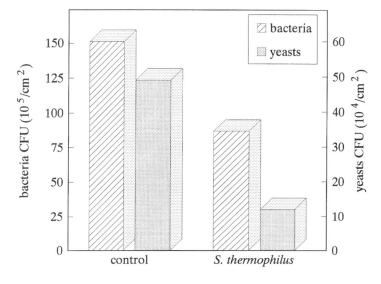

FIGURE 4 Number of bacterial and yeast CFU/cm^2 of valve area isolated from Groningen button voice prostheses after biofilm formation in a modified Robbins device. The standard deviation for the control and for the device perfused by *S. thermophilus* suspension is $\pm 30\%$ over three buttons in one run for both bacterial and yeast counts.

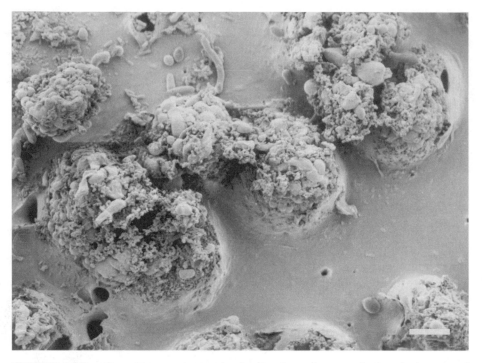

FIGURE 5 Scanning electron micrograph of a Groningen button voice prosthesis removed from the modified Robbins device after perfusion three times daily with a thermophilic streptococcal suspension. Bar, 10 μm.

mechanism by which biosurfactant-releasing strains may interfere with the adhesion of other microorganisms is schematically depicted in Fig. 6 and is concurrent with hypotheses by Neu (16).

Whereas our previous study on thermophilic streptococcal interference on voice prosthetic materials was confined to initial adhesion of yeasts, this study extends into the growth phase of biofilm formation. Also at the growth phase, distinct effects of the presence of biosurfactant-releasing streptococci on bio-

film formation were observed. The role of biosurfactant release and adsorption is emphasized by the observation that no *S. thermophilus* cells were isolated from the biofilms formed. Clinically, these results provide evidence supporting suggestions that the consumption by laryngectomees of Turkish yogurt containing *S. thermophilus* strains prolongs the lifetime of their prostheses. Earlier, a study similar to that performed here (5), provided evidence supporting suggestions within the laryngectomized community in the Netherlands that

FIGURE 6 Generalized model for the interference by biosurfactant-releasing microorganisms with the adhesion of other strains.

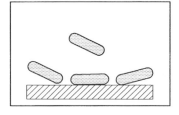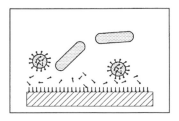

consumption of buttermilk, containing probiotic *L. lactis*, prolongs the lifetime of their voice prostheses.

In summary, interference by biosurfactant-releasing, thermophilic streptococci on initial adhesion of yeasts to silicone rubber observed on a reductionistic basis in the parallel plate flow chamber extends to a teleological effect on the formation of a mixed fungal/bacterial biofilm on silicone rubber voice prostheses in the modified Robbins device. In addition, in vitro interference by biosurfactant-releasing, thermophilic streptococci with oropharyngeal biofilm formation is accompanied by clinical observations that consumption of yogurt containing these organisms by laryngectomees prolongs the lifetime of voice prostheses.

REFERENCES

1. **Batish, V. K., R. Lal, and H. Chander.** 1990. Effects of nutritional factors on the production of antifungal substance by *Lactococcus lactis* spp. *lactis biovar diacetylactis. Aust. J. Dairy Technol.* **45**:74–76.

2. **Blomberg, L., A. Hendriksson, and P. L. Conway.** 1993. Inhibition of adhesion of *Escherichia coli* K88 to piglet ileal mucus by *Lactobacillus* spp. *Appl. Environ. Microbiol.* **59**:34–39.

3. **Bouman, S., D. B. Lund, F. M. Driessen, and D. G Schmidt.** 1982. Growth of thermoresistant streptococci and deposition of milk constituents on plates of heat exchangers during long operating times. *J. Food Prot.* **45**:806–812.

4. **Busscher, H. J., M. N. Bellon-Fontaine, N. Mozes, H. C. van der Meij, J. Sjollema, O. Cerf, and P. G. Rouxhet.** 1990. Deposition of *Leuconostoc mesenteroides* and *Streptococcus thermophilus* to solid substrata in a parallel plate flow cell. *Biofouling* **2**:55–63.

5. **Busscher, H. J., G. Bruinsma, R. van Weissenbruch, C. Leunisse, H. C. van der Mei, F. Dijk, and F. W. J. Albers.** Consumption of buttermilk delays biofilm formation on silicone rubber voice prostheses in an artificial throat. *Eur. Arch. Oto-Rhino. Laryngol.*, in press.

6. **Busscher, H. J., C. E. de Boer, G. J. Verkerke, R. Kalicharan, H. K. Schutte, and H. C. van der Mei.** 1994. In vitro ingrowth of yeasts into medical grade silicone rubber. *Int. Biodeterior Biodegrad.* **33**:383–390.

7. **Busscher, H. J., G. I. Geertsema-Doornbusch, E. P. J. M. Everaert, G. J. Verkerke, B. van de Belt-Gritter, R. Kalicharan,**

and **H. C. van der Mei.** 1996. Biofilm formation and silicone rubber surface modification in the development of a total artificial larynx, p. 47–52. *In* J. Algaba (ed.), *Surgery and Prosthetic Voice Restoration after Total and Subtotal Laryngectomy.* Elsevier Science BV, Amsterdam, the Netherlands.

8. **Busscher, H. J., T. R. Neu, and H. C. van der Mei.** 1994. Biosurfactant production by thermophilic dairy streptococci. *Appl. Microbiol. Biotechnol.* **41**:4–7.

9. **Busscher, H. J., M. van der Kuijl-Booij, and H. C. van der Mei.** 1996. Biosurfactants from thermophilic dairy streptococci and their potential role in the fouling control of heat exchanger plates. *J. Ind. Microbiol.* **16**:15–21.

10. **Busscher, H. J., C. G. van Hoogmoed, G. I. Geertsema-Doornbusch, M. van der Kuijl-Booij, and H. C. van der Mei.** 1997. *Streptococcus thermophilus* and its biosurfactants inhibit adhesion by *Candida* spp. on silicone rubber. *Appl. Environ. Microbiol.* **63**:3810–3817.

11. **Fuller, R.** 1995. Probiotics: their development and use, p. 1–8. *In* R. Fuller, P. J. Heidt, V. Rusch, and D. van der Waaij (eds.), *Probiotics: Prospects of Use in Opportunistic Infections.* Institute for Microbiology and Biochemistry, Herborn-Dill, Germany.

12. **Havenaar, R., and J. H. J. Huis in't Veld.** 1992. Probiotics: a general view, p. 151–170. *In* B. J. B. Wood (ed.), *The Lactic Acid Bacteria in Health and Disease.* Elsevier, London.

13. **Hawthorn, L. A., and G. Reid.** 1990. Exclusion of uropathogen adhesion to polymer surfaces by *Lactobacillus acidophilus. J. Biomed. Mater. Res.* **24**:39–46.

14. **Mahieu H. F., H. K. F. van Saene, H. J. Rosingh, and H. K. Schutte.** 1986. *Candida* vegetations on silicone voice prostheses. *Arch. Otolaryngol. Head Neck Surg.* **112**:321–325.

15. **Mahieu, H. F., J. J. M. van Saene, J. den Besten, and H. K. F. van Saene.** 1986. Oropharynx decontamination preventing *Candida* vegetation on voice prostheses. *Arch. Otolaryngol. Head Neck Surg.* **112**:1090–1092.

16. **Neu, T. R.** 1996. Significance of bacterial surface-active compounds in interaction of bacteria with interfaces. *Microbiol. Rev.* **60**:151–166.

17. **Neu, T. R., H. C. van der Mei, H. J. Busscher, F. Dijk, and G. J. Verkerke.** 1993. Biodeterioration of medical-grade silicone rubber used for voice prostheses: a SEM study. *Biomaterials* **14**:459–464.

18. **Reid, G., A. W. Bruce, J. A. McGroarty, K.-J. Cheng, and J. W. Costerton.** 1990. Is

there a role for lactobacilli in prevention of urogenital and intestinal infections? *Clin. Microbiol. Rev.* **3:**335–344.

19. **Rolla, G., S. M. Waaler, and V. Kjaerheim.** 1998. Concepts in dental plaque formation, p. 1–17. *In* H. J. Busscher and L. V. Evans (ed.), *Oral Biofilms and Plaque Control.* Harwood Academic Publishers, India.

20. **Sanders, M. E.** 1995. Lactic acid bacteria and human health, p. 126–140. *In* R. Fuller, P. J. Heidt, V. Rusch, and D. van der Waaij (ed.), *Probiotics: Prospects of Use in Opportunistic Infections.* Institute for Microbiology and Biochemistry, Herborn-Dill, Germany.

21. **Van den Hoogen, F. J. A., M. J. Oudes, G. Hombergen, H. F. Nijdam, and J. J. Manni.** 1996. The Groningen, Nijdam and Provox Voice prostheses: a prospective clinical comparison based on 845 replacements. *Acta Otolaryngol.* **116:** 119–124.

22. **Van Loosdrecht, M. C. M., J. Lyklema, W. Norde, and A. B. J. Zehnder.** 1990. Influence of interfaces on microbial activity. *Microbiol. Rev.* **54:**75–87.

23. **Velraeds, M. C. M., H. C. van der Mei, G. Reid, and H. J. Busscher.** 1996. Physicochemical and biochemical characterization of biosurfactants released by *Lactobacillus* strains. *Coll. Surf. B: Biointerfaces* **8:**51–61.

24. **Wagner, R. D., C. Pierson, T. Warner, M. Dohnalek, J. Farmer, L. Roberts, M. Hilty, and E. Balish.** 1997. Biotherapeutic effects of probiotic bacteria on candidiasis in immunodeficient mice. *Infect. Immun.* **65:**4165–4172.

CONFOCAL MICROSCOPY IN THE STUDY OF THE INTERACTIONS BETWEEN MICROORGANISMS AND CELLS

Ilan Tsarfaty, Rom T. Altstock, Leonid Mittelman,
Hana Sandovsky-Losica, Jeries Jadoun, Ina Fabian,
Ester Segal, and Shlomo Sela

6

The interactions between microorganisms and mammalian cells are very complex and involve changes in both the cell and microorganism. To understand the molecular and cellular mechanisms involved in these processes, a combined effort of researchers and techniques from the fields of microbiology and cellular biology is required. Fluorescence microscopy has become a powerful tool for studying both the localization of cellular components and microorganisms, with use of target-specific fluorescent probes and labeled antibodies in fixed and living cells (11). In recent years, confocal ("having the same foci") laser scanning microscopy (CLSM) has contributed to the substantial improvement in fluorescent imaging and analysis, offering a powerful tool for studying the interactions between microorganisms and cells in situ (14, 17).

CLSM produces sharp images even when performed on thick specimens. This can be achieved at various depths by rejecting the out-of-focus information and allowing only the plane of interest to be detected (1). The CLSM imaging system achieves out–of-focus rejection essentially by use of two strategies: (i) illumination of a single point in the specimen at a time, with a focused laser beam, so that illumination intensity drops off rapidly above and below the plane of focus, in addition to minimizing the illumination of the surrounding area and (ii) a "pinhole" aperture that blocks the light emitted from anywhere but the focal plane from reaching the detector. A confocal microscope can be used in reflection mode and still exhibit the same out-of-focus rejection performance. These strategies allow CLSM optics to improve by 1.4 times the resolution obtained with a conventional light microscope (reviewed in reference 10 and references within).

Most CLSM biomedical applications are in the detection and analysis of fluorescently-labeled molecules. Fluorescence is a property of certain molecules (called fluorophores or fluorescent dyes) that as a consequence of excitation by light with specific wavelength emit light at a longer wavelength. Fluorescence is the result of a three-stage process: (i) excitation of the fluorophores by an external source (such as a laser), (ii) absorption of the light

Ilan Tsarfaty, Rom T. Altstock, Hana Sandovsky-Losica, Jeries Jadoun, Ester Segal, and Shlomo Sela, Department of Human Microbiology, Sackler School of Medicine, Tel Aviv University, Tel Aviv 69978, Israel. *Leonid Mittelman,* Interdepartmental Core Facility, Sackler School of Medicine, Tel Aviv University, Tel Aviv 69978, Israel. *Ina Fabian,* Department of Cell Biology and Histology, Sackler School of Medicine, Tel Aviv University, Tel Aviv 69978, Israel.

Microbial Ecology and Infectious Disease, Edited by Eugene Rosenberg
©1999 American Society for Microbiology, Washington, D.C.

(energy) by the fluorophore, and (iii) emission of light with a longer wavelength than the excitation light (6).

CLSM uses a laser beam as a light source because a laser provides high intensity, low divergence, and superior focusing ability for illuminating individual points within a specimen. The most common lasers used in confocal microscopes are UV (363 nm), HeNe (633 nm), and KrAr (448, 568, 647 nm). Up to three different lasers can be applied simultaneously (one for each channel). The lasers that best match the excitation properties of the fluorescent dye(s) are used to achieve an optimal signal. The laser beam scans across the specimen, thus causing a light signal to be emitted (fluorescence) or reflected and subsequently detected by the photomultiplier (photodetector). The photomultiplier measures the intensity of the fluorescent light for each point and produces a corresponding analog signal. A subsystem is used to capture the detector's analog signal, reduce the noise, and convert the analog signal to a digital signal, which in turn is used to generate a digital image. In this image, the fluorescent light intensity of each point is represented by a corresponding pixel with a value ranging from 0 to 255. The digital image is monochromatic. Colors can be assigned to the 256 values. This can be used to produce pseudocolor images. In other words, CLSM images originally contain no color data but are often "colored" for presentation purposes by use of pseudocolors (look-up tables). For example, CLSM images of specimens with rhodamine-labeled molecules are often assigned a red hue according to relative intensities, while fluorescein is commonly assigned green hues.

Most CLSMs are commonly provided with three distinct channels (photomultipliers) for detecting and displaying three separate individual images. Three different fluorescence signals can therefore be recorded simultaneously with full resolution. Often one channel (detector) is used to acquire a nonconfocal transmitted laser light-scanned image (e.g., differential interference contrast [DIC] or phase contrast). Fluorescence images acquired in combination with these nonconfocal images are subsequently superimposed, producing an image that allows viewing of the fluorescence signal location within the cellular structure. A specimen can also be analyzed at different depths by changing the plane of focus. The plane of focus (Z plane) is selected by moving the microscope stage up and down by means of a computer-controlled stepping motor. The typical precision of the focus stepping motor on a CLSM is as little as 0.1 μm. Three-dimensional (3D) reconstruction of the fluorescence pattern can be computer generated by recording a series of two-dimensional (2D) optical sections (Z planes) at specific depth intervals (e.g., every 5 μm). Dynamic changes in live systems over time can also be analyzed by CLSM (12). For this technique, the focal plane remains in the same position of the specimen and images are recorded at specific time intervals.

This chapter demonstrates the benefits of fluorescence labeling, confocal microscopy, and computerized image analysis in the study of actin cytoskeleton alteration during microbial-human cell interactions. Actin is a ubiquitous eukaryotic cytoskeletal protein, critical for many aspects of cell activity. In addition to maintaining cell morphology, it is required for cell motility, cell division, and intracellular transport (15). Actin reorganization is rapidly induced by a large variety of extracellular factors (13, 15, 20). To study the role actin plays in a variety of biological functions, researchers have often employed molecules that modify actin polymerization or depolymerization. One such molecule is jaspamide, a naturally occurring cyclic peptide isolated from the marine sponge *Hemiastrella minor*. Jaspamide interacts directly with purified actin to induce actin polymerization (2).

In this chapter we present CLSM techniques using fluorescent labels for both microorganisms and cellular actin to discriminate between attached and internalized bacteria or yeasts. Using these techniques, we show actin cytoskeleton involvement in microorganism internalization and the inability of jaspamide-induced actin aggregation to inhibit the internalization of microorganisms.

CELL CULTURE, ANTIBODIES, AND TREATMENTS

HEp2 human larynx epithelial cells were maintained in Dulbecco's modified Eagle medium (DMEM) with 2 mM L-glutamine and 10% fetal bovine serum (FBS; Biological Industries, Israel) supplemented with 200 μg of streptomycin and 200 IU of penicillin per ml.

For purification of human blood monocytes, heparinized blood obtained with informed consent from healthy donors was layered on Ficoll-Hypaque (Pharmacia Fine Chemicals, Uppsala) and centrifuged at 400 × g for 30 min at room temperature, and subsequently the mononuclear cell layer was collected. The cells were resuspended in IMDM containing 10% FBS and plated at a concentration of 5 × 10^6/ml in 75-cm² flasks. Following a 24-h incubation at 37°C, the cells were washed with phosphate-buffered saline (PBS) to remove nonadherent cells, and the adherent cells were detached by vigorous washing with cold Ca^{2+}-Mg^{2+}-free PBS and resuspended in IMDM containing 10% FBS as previously described (9). Jaspamide (Molecular Probes, Eugene, Oreg.) stock solution of 10^{-3} M was prepared in dimethyl sulfoxide and stored at −20°C. The drug was diluted with IMDM or DMEM to the required concentrations before use. Cells (5 × 10^5/ml) were treated with different concentrations (10^{-8} to 10^{-6} M) of jaspamide for 1 to 48 h.

IMMUNOSTAINING, F-ACTIN STAINING, AND CLSM ANALYSIS

Immunostaining was carried out as previously described (19). In brief, cells were fixed with ice-cold 100% methanol and 100% acetone (10 min each). Following washing, cells were blocked (1% normal donkey serum and 0.1% bovine serum albumin in PBS) for 1 h, incubated with rabbit anti-*Streptococcus pyogenes* (7) (diluted 1:100) for 1 h, and subsequently labeled with fluorescein isothiocyanate

(FITC)-conjugated donkey anti-rabbit antibodies (diluted 1:100) for 1 h. All steps were carried out at room temperature.

F-actin was detected by use of rhodamine phalloidin (Rh-phalloidin) (Molecular Probes) as suggested by the manufacturer (simultaneous fixation protocol). In brief, treated and untreated cells were incubated for 20 min with 3.7% formaldehyde containing 100 μg/ml lysophosphatidyl choline (Sigma, St. Louis, Mo.) and 0.3 μM Rh-phalloidin and then washed. Coverslips were mounted using Gel Mount (Biomeda, Foster City, Calif.).

Images of fluorescently labeled cells were obtained using a Zeiss CLSM. The Zeiss (Oberkochen, Germany) LSM 410 microscope is equipped with a 25-mW krypton-argon laser (488, 568, 647 nm) and a 10-mW HeNe laser (633 nm); images were stored on an optical disk drive and printed using a Codonics NP1600 printer (Codonics, Middleburg Heights, Ohio).

PHAGOCYTOSIS OF C. ALBICANS

Candida albicans was grown in Sabouraud dextrose broth for 5 days, washed twice in saline, and resuspended in Hanks balanced salt solution (HBSS) to a concentration of 2 × 10^7 yeast particles per ml as previously described (4). Fluorescence labeling of F-actin and phagocytosed *C. albicans* in experiments requiring simultaneous visualization was carried out in two stages: *C. albicans* cells (2 × 10^7) were centrifuged at 2,000 rpm for 10 min, and the yeast pellet was stained with PKH2 green fluorescent general cell linker kit (Sigma) according to the manufacturer's instructions. Monocytes preincubated with 10^{-7} M jaspamide were incubated for 30 min with the stained *C. albicans* as described above. Subsequently, cells were washed with HBSS and stained with Rh-phalloidin as described above.

FITC LABELING OF BACTERIA AND C. ALBICANS

FITC labeling was performed as previously described (7) with the following modifications: *S. pyogenes* (JRS4) or *C. albicans* cells incubated at a concentration of 10^9/ml with 0.1 mg of FITC per ml (Sigma) in 50 mM NaHCO$_3$ in 100 mM NaCl (buffer, pH 9.0) for 20 h at room temperature in the dark. The bacteria or yeasts were then washed twice with PBS to remove free FITC and resuspended in PBS to a concentration of 10^8 bacteria per ml.

HOW IS A CONFOCAL IMAGE GENERATED?

Confocal microscopy allows accurate and nondestructive optical sectioning in a plane perpendicular or parallel to the optical axis of the microscope. A scanning laser-beam is focused to a small spot by an objective lens. The mixture of reflected light and emitted fluorescent light is captured by the same objective and is focused onto a photodetector (photomultiplier). A scheme representing a simplified CLSM light path of reflected and emitted (fluorescence) light is shown in Fig. 1. A confocal aperture (pinhole) is placed in front of the photodetector. The fluorescence from points on the specimen that are above (red in Fig. 1) or below (blue in Fig. 1) the focal plane where the laser beam was focused (out–of–focus light) will be largely obstructed and will not pass through the pinhole. Light reflected or fluorescence originating from points in the focal plane will pass through the pinhole (green in Fig. 1). This becomes especially important when dealing with thick specimens.

CLSM'S CONFOCAL MODE FOR IMPROVING RESOLUTION AND CONTRAST OF FLUORESCENTLY LABELED SPECIMENS

To demonstrate the ability of the CLSM to increase resolution, internalized bacteria and cellular actin were costained and subjected to CLSM analysis. *S. pyogenes* was incubated with HEp2 cells for 2 h, cells were fixed, and double immunofluorescence staining was performed. The bacteria were stained with rabbit antibacteria antibody and FITC-labeled don-

key anti-rabbit secondary antibody (green) (Fig. 2A) and the cells were stained with anti-actin antibody (Boehringer Mannheim) and rhodamine-labeled anti-mouse secondary antibody (red) (Fig. 2C) as described above. The image acquired in nonconfocal mode (Fig. 2, panels A to C, outer square) was compared with the image acquired in confocal mode (Fig. 2, panels A–C, inner square). In the area of the image acquired in nonconfocal mode, the resolution is very poor. The image appears blurry, and no fine details can be perceived from the images of both green and red signals (Fig. 2, outer square). In contrast, the images acquired in confocal mode exhibit improved resolution with enhanced detail of both the filamentous structure of the cellular actin and the bacteria. In addition, background noise is extensively reduced (Fig. 2, panels A and C, inner square, respectively). These results demonstrate that omitting out-of-focus signal as accomplished by the CLSM significantly increases signal-to-noise ratio. These attributes enable study of the interaction between the actin cytoskeleton and bacteria in greater detail.

Colocalization of two proteins is very important and may indicate the association between these proteins. To study the colocalization of the bacterial antigens (Fig. 2A) and cellular F-actin (Fig. 2C), the green and the red images were overlaid (Fig 2B). The yellow color indicates colocalization of the molecules labeled with green and red staining. In the nonconfocal mode (Fig. 2, outer square) the colocalized signal (yellow) surrounds all the bacterial staining. The colocalization is not precise and can result from signals that do not originate from the focal plane. Due to the poor resolution and out-of-focus signals, a false colocalization is observed in the margins of the bacteria. In contrast, the colocalization in confocal mode exhibits improved resolution, and the yellow signal is restricted to precise regions in the same focal plane, in which actin associates with bacteria (Fig. 2B, inner square).

CLSM Z SECTIONS AND COLOCALIZATION ANALYSIS IN THE DETECTION OF MICROORGANISM INTERNALIZATION INTO MAMMALIAN CELLS

The major challenge in microscopic detection of microorganism internalization into mammalian cells is distinguishing between adherent and internalized microorganisms. The capabilities of CLSM to resolve specimens in different focal plane angles provide simple tools for identifying internalized microorganisms. Moreover, CLSM's enhanced resolution enables subcellular localization of the internalized microorganisms.

These capabilities of CLSM are demonstrated by incubating HEp2 cells with FITC-labeled *C. albicans* for 4 h. Subsequently, the cells were fixed and stained for F-actin by use of Rh-phalloidin. Stained cells were analyzed by CLSM. Control HEp2 cells that were not incubated with *C. albicans* exhibit only red staining (F-actin) (Fig. 3A). Internalization of the FITC-labeled *C. albicans* into HEp2 cells is demonstrated by intercalation of the *C. albicans* into F-actin fibers located inside the cells (Fig. 3B). Measuring one focal plane and showing that the *C. albicans* and the F-actin reside within the same focal plane is not sufficient to conclude that the *C. albicans* is internalized. *C. albicans* in a membrane invagination will produce a similar image that cannot be distinguished from internalized *C. albicans* by this analysis alone.

By default, CLSM scans a specimen horizontally, producing a cross section (X-Y plane). However, CLSM can also scan the specimen perpendicularly, along either the Z-X or Z-Y planes, without having to rotate the specimen. To facilitate the explanation, a schematic representation of the specimen and possible laser-scanned planes is provided. The box represents a specimen, while laser-beam scanning planes are shown as blue planes (Fig. 3D). The dark blue plane depicts the default X-Y plane, which is representative of the type of scanning used to obtain the CLSM image shown in Fig. 3C. The light blue plane (shown on the Z-X plane) depicts a perpendicular scan (Z-section), which illustrates the type of scanning used to obtain the CLSM image shown in Fig. 3E.

Whereas the single scan of X-Y alone is not sufficient to conclude internalization, when used in combination with a Z-section scanning, internalization can be clearly determined. This is demonstrated by use of the same specimen described above subjected to CLSM analysis at a greater magnification (Fig. 3C). An HEp2 cell appearing to contain two internalized *C. albicans* and one extracellular adherent particle was subjected to CLSM analysis (Fig. 3C). A Z section of the above specimen, in which the scan plane is depicted by a purple line (Fig. 3C), was carried out. The image generated from this focal plane (Fig. 3E) shows two *C. albicans* (yellow/green) that are intercalated with the F-actin cytoskeleton (red). Taken together, these results indicate that those two yeast particles are internalized, while the third *C. albicans* particle (green) appearing on the left side of the image (Fig. 3E) is not internalized. Association with bacterial internalization has been shown for several species (8). Moreover, direct association between internalized bacteria and cellular F-actin in the shape of a cup was previously reported for several bacteria (16). However, cytochalasin D does not inhibit internalization of *Proteus mirabilis*, suggesting that the latter species enters the cells by a mechanism that does not depend on actin polymerization (3). To investigate whether a similar pattern of association occurs during *C. albicans* internalization to HEp2 cells, a colocalization analysis was performed.

Colocalization is an important analysis option made available by CLSM because of its focal and multiple label detection abilities. After scanning a specimen for each label, colocalization can be analyzed by several methods. The most common method is overlaying of pseudocolored images, usually one red and the other green, to produce one image in which a yellow color appears where colocalization

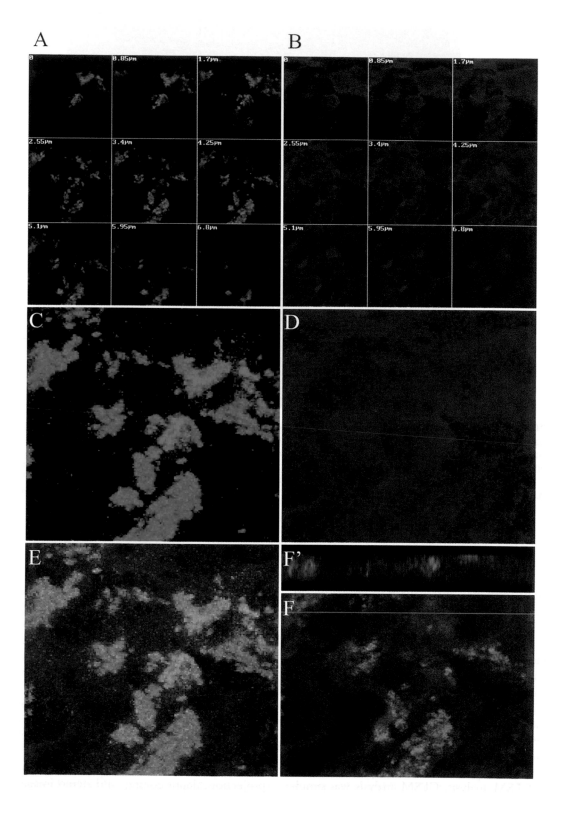

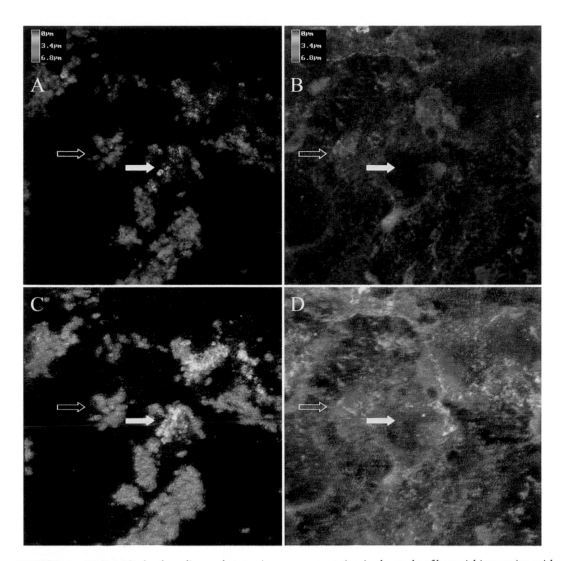

FIGURE 6 CLSM 3D depth coding and stereo image representation in the study of bacterial interaction with cellular F-actin. HEp2 cells were treated with jaspamide, incubated with the bacteria, and costained for bacterial antigen and F-actin. Nine focal planes were generated for each staining (see Fig. 5). Depth coding analysis for the (A) bacteria and (B) cellular actin and stereo image representation of the (C) bacteria and (D) cellular actin were performed. Panels C and D should be viewed using red/green filtered glasses (left, red; right, green). Magnification panels A–D, ×1,200.

←

FIGURE 5 CLSM 3D image analysis in the study of bacterial interaction with cellular F-actin. HEp2 cells were treated with jaspamide, incubated with the bacteria, costained for bacterial antigen and F-actin, and subjected to CLSM analysis. CLSM analysis was simultaneously performed for (A) bacterial staining and (B) cellular actin staining at nine different focal planes and 3D projection with −4° projection angle for the (C) bacterial-staining, (D) F-actin–staining, and (E) the red-green overlaid images. (F′) A Z section was performed on (F) a single plane of the overlaid image across the green line. Magnification: panels A and B, ×400; panels C–F′, ×1,200.

Projection is the transformation of 3D data into a 2D image that portrays the 3D organization of the specimen. Perspective projection includes the concept of distance from the viewer by scaling the projected image of objects by an amount related to their distance from the view reference point. Calculation of projection transformation is performed in several stages as follows. First, a viewpoint (eye position) and a view direction are specified. Next, the x and y coordinates are rotated. Finally, the x and y coordinates are scaled by a factor based on the z coordinate (which represents the distance from the viewpoint). The projected image can rotate to all conceivable angles. An animation of the different projections will result in a 3D animation of the object. Using the Zeiss CLSM 3D projection program, an image that portrays the volumetric data derived from all nine focal planes in Fig. 5A was generated and visualized with a $-4°$ projection angle. Projection was performed for the bacterial staining (Fig. 5C), the F-actin staining (Fig. 5D), and the overlaid images (Fig. 5E). This analysis demonstrates that some of the bacteria are intercalated into the cellular F-actin.

To further substantiate this observation, green and red images of the same focal plane from approximately the middle of the cell were superimposed. The resulting image exhibits colocalization of several bacterial groups with cellular F-actin as described above (Fig. 5E). The yellow regions indicate colocalization between the actin and the bacterial antigen (Fig. 5, E and F). A Z section of the same region was performed as described previously for *C. albicans*. This analysis shows that some of the bacteria are intercalated within the F-actin fibers, and in several locations, colocalization between the green and red signals indicates the association between bacterial proteins and cellular F-actin (Fig. 5F′).

Height-color-coded depth of focus is a common way to visualize 3D structure. In this method each focal plane of a series is assigned a color according to its depth and the color-coded images are superimposed. The resulting image is a "map" that contains information about the Z position of the scanned structures. As on a conventional map, the elevations are coded in red and the depressions are blue. To enable direct evaluation, a color scale is displayed specifying the relative height associated with the colors (21). The major disadvantage of this method of 3D visualization is that the intensity of the signal is not thoroughly represented. Nevertheless, this visualization can facilitate the understanding of the 3D distribution of the labeled molecules with higher-intensity signal within the specimen. The depth-coded image assembled from the image series in Fig. 5A shows that several groups of bacteria (Fig. 6A, open arrow) have the same color (blue-green) as the cellular F actin (Fig. 6B, open arrow), indicating that the bacteria and the actin reside in the same focal plane. A different group of bacteria (Fig. 6A, solid arrow) are colored red, while the actin at the same coordinates is colored blue-green, indicating that they are not located on the same plane.

The human visual system gauges the relative depth of objects in 3D space by weighing minute positional differences between left and right images (eyes). The 3D visualization method of stereo images uses this phenomenon to generate pictures that allow a 3D perception of an object. To achieve 3D visualization by this method, two different images with slightly different perspectives (horizontal displacement) of the same subject are generated. The brain perceives these images as 3D images if the left image is directed only to the left eye and the right image directed only to the right eye. There are several ways to direct the images to the appropriate eye. One of the most common methods of stereo imaging is called anaglyphs. In the anaglyph method the "left" view of an image is encoded in red and the "right" view is encoded in green. The two images are superimposed, forming a single image. The image is viewed with red/green filtered glasses (left, red; right, green) that direct the "right image" to the right eye and "left image" to the left eye.

Stereo images were generated from the series presented in Fig. 5 for both the bacteria (Fig. 6C) and the cellular F-actin (Fig. 6D). Internalization of the bacteria is observed by comparing the bacterial stereo images with the actin stereo images. The same group of bacteria shown to be internalized by the depth coding occupies the same space (Fig. 6C, open arrow) as the cellular F-actin (Fig. 6D, open arrow). These results demonstrate that the bacteria are inside the cell, surrounded by the cellular F-actin. A second group of bacteria (Fig. 6C, solid arrow) is localized above the F-actin (Fig. 6D, solid arrow), indicating that the bacteria are not internalized.

These 3D analyses demonstrate the power of confocal microscopy to study the interaction between cells and microorganisms. CLSM technology is still young, and future advances in both biological experiments and 3D computation will enable a closer look and a better understanding of the interaction between microorganisms and human cells.

CLSM—THE FUTURE

CLSM is most frequently employed to record images and determine subcellular localization of fluorescently labeled molecules in cells, both fixed and living. These constitute only a limited scope of CLSM capabilities. To further exploit CLSM's potential as an analytical tool for measuring intensities, applicable mathematical algorithms must be developed. Current CLSM procedures are user interactive and very time consuming. The techniques applied to most systems to automate CLSM procedures are fundamentally operator dependent. Image-analysis algorithms for identifying structures in digital images of biological specimens are currently under development. One hopes that these algorithms will be used to develop improved automatic data acquisition and analysis. This will allow automated reconstruction of specimens in 3D images with calculated relative intensities and volume

manifestation, all presented in a comprehensible fashion on a graphics workstation (5).

REVIEWS AND KEY PAPERS

Finlay, B. B., and S. Falkow. 1997. Common themes in microbial pathogenicity revisited. *Microbiol Mol. Biol. Rev.* **61:**136–169.

Pujol, C., E. Eugene, L. de Saint Martin, and X. Nassif. 1997. Interaction of Neisseria meningitidis with a polarized monolayer of epithelial cells. *Infect Immun.* **65:**4836–4842.

Sanger, J. M., J. W. Sanger, and F. S. Southwick. 1992. Host cell actin assembly is necessary and likely to provide the propulsive force for intracellular movement of Listeria monocytogenes. *Infect. Immun.* **60:**3609–3619.

REFERENCES

1. Amos, W. B., J. G. White, and M. Fordham. 1987. Use of confocal imaging in the study of biological structures. *Appl. Optics* **26:**3239–3243.
2. Bubb, M. R., A. M. Senderowicz, E. A. Sausville, K. L. Duncan, and E. D. Korn. 1994. Jasplakinolide, a cytotoxic natural product, induces actin polymerization and competitively inhibits the binding of phalloidin to F-actin. *J. Biol. Chem.* **269:**14869–14871.
3. Chippendale, G. R., J. W. Warren, A. L. Trifillis, and H. L. Mobley. 1994. Internalization of Proteus mirabilis by human renal epithelial cells. *Infect. Immun.* **62:**3115–3121.
4. Fabian, I., M. Lass, Y. Kletter, and D. W. Golde. 1992. Differentiation and functional activity of human eosinophilic cells from an eosinophil HL-60 subline: response to recombinant hematopoietic growth factors. *Blood* **80:**788–794.
5. Golish, S. R., and D. A. Zarling. 1992. Measurements in cell nuclei using automated CLSM. Presented at the 3D Imaging Sciences in Microscopy, Amsterdam.
6. Haugland, R. P. 1996. *Handbook of Fluorescent Probes and Research Chemicals*, 6th ed. Molecular Probes Inc., Eugene, Oreg.
7. Kabha, K., J. Schmegner, Y. Keisari, H. Parolis, J. Schlepper Schaeffer, and I. Ofek. 1997. SP-A enhances phagocytosis of Klebsiella by interaction with capsular polysaccharides and alveolar macrophages. *Am. J. Physiol.* **272:**L344–352.
8. Miliotis, M. D., B. D. Tall, and R. T. Gray. 1995. Adherence to and invasion of tissue culture cells by Vibrio hollisae. *Infect. Immun.* **63:**4959–4963.
9. Mor, S., A. Nagler, V. Barak, Z. T. Handzel, C. Geller Bernstein, and I. Fabian. 1995. Histamine enhances granulocyte-macrophage

colony-stimulating factor and interleukin-6 production by human peripheral blood mononuclear cells. *J. Leukocyte Biol.* **58**:445–450.

10. **Pawley, J. B.** 1995. *Handbook of Biological Confocal Microscopy*, 2nd ed. Plenum Press, New York.

11. **Pedley, K. C.** 1997. Applications of confocal and fluorescence microscopy. *Digestion* **58** (Suppl. 2):62–68.

12. **Petroll, W. M., J. V. Jester, and H. D. Cavanagh.** 1994. In vivo confocal imaging: general principles and applications. *Scanning* **16**:131–149.

13. **Pollard, T. D., and J. A. Cooper.** 1986. Actin and actin-binding proteins. A critical evaluation of mechanisms and functions. *Annu. Rev. Biochem.* **55**:987–1035.

14. **Pujol, C., E. Eugene, L. de Saint Martin, and X. Nassif.** 1997. Interaction of Neisseria meningitidis with a polarized monolayer of epithelial cells. *Infect Immun.* **65**:4836–4842.

15. **Ridley, A. J.** 1995. Rho-related proteins: actin cytoskeleton and cell cycle. *Curr. Opin. Genet. Dev.* **5**:24–30.

16. **Rosenshine, I., S. Ruschkowski, M. Stein, D. J. Reinscheid, S. D. Mills, and B. B. Finlay.** 1996. A pathogenic bacterium triggers epithelial signals to form a functional bacterial receptor that mediates actin pseudopod formation. *EMBO J.* **15**:2613–2624.

17. **Sanger, J. M., J. W. Sanger, and F. S. Southwick.** 1992. Host cell actin assembly is necessary and likely to provide the propulsive force for intracellular movement of Listeria monocytogenes. *Infect. Immun.* **60**:3609–3619.

18. **Sato, N., N. Funayama, A. Nagafuchi, S. Yonemura, S. Tsukita, and S. Tsukita.** 1992. A gene family consisting of ezrin, radixin and moesin. Its specific localization at actin filament/plasma membrane association sites. *J. Cell Sci.* **103**:131–143.

19. **Tsarfaty, I., J. H. Resau, S. Rulong, I. Keydar, D. L. Faletto, and G. F. Vande Woude.** 1992. The met proto-oncogene receptor and lumen formation. *Science* **257**:1258–1261.

20. **Wessells, N. K., B. S. Spooner, J. F. Ash, M. O. Bradley, M. A. Luduena, E. L. Taylor, J. T. Wrenn, and K. Yamaa.** 1971. Microfilaments in cellular and developmental processes. *Science* **171**:135–143.

21. **Zeiss.** 1995. *LSM 410 Invert Laser Scan Microscope: Operating Manual.* Zeiss Gruppe, Jena, Germany.

CROSS-TALK BETWEEN ENTEROPATHOGENIC *ESCHERICHIA COLI* AND HOST EPITHELIAL CELLS

Ilan Rosenshine and Yuan Fang

7

PATHOGENIC STRAINS OF *E. COLI*

The life cycle of pathogenic *Escherichia coli* and related gram-negative enteropathogens consists of two stages: life outside of the host, in most cases in a relatively cool and nutrient-depleted environment, and life within the host. The host environment is usually warmer (37°C) and richer in nutrients. However, the host environment also contains several mechanisms that act specifically to kill bacteria and to restrict their growth. Pathogens must therefore maintain genes that enable survival in, and exploitation of, the host. These specific genes, the virulence genes, are absolutely essential for successful colonization by the pathogen, and in most cases, they cannot be found in related nonpathogenic strains.

Most *E. coli* strains are nonpathogenic and are among the normal gut flora. Other strains are pathogenic and can cause either bladder infection, meningitis, or diarrhea. At least five different classes of diarrheagenic *E. coli* exist, including enterotoxigenic *E. coli* (ETEC), enterohemorragic *E. coli* (EHEC), enteroaggregative *E. coli* (EAEC), enteroinvasive *E. coli* (EIEC), and enteropathogenic *E. coli* (EPEC). These *E. coli* strains cause symptoms ranging from cholera-like bowel disturbances to extreme colitis. Each class of diarrheagenic *E. coli* possesses a distinct set of virulence factors including specific adhesins, invasins, and/or toxins, which are responsible for causing a specific type of diarrhea.

TYPE III SECRETION SYSTEMS

A recent exciting development in the field of bacterial pathogenesis is the discovery of the type III protein secretion mechanism in plant and animal pathogens (26). These type III systems secrete key virulence factors, some of which are injected (translocated) directly from the pathogen's cytoplasm into the host cell cytoplasm (26). The type III secretion pathway is independent of the *sec* system, and proteins are secreted without forming a periplasmic intermediate. The secretory signals that mediate secretion by the type III system have not been clearly identified, and secretion requires the involvement of a large number of accessory proteins. So far, type III secretion systems have been identified as playing an essential role in the virulence of *Salmonella*, *Shigella*, and *Yersinia* spp., EIEC, EHEC, EPEC, *Hafnia alvei*, *Cytobacter rodantium*, *Chlamydia* spp., and *Pseudomonas aeruginosa* (16, 26). Type III secretion

Ilan Rosenshine and Yuan Fang, Department of Molecular Genetics and Biotechnology, The Hebrew University Faculty of Medicine, P.O. Box 12272, Jerusalem 91120, Israel.

Microbial Ecology and Infectious Disease, Edited by Eugene Rosenberg
©1999 American Society for Microbiology, Washington, D.C.

systems are also essential for the virulence of several plant pathogens including *Pseudomonas solanacearum*, *Pseudomonas syringae*, and *Xanthomonas capestris* (2). As research progresses, it is expected that type III secretion systems will be detected in many other animal and plant pathogens.

Type III secretion systems are usually encoded by genetic elements 30 to 40 kbp in size that are located either on large plasmids or as a pathogenicity island in the chromosome (26). In several cases, the G + C content of the DNA of these elements is low in comparison with the G + C of the rest of the genome, and some pathogenicity islands appear as large insertions within genes. Therefore, it appears that some of these pathogenicity islands are mobile genetic elements and that pathogens acquire these elements by horizontal DNA transfer. More than one of these type III secretion systems may be involved in the virulence of a given pathogen. *Salmonella* spp. for instance, appear to acquire several pathogenicity islands during their evolution, and two of them encode distinct type III secretion systems (13).

THE PATHOGENICITY OF EPEC

EPEC was the first of the *Escherichia* species to be identified as a causative agent of diarrhea (5). EPEC causes a persistent, watery diarrhea that can lead to dehydration and death. Vomiting and fever usually accompany fluid loss. EPEC is a predominant cause of infantile diarrhea worldwide. In developed countries, it is involved in sporadic outbreaks of diarrheal disease in day-care centers and nurseries (35). EPEC, however, poses a major endemic health threat to young children (less than 6 months) in developing countries. Within these countries, neonatal diarrhea due to EPEC still has a high mortality rate (27, 42).

EPEC colonizes the small intestinal mucosa and produces a typical histopathological feature known as the attaching and effacing (AE) lesion (34). The AE lesion is characterized by localized destruction of brush border microvilli, intimate bacterial attachment to the host

cell membrane, and formation of an underlying pedestal-like structure in the host cell. This structure consists of polymerized actin and several actin-binding proteins (9, 23). In addition, some of the infecting EPEC invade the entrocytes and penetrate the epithelial monolyer.

AE lesions are also produced by EPEC in a variety of tissue culture cell lines (23). EPEC invades these cell lines and penetrates polarized epithelial monolyers in vitro. In a pioneering study, Donnenberg et al. (7) utilized the invasion phenotype to screen for noninvasive EPEC mutants. Several of these mutants were also incapable of forming AE lesions. Later, the mutated genes were identified as encoding components of a type III secretion system (17). In vitro studies employing infection of cultured epithelial cells with defined EPEC mutants support a three-stage model of AE lesion formation: (i) initial non-intimate attachment, (ii) signal transduction and cytoskeletal rearrangements in host cells, and (iii) intimate bacterial adhesion, actin accumulation, and pedestal formation (8).

The two later stages depend on EPEC's type III secretion system that is encoded by a 35-kbp chromosomal pathogenicity island, designated LEE (for *locus* for *enterocyte effacement*). The LEE contains all the genes required to produce AE lesions (30, 31), including those that encode the secretion apparatus; several secreted proteins including EspA, EspB, and EspD; an adhesin termed intimin, for the translocated intimin receptor (Tir); and regulatory proteins. Tir is translocated by EPEC into the host cell plasma membrane, where it forms a transmembrane intimin receptor (19). Intimin-Tir interaction is required for intimate attachment of EPEC to host cells (19) and for organization of polymerized actin into a cuplike pedestal beneath an attached bacterium (8). EspB, EspA, and EspD appear to be part of the apparatus that acts in concert with the secretion machinery to mediate protein translocation into infected host cells. Strains with *espA*, *espB*, and *espA* mutations still secrete proteins via the type III system but are unable to translocate proteins into the host cell (24, 45) and do not mediate signal transduction (10, 21, 25).

The first stage in EPEC infection, nonintimate adherence, is mediated by type IV pili termed the bundle-forming pili (BFP) and possibly by other factors (8). The BFP are encoded in a large operon located on a 70-kbp plasmid. This plasmid also contains the *per* locus that encodes a positive transcriptional regulator of BFP and of several LEE genes including the intimin gene *eae* (12, 44).

ENVIRONMENTAL FACTORS THAT REGULATE EXPRESSION OF LEE GENES

Temperature is a typical environmental signature of the host. Several pathogens, including EPEC, use a temperature shift to 37°C as the signal to activate virulence mechanisms (32). The ability of EPEC to induce formation of AE lesions is strictly dependent on growth at 37°C (39). Cultures grown at 27°C cannot induce formation of AE lesions even when infection is carried out at 37°C. Cultures grown at 37°C induce rapid formation of AE lesions even when infection is carried out at 27°C. This indicates that the production of components of the type III secretion system is thermoregulated. In accordance with this, EspB and intimin are produced at 37°C but not at 27°C (22). JPN15 is an EPEC strain cured of the large plasmid that encodes BFP and the Per positive regulator. JPN15 still induces formation of AE lesions, and as in the wild-type strain, this process is still thermoregulated. Thus, the temperature-sensing machinery appears to be independent of the *per* locus.

A second factor that strongly affects the ability of EPEC to induce formation of AE lesions is the growth phase. EPEC induces rapid formation of AE lesions when in mid-logarithmic growth phase, and it becomes inactive in late-logarithmic growth phase and upon entering the early stationary phase (39). Using transcriptional fusions with the *gfp* reporter gene, we determined that transcription of several LEE genes including *eae::gfp*, *sepD::*

gfp, is induced in early to mid-logarithmic growth phase (culture density of 0.1 to 0.4 OD_{600}) and is repressed later, when cultures reach a density above 0.5 OD_{600}. Accordingly, the levels of several proteins encoded in LEE genes, including intimin and EspA, appear to be high in the early logarithmic growth phase and reduced at a later growth phase (22, 24). The molecular mechanism behind this growth phase regulation is still not known.

In addition to dependency on temperature and growth phase, optimal "activation" of EPEC also depends upon the composition of the culture media. Activation is more efficient when EPEC is grown in minimal medium that contains glucose as a carbon source and is at pH 7.2 (20). Activation is less efficient in richer media or upon growth at pH 8.0 or at pH 6.0 (20). Production of BFP was also shown to be subject to growth phase and thermoregulation (37). In the stationary growth phase, EPEC appear as motile single cells. In the mid-logarithmic growth phase at 37°C, EPEC produces the BFP that in turn mediate massive bacterial aggregation. The bacterial aggregates dissociate to single cells after entering the stationary growth phase (37). It is not yet known whether or not common factors mediate the growth phase and thermoregulation of both the BFP and the LEE genes.

TYPE III SECRETION SYSTEM ACTIVATION BY CONTACT WITH THE HOST CELL

EPEC grown in Dulbecco's modified Eagle medium (DMEM) at 37°C to mid-logarithmic growth phase was termed "activated." Activated EPEC execute rapid and complex interactions with host cells immediately upon infection. The activated culture expresses a mature type III secretion system; however, this system exhibits only basal levels of secretion activity. Contact of the activated EPEC with the host cell activates this preformed secretion system to secrete and translocate proteins into the host cell, including EspB and Tir. The BFP of EPEC appear to play an important role in activating the type

III system by mediating rapid initial bacterial contact with the host cells. Contact induction of the type III secretion system is attenuated in mutants that do not produce BFP. The molecular basis for this contact activation of the type III secretion system is not yet clear.

Contact activation of the type III secretion system was inhibited by chloramphenicol. Chloramphenicol also inhibited formation of AE lesions by activated EPEC culture (39). Moreover, increased levels of EspB in infecting EPEC indicate that contact of EPEC with the host cell induces *espB* expression or greater stability of EspB (45). Taken together these results indicate that activation of the type III secretion system depends on de novo protein synthesis in EPEC upon contact with the host cell. It is not yet clear whether this dependency on de novo protein synthesis involves transcriptional activation of a specific gene(s) upon contact with the host cell or whether it enables replacement of a very labile protein.

Contact activation of the type III secretion system was reported also in *Salmonella, Shigella*, and *Yersinia* spp (33, 36, 46). However the activation of the type III secretion systems in *Salmonella* and *Shigella* is independent of *de novo* protein synthesis (30, 46). In contrast, expression of *yopE*, which encodes one of the translocated effectors of *Yersinia*, is induced upon contact with host cells (36). The molecular mechanism behind the contact induction of the type III secretion systems has not been determined.

TWO FUNCTIONS OF EspB: BEING TRANSLOCATED AND BEING A TRANSLOCATOR

Immediately upon infection, the type III secretion system of EPEC mediates translocation of EspB into the host cell (45). The translocated EspB has been localized to both the membrane and the cytosol of the host cell. One of the techniques used to generate these data utilizes the adenylate cyclase (*cyaA*) reporter gene (43). We have constructed a protein fusion between the catalytic domain of *Bordetella pertussis* AC toxin (CyaA) and EspB. CyaA is a calmodulin-dependent enzyme, and

thus it is activated only in the host cell cytoplasm, which contains calmodulin. Hence, increased levels of cAMP in the host cell would indicate that EspB mediates translocation of the fused CyaA domain into the host cell. Indeed, the fusion protein EspB–CyaA was efficiently secreted and translocated into the host cell by the EPEC wild type but not by mutants deficient in components of the type III secretion system (45).

Interestingly, a Δ*espB* mutant still secretes EspB–CyaA but fails to translocate it. This, together with other results, indicates that EspB, in addition to being translocated, functions as translocator of itself, of Tir, and possibly of other proteins (45). In agreement, EspB shows low homology to YopB, a pore-forming protein that acts as a protein translocator in the type III secretion system of *Yersinia* spp. (14). In analogy with YopB, EspB may also be involved in forming a channel in the plasma membrane of the host cell. The EspB–CyaA fusion protein was not active as a translocator. This indicates that being translocated itself and translocating other proteins are two different functions of EspB, which are probably located at different domains. Further work is needed to define these domains.

EspA IS REQUIRED FOR EspB TRANSLOCATION

Translocation, but not secretion, of EspB appears to be mediated by fragile filaments that bridge between the bacteria and the host cell surface. One of the components of these filaments is EspA (24). Assembly of fully mature EspA filaments appears to depend also on some function of EspD (24). Thus, mutants in *espA* that do not form the filaments or mutants in *espD* that produce modified filaments do not translocate EspB and Tir and do not induce formation of AE lesions (24). In contrast, these mutants still secret EspB, Tir, and other proteins (21, 25).

INTIMATE ATTACHMENT STRONGLY ENHANCES TRANSLOCATION

Successful EspB translocation is associated with rapid translocation of Tir. The translocated Tir transverses the plasma membrane of the host cell. The cytosolic domain of Tir becomes tyrosine phosphorylated upon entering the host cell, and an exposed surface domain forms an attachment site for the EPEC adhesin intimin. Interaction of intimin with Tir leads to rapid recruitment of Tir beneath the attached bacterium and to intimate attachment. Intimate attachment strongly enhanced the efficiency of further protein translocation via the type III secretion system. This translocation enhancement is possibly due to stabilization of the EspA filaments by facilitation of host-pathogen bridging with very short filaments. Thus, it appears that EspA/EspB and intimin/Tir are involved in a positive-feedback circuit between translocation and intimate attachment. This may also explain the typical localized adherence of EPEC wild type (8) or of EPEC mutants that do not produce BFP (12). It appears that an excess of Tir that was translocated by, and is localized around, the first intimately attached EPEC acts as an intimin receptor for other individual EPECs. Thus EPEC cells appear to cooperate in the process of signaling and attachment to the host cell. An analogous cooperative process is evident during *Salmonella* invasion of host cells. The first invading *Salmonella* cells induce localized but extensive membrane "ruffles" that mediate uptake of additional bacteria that are trapped within the ruffles (11).

The estimated time frame for an individual activated EPEC to form the initial attachment, to establish a positive-feedback circuit of translocation and intimate attachment, to recruit actin filaments, and to initiate the formation of actin pedestals is less than 10 min (39).

MOLECULAR COMPOSITION OF THE ACTIN PEDESTAL

EPEC-induced actin pedestals are composed of actin filaments and several actin-binding proteins. The typical morphology of these actin structures evolves within a few hours from flat, cuplike structures into a short actin pedestal and then into elongated pedestals (40, 41). These pedestals can grow longer or

shorter while remaining tethered in place on the cell surface (41). Alternatively, these actin stalks propel attached extracellular EPEC along the cell surface, reaching a speed of up to 0.07 μm/s (41). The base of the pedestals is rich in myosin and tropomyosin (29, 41), while actin filaments, villin, and a-actinin are distributed uniformly along it (9, 23, 41). The tip of this structure is rich in tyrosine-phosphorylated Tir (19, 40). High concentrations of ezrin, plastin, and tailin within the pedestals were also reported (1, 9), but the distribution of these proteins along the stalk was not examined.

FORMATION OF THE ACTIN PEDESTAL

EPEC must induce several processes to form the actin pedestals, including localized actin polymerization, bundling of the newly polymerized actin filaments, and organization of the polymerized bundles beneath attached bacteria. Not much is known about any of the above processes. Genetic analysis indicates that Tir and intimin are needed to organize the pedestal beneath attached bacteria. Mutants in either *eae* or *tir* fail to focus the actin structure beneath the bacterium (18, 19, 38, 40). We speculate that the intracellular domain of Tir may be associated with the actin bundles and therefore association of the extracellular domain of Tir with intimin provides a physical link between the extracellular EPEC and the actin bundles. However, direct or indirect interaction of actin with Tir has yet to be shown.

Less is known about EPEC activities that induce actin polymerization and bundling. Regulation of actin polymerization and bundling in epithelial cells is often mediated by several small GTP-binding proteins including Rho, Rac, and Csdc42 (15). However, we recently demonstrated that these GTP-binding proteins are not involved in formation of the EPEC-induced actin pedestals (3). Several signal transduction activities are mediated by the infecting EPEC, including activation of PLC-γ (20); a flux of inositol phosphate (including mono-, di-, and triphosphates (10); an increase in the intracellular Ca^{2+} concentration (4); activation of protein kinase C (6), and serine/threonine phosphorylation of several proteins including light-chain myosin (28). These signaling events appear to depend on the type III protein secretion system of EPEC. However, it is not yet clear how these events are triggered and whether these are primary or secondary events during the formation of the actin pedestals.

UNANSWERED QUESTIONS

Many basic aspects of EPEC infection remain elusive. These include the mechanism of host specificity of EPEC and related AE-causing pathogens, the biological significance of the formation of AE lesions, and the direct cause of the diarrhea induced by the pathogen. In addition, we would like to know more about the molecular mechanisms that are involved in virulence. Some of these unanswered questions are listed below.

1. The regulatory network that controls the expression of the LEE gene in response to contact with the host cell, growth phase, temperature, pH, and perhaps other environmental factors are not known; nor is the molecular mechanism behind this putative transcriptional regulation.

2. It is not known how EPEC's type III secretion system is induced upon contact with the host cell, how EPEC "senses" the host cell, or what host and bacterial factors are involved. It would be interesting to determine whether the specific recognition of the host cell that results in activation of the type III secretion system is also involved in the host specificity of EPEC and related pathogens.

3. We still know very little about the molecular mechanism of protein secretion and translocation by any of the type III secretion systems. This includes the structure and function of the many proteins that are involved in the formation of the secretion/translocation apparatus. The amount of information about recognition between the secretion system and the secreted proteins is also very limited.

4. We believe that, in addition to EspB and Tir, EPEC translocates other effectors that are involved in the formation of the actin pedestals. These factors have yet to be identified.

5. The biological significance of the tyrosine phosphorylation of Tir is not clear. It is also unclear whether, and how, Tir interacts with actin or actin-binding proteins.

6. The mechanism of DNA transfer that is involved in the horizontal spread of LEE and related genetic elements has yet to be elucidated.

ACKNOWLEDGMENT

Work at I.R.'s laboratory is supported by grants from the Israeli Academy of Science, the Israel-United States Binational Foundation, the State of Niedersachsen, and the Israeli Ministry of Health.

REVIEWS AND KEY PAPERS

Donnenberg, M. S., J. B. Kaper, and B. B. Finlay. 1997. Interactions between enteropathogenic *Escherichia coli* and host epithelial cells. *Trends Microbiol.* **5:**109–114.

Kenny, B., R. DeVinney, M. Stein, D. J. Reinscheid, E. A. Frey, and B. B. Finlay. 1997. Enteropathogenic *E. coli* (EPEC) transfers its receptor for intimate adherence into mammalian cells. *Cell* **91:**511–520.

Knutton, S., I. Rosenshine, M. J. Pallen, I. Nisan, B. C. Neves, C. Bain, C. Wolff, G. Dougan, and G. Frankel. 1998. A novel EspA-associated surface organelle of enteropathogenic *Escherichia coli* involved in translocation of EspB into eukaryotic cells. *EMBO J.* **17:**2166–2176.

McDaniel, K. T., and J. B. Kaper. 1997. A cloned pathogenicity island from enteropathogenic *Escherichia coli* confers the attaching and effacing phenotype on *E. coli* K-12. *Mol. Microbiol.* **23:**399–407.

Wolff C., I. Nisan, E. Hanski, G. Frankel, and I. Rosenshine. 1998. Protein translocation into host epithelial cells by infecting enteropathogenic *Escherichia coli*. *Mol. Microbiol.* **28:**143–156.

REFERENCES

1. **Adam, T., M., Arpin, M. C. Prevost, P. Gounon, and P. J. Sansonetti.** 1995. Cytoskeletal rearrangements and the functional role of T-plastin during entry of *Shigella flexneri* into HeLa cells. *J. Cell Biol.* **129:**367–381.

2. **Alfano, J. R., and M. Collmer.** 1997. The type III (Hrp) secretion pathway of plant pathogenic bacteria: trafficking harpins, Avr proteins, and death. *J. Bacteriol.* **179:**5655–5662.

3. **Ben-Ami, G., V. Ozeri, E. Hanski, F. Hofmann, K. Aktories, K. M. Hahn, G. M. Bokoch, and I. Rosenshine.** 1998. Agents that inhibit Rho, Rac and Cdc42 do not block formation of actin pedestals in HeLa cells infected with enteropathogenic *Escherichia coli. Infect. Immun.* **66:**1755–1758.

4. **Baldwin, T. J., W. Ward, A. Aitken, S. Knutton, and P. H. Williams.** 1991. Elevation of intracellular free calcium levels in HEp-2 cells infected with enteropathogenic *Escherichia coli. Infect. Immun.* **59:**1599–1604.

5. **Bray, J.** 1945. Isolation of antigenically homogeneous strains of Bact. coli neopolitanum from summer diarrhoea of infants. *J. Pathol. Bacteriol.* **57:**239–247.

6. **Crane, J. K., and J. S. Oh.** 1997. Activation of host protein kinase C by enteropathogenic *Escherichia coli. Infect. Immun.* **65:**3277–3285.

7. **Donnenberg, M. S., S. B. Calderwood, R. A. Donohue, G. T. Keusch, and J. B. Kaper.** 1990. Construction and analysis of Tn*phoA* mutants of enteropathogenic *Escherichia coli* unable to invade HEp-2 cells. *Infect. Immun.* **58:**1565–1571.

8. **Donnenberg, M. S., J. B. Kaper, and B. B. Finlay.** 1997. Interactions between enteropathogenic *Escherichia coli* and host epithelial cells. *Trends Microbiol.* **5:**109–114.

9. **Finlay, B. B., I. Rosenshine, M. S. Donnenberg, and J. B. Kaper.** 1992. Cytoskeletal composition of attaching and effacing lesions associated with enteropathogenic *Escherichia coli* adherence to HeLa cells. *Infect. Immun.* **60:**2541–2543.

10. **Foubister, V., I. Rosenshine, M. S. Donnenberg, and B. B. Finlay.** 1994. The *eaeB* gene of enteropathogenic *Escherichia coli* is necessary for signal transduction in epithelial cells. *Infect. Immun.* **62:**3038–3040.

11. **Francis, C. L., T. A. Ryan, B. D. Jones, S. J. Smith, and S. Falkow.** 1993. Ruffles induced by *Salmonella* and other stimuli direct macropinocytosis of bacteria. *Nature* **364:**639–642.

12. **Gomez-Duarte, O. G., and J. B. Kaper.** 1995. A plasmid-encoded regulatory region activates chromosomal *eaeA* expression in enteropathogenic *Escherichia coli. Infect. Immun.* **63:** 1767–1776.

13. **Groisman, E. A., and H. Ochman.** 1997. How *Salmonella* became a pathogen. *Trends Microbiol.* **5:**343–349.

14. **Håkansson, S., K. Schesser, C. Persson, E. E. Galyov, R. Rosqvist, F. Homble, and H. Wolf-Watz.** 1996. The YopB protein of *Yersinia pseudotuberculosis* is essential for the translocation of Yop effector proteins across the target cell plasma membrane and displays a contact-dependent membrane disrupting activity. *EMBO J.* **15:**5812–5823.

15. **Hall, A.** 1998. Rho GTPases and actin cytoskeleton. *Science* **279:**509–514.

16. **Hsia, R. C., Y. Pannekoek, E. Ingerowski, and P. M. Bovaoil.** 1997. Type III secretion genes identify a putative virulence locus in *chlamydia. Mol. Microbiol.* **25:**351–359.

17. **Jarvis, K. G., J. A. Giron, A. E. Jerse, T. K. McDaniel. M. S. Donnenberg, and J. B. Kaper.** 1995. Enteropathogenic *Escherichia coli* contains a specialized secretion system necessary for the export of proteins involved in attaching and effacing lesions formation. *Proc. Natl. Acad. Sci. USA* **92:**7996–8000.

18. **Jerse, A. E., J. Yu, B. D. Tall, and J. B. Kaper.** 1990. A genetic locus of enteropathogenic *Escherichia coli* necessary for the production of attaching and effacing lesions on tissue culture cells. *Proc. Natl. Acad. Sci. USA* **87:**7839–7843.

19. **Kenny, B., R. DeVinney, M. Stein, D. J. Reinscheid, E. A. Frey, and B. B. Finlay.** 1997. Enteropathogenic *E. coli* (EPEC) transfers its receptor for intimate adherence into mammalian cells. *Cell* **91:**511–520.

20. **Kenny, B., and B. B. Finlay.** 1997. Intimin-dependent binding of enteropathogenic *Escherichia coli* to host cells triggers novel signaling events, including tyrosine phosphorylation of phospholipase C-γ1. *Infect. Immun.* **65:**2528–2536.

21. **Kenny, B., L. C. Lai, B. B. Finlay, and M. S. Donnenberg.** 1996. EspA, a protein secreted by enteropathogenic *Escherichia coli*, is required to induce signals in epithelial cells. Mol. Microbiol. **20:**313–323.

22. **Knutton, S., J. Adu-Bobie, C. Bain, A. D. Phillips, G. Dougan, and G. Frankel.** 1997. Down regulation of intimin expression during attaching and effacing enteropathogenic *Escherichia coli* adhesion. *Infect. Immun.* **65:**1644–1652.

23. **Knutton, S., T. Baldwin, P. H. Williams, and A. S. McNeish.** 1989. Actin accumulation at sites of bacterial adhesion to tissue culture cells: basis of a new diagnostic test for enteropathogenic and enterohemorrhagic *Escherichia coli. Infect. Immun.* **57:**1290–1298.

24. **Knutton, S., I. Rosenshine, M. J. Pallen, I. Nisan, B. C. Neves, C. Bain, C. Wolff, G. Dougan, and G. Frankel.** 1998. A novel EspA associated surface organelle of enteropathogenic

Escherichia coli involved in translocation of EspB into eukaryotic cells. *EMBO J.* **17:**2166–2176.

25. **Lai, L. C., L. A. Wainwright, K. D. Stone, and M. S. Donnenberg.** 1997. A third secreted protein that is encoded by the enteropathogenic *Escherichia coli* pathogenicity island is required for transduction of signals and for attaching and effacing activities in host cells. *Infect. Immun.* **65:**2211–2217.

26. **Lee, A. C.** 1997. Type III secretion systems: machines to deliver bacterial proteins into eukaryotic cells? *Trends Microbiol.* **5:**148–156.

27. **Levine, M. M., and R. Edelman.** 1984. Enteropathogenic *Escherichia coli* of classic serotypes associated with infant diarrhea: epidemiology and pathogenesis. *Epidemiol. Rev.* **6:**31–51.

28. **Majarrez-Hernandez, H. A., B. Amess, L. Selers, T. J. Baldwin, S. Knutton, P. H. Williams, and A. Aitken.** 1991. Purification of a 20-kDa phosphoprotein from epithelial cells and identification as a myosin light chain phosphorylation induced by enteropathogenic *Escherichia coli* and phorbol ester. *FEMS Lett.* **292:**121–127.

29. **Manjarrez-Hernandez, H. A., T. J. Baldwin, A. Aitken, S. Knutton, and P. H. Williams.** 1992. Intestinal epithelial cell protein phosphorylation in enteropathogenic *Escherichia coli* diarrhoea. *Lancet* **339:**521–523.

30. **McDaniel, T. K., K. G. Jarvis, M. S. Donnenberg, and J. B. Kaper.** 1995. A genetic locus of enterocyte effacement conserved among diverse enterobacterial pathogens. *Proc. Natl. Acad. Sci. USA* **92:**1664–1668.

31. **McDaniel, K. T., and J. B. Kaper.** 1997. A cloned pathogenicity island from enteropathogenic *Escherichia coli* confers the attaching and effacing phenotype on *E. coli* K-12. *Mol. Microbiol.* **23:**399–407.

32. **Mekalanos, J. J.** 1992. Environmental signals controlling expression of virulence determinants in bacteria. *J. Bacteriol.* **174:**1–7.

33. **Menard, R., P. Sansonetti, and C. Parsot.** 1994. The secretion of the *Shigella flexneri* Ipa invasins is activated by epithelial cells and controlled by IpaB and IpaD. *EMBO J.* **13:**5293–5302.

34. **Moon, H. W., S. C. Whipp, R. A. Argenzio, M. M. Levine, and R. A. Giannella.** 1983. Attaching and effacing activities of rabbit and human enteropathogenic *Escherichia coli* in pig and rabbit intestines. *Infect. Immun.* **41:**1340–1351.

35. **Paulozzi, L. J., K. E. Johnson, L. M. Kamahele, C. R. Clausen, L. W. Riley, and S. D. Helgerson.** 1986. Diarrhea associated with adherent enteropathogenic *Escherichia coli* in an infant and toddler center, Seattle, Washington. *Pediatrics* **77:**296–300.

36. **Pettersson, J., R. Nordfelth, E. Dubinina, T. Bergman, M. Gustafsson, K. E. Magnusson, and H. Wolf-Watz.** 1996. Modulation of virulence factor expression by pathogen target cell contact. *Science* **273:**1231–1233.

37. **Puente, J. L., D. Bieber, S. W. Ramer, W. Murray, and G. K. Schoolnik.** 1996. The bundle-forming pili of enteropathogenic *Escherichia coli*: transcriptional regulation by environmental signals. *Mol. Microbiol.* **20:**87–100.

38. **Rosenshine, I., M. S. Donnenberg, J. B. Kaper, and B. B. Finlay.** 1992. Signal transduction between enteropathogenic *Escherichia coli* (EPEC) and epithelial cells: EPEC induces tyrosine phosphorylation of host cell proteins to initiate cytoskeletal rearrangement and bacterial uptake. *EMBO J.* **11:**3551–3560.

39. **Rosenshine, I., S. Ruschkowski, and B. B. Finlay.** 1996. Expression of attaching/effacing activity by enteropathogenic *Escherichia coli* depends on growth phase, temperature, and protein synthesis upon contact with epithelial cells. *Infect. Immun.* **64:**966–973.

40. **Rosenshine, I., S. Ruschkowski, M. Stein, D. Reinsceid, D. S. Mills, and B. B. Finlay.** 1996. A pathogenic bacterium triggers epithelial signals to form a functional bacterial receptor that mediates pseudopod formation. *EMBO J.* **15:**2613–2624.

41. **Sanger, J. M., R. Chang, F. Ashton, J. B. Kaper, and J. W. Sanger.** 1996. Novel form of actin-based motility transports bacteria on the surfaces of infected cells. *Cell Motil. Cytoskeleton* **34:**279–287.

42. **Senerwa, D., Ø. Olsvik, L. N. Mutanda, K. J. Lindqvist, J. M. Gathuma, K. Fossum, and K. Wachsmuth.** 1989. Enteropathogenic *Escherichia coli* serotype O111:HNT isolated from preterm neonates in Nairobi, Kenya. *J. Clin. Microbiol.* **27:**1307–1311.

43. **Sory, M. P., and G. R. Cornelis.** 1994. Translocation of a hybrid YopE-adenylate cyclase from *Yersinia enterocolitica* into HeLa cells. *Mol. Microbiol.* **14:**538–594.

44. **Tobe, T., G. K. Schoolnik, I. Sohel, V. H. Bustamante, and J. L. Puente.** 1996. Cloning and characterization of *bfpTVW*, genes required for the transcriptional activation of *bfpA* in enteropathogenic *Escherichia coli*. *Mol. Microbiol.* **21:**963–975.

45. **Wolff, C., I. Nisan, E. Hanski, G. Frankel, and I. Rosenshine.** 1998. Protein translocation into host epithelial cells by infecting enteropathogenic *Escherichia coli*. *Mol. Microbiol.* **28:**143–156.

46. **Zierler, M. K., and J. E. Galan.** 1995. Contact with cultured epithelial cells stimulates secretion of *Salmonella typhimurium* invasion protein InvJ. *Infect. Immun.* **63:**4024–4028.

PORE FORMATION BY ANTHRAX PROTECTIVE ANTIGEN

Ericka L. Benson, Paul D. Huynh, Alan Finkelstein, and R. John Collier

8

Many bacterial strains have evolved the ability to produce proteinaceous toxins that act either on selected eukaryotic cells (and presumably provide an advantage for survival in a eukaryotic host) or on other prokaryotes (providing a selective advantage in competing for an environmental niche). The activity of most toxins is directed at a cellular component and requires interaction in some fashion with the membrane of the target cell. This interaction may serve to elicit a transmembrane signal, form a pore in a membrane, or transport an enzymatically active moiety of the toxin across a membrane into the cytosolic interior. Medically important toxins have been most extensively studied, and the most potent among them are those that act by enzymically modifying an intracellular substrate. Currently it is not understood in detail for any toxin how the enzymic moiety crosses a membrane.

Intracellularly acting toxins are generally bipartite entities, which have been termed A-B toxins. The B moiety of these toxins is re-sponsible for binding the toxin to the target cell and, in some cases, translocating the enzymatically active A moiety across the membrane into the cytosol (11). Within the cytosol, the A moiety carries out enzymatic activity to disrupt cellular function, such as by ADP-ribosylating (and inactivating) factors involved in protein synthesis, cAMP production, or actin polymerization; by exhibiting adenylyl cyclase activity and perturbing cAMP-dependent signaling pathways; or by proteolytically inactivating proteins involved in other cellular functions (Table 1). The A and B moieties either inhabit separate domains (or combinations of domains) within a single polypeptide (e.g., diphtheria, tetanus toxins); constitute separate polypeptides within an oligomeric protein assembled prior to release from the bacteria (e.g., cholera toxin); or are separate proteins that interact and undergo self-assembly to form a toxin-like oligomer at the surface of target cells (e.g., anthrax toxin).

For some intracellularly acting toxins, membrane translocation of the A moiety depends upon insertion of the B moiety into the host membrane, forming an ion-conducting pore. X-ray crystal structures have been solved for the water-soluble forms of two pore-forming A-B toxins, diphtheria toxin and anthrax protective antigen, and also of other

Ericka L. Benson and R. John Collier, Department of Microbiology and Molecular Genetics, Harvard Medical School, Boston, MA 02115. *Paul D. Huynh and Alan Finkelstein*, Department of Physiology and Biophysics, Albert Einstein College of Medicine, Bronx, NY 10461.

Microbial Ecology and Infectious Disease, Edited by Eugene Rosenberg
©1999 American Society for Microbiology, Washington, D.C.

TABLE 1 Representative A-B toxins

Toxin	Domain organization A | B	Activity	Target	Effect	Channel
Diphtheria toxin		ADP-ribosylation	EF-2	Inhibition of protein synthesis	Y
Exotoxin A		ADP-ribosylation	EF-2	Inhibition of protein synthesis	?
Cholera toxin		ADP-ribosylation	G_s	↑cAMP	N
E. coli LT		ADP-ribosylation	G_s	↑cAMP	N
Pertussis toxin		ADP-ribosylation	G_i	↑cAMP	N
Iota toxin		ADP-ribosylation	Actin	Inhibition of actin polymerization	?
B. pertussis adenylate cyclase toxin		Adenylate cyclase	ATP	↑cAMP	Y
Botulinum toxin		Protease	VAMP, syntaxin, SNAP-25	Inhibition of neurotransmitter release	Y
Tetanus toxin		Protease	VAMP	Inhibition of neurotransmitter release	Y
Anthrax toxin		Adenylate cyclase Protease	ATP MAPKK	↑cAMP Cytokine release	Y

toxins that function simply by forming pores at the cell surface (5, 23, 24, 30, 31 , 33). In one case, the crystal structure of a pore-forming toxin has been solved in its membrane-inserted form (37). Membrane insertion by these water-soluble proteins involves conformational changes to expose or generate new surfaces that can penetrate hydrophobic membrane barriers. In the case of pore-forming A-B toxins, it is unclear whether the pore formed by the B moiety serves as a conduit for translocation or is a nonphysiological byproduct of membrane penetration.

The best-studied category of membrane-inserting toxins consists of proteins that contain a fundamentally hydrophobic interior that becomes exposed upon insertion into the membrane. Prototypes of this group are the B moiety of diphtheria toxin and channel-forming colicins, which disrupt the ionic balance of target bacterial membranes. The X-ray crystal structures of these proteins indicate similar membrane-interacting domains, consisting of three "layers" of two or more antiparallel α-helices (5, 8, 43). The two outer layers are composed of amphipathic helices oriented with polar residues facing outward and surround a middle layer of hydrophobic helices. Membrane insertion is achieved by a conformational change that exposes the hydrophobic helices, allowing them to partition into the lipid bilayer (Fig. 1A). These conformational changes are triggered by partial unfolding at the appropriate membrane surface, induced by conditions such as (in diphtheria toxin, for example) proximity to negatively charged lipids and a low pH environment such as that found in an endosomal compartment (6, 26, 35, 40).

A second group of membrane-inserting toxins contain B moieties that are devoid of significant stretches of hydrophobic sequences as judged by hydrophobicity plots and, consequently, need to assemble new hydrophobic surfaces sufficient to span the membrane. The known water-soluble structures of these toxins consist primarily of β-sheet, with very little α-helical content and no regions of significant hydrophobicity to span a membrane (23, 30, 33, 34, 37). Membrane insertion of these toxins involves an oligomerization step for effective multiplication of small regions of hydrophobicity in the monomer to create a new substantially hydrophobic membrane-spanning surface. The X-ray crystal structure of one of these toxins, the alpha-hemolysin

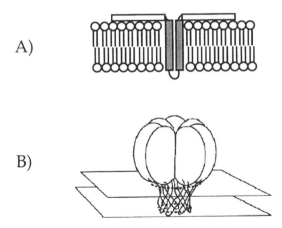

FIGURE 1 Models for membrane penetration by bacterial toxins. (A) Insertion of hydrophobic α-helices. Conditions near the membrane promote unfolding of protein that enables interior hydrophobic α-helices (shaded boxes) to enter the membrane. (B) β-Barrel–mediated insertion. The membrane-contiguous face, composed of hydrophobic residues, is assembled from numerous monomeric β segments.

from *Staphylococcus aureus*, has been solved in its membrane-inserted form (37). In this pore structure, the transmembrane motif consists of a porinlike 14-stranded β-barrel formed from seven β-hairpins (Fig. 1B). One β-hairpin is contributed by each of the protomers, and each hairpin is in turn derived from a Gly-rich amphipathic loop of the monomeric water-soluble protein. The loop contains alternating hydrophilic and hydrophobic residues. Once assembled into the membrane-penetrant β-barrel, the hydrophilic residues face the aqueous lumen of the pore, and the hydrophobic residues form the exterior, membrane-contiguous surface of the barrel. It is thought that variations on the theme of β-barrel formation will be a common mechanism of insertion of other fundamentally hydrophilic toxins (13, 22).

ANTHRAX TOXIN

We have recently focused effort on understanding the mechanism by which anthrax toxin translocates across membranes. In anthrax toxin, the A and B moieties are separate proteins that self-assemble at the mammalian cell surface to form a hetero-oligomeric complex. The B moiety, protective antigen (PA), mediates the translocation of two alternative A moieties, edema factor (EF) and lethal factor (LF), into the cytosol. Under the current model for anthrax intoxication (Fig. 2), PA first binds to a ubiquitous cell surface receptor (9) and is then cleaved by furin or a furinlike protease (16). Removal of the N-terminal 20-kDa fragment enables the remaining receptor-bound 63-kDa fragment (PA$_{63}$) to form a heptameric prepore (29) and to bind EF or LF (21). The entire complex is then trafficked to the endosome, where the low pH environment induces the PA$_{63}$ heptamer to insert and form channels within membranes and to translocate EF and LF to the cytosol (10, 12). Within the cytosol, EF functions as a calmodulin-dependent adenylate cyclase (20). LF only yields an effect within macrophages, where it induces cytokine release (15, 18). Recently, LF has been shown to function as

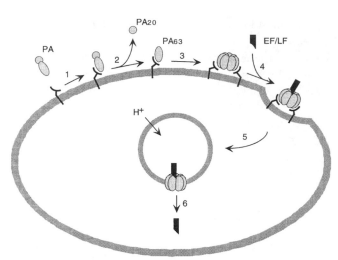

FIGURE 2 Model of anthrax toxin entry into cells. 1, Binding of PA to its receptor. 2, Proteolytic activation of PA and dissociation of PA_{20}. 3, Self-association of monomeric PA_{63} to form the heptameric prepore. 4, Binding of EF or LF to the prepore. 5, Endocytosis of the receptor: PA_{63}:ligand complex. 6, pH-dependent insertion of PA_{63} and translocation of the ligand.

a metalloprotease that is capable of cleaving MAP-kinase-kinase (7).

Under low-pH conditions, correlating with the environment in an acidic intracellular compartment, PA_{63} forms cation-selective channels within artificial or cellular membranes (3, 19, 28). Insertion of the PA_{63} heptamer into the endosomal membrane is believed to mediate translocation of EF and LF, and elucidation of the insertion mechanism is crucial for understanding the translocation process. In the hope of gaining insight into the mechanism by which PA penetrates membranes, much attention has been paid to the recent X-ray crystal structures of PA in its water-soluble monomeric (PA_{83}) and heptameric (PA_{63}) forms (Fig. 3) (33). Monomeric PA can be divided into four distinct domains. Domain 1 (residues 1–249) contains the site for proteolytic activation. Upon proteolysis and removal of the N-terminal PA_{20} fragment, the remainder of this domain (domain 1b) is stabilized by coordination of two calcium ions and may be involved in binding EF and LF. Domain 2 (residues 250–487) is the largest domain and mediates monomer-monomer contacts in the PA_{63} heptamer. The function of the smallest domain, domain 3 (residues 488–594) is unclear, but studies with monoclonal antibodies have implicated it, along

with domain 1b, in binding of EF and LF (25). Domain 4 (residues 595–735) binds to the cell surface receptor, as shown by deletion mutagenesis and monoclonal antibodies that prevent receptor binding (25, 36).

The water-soluble PA_{63} heptamer is in the form of a hollow ring with a lumen diameter of 20 to 35 Å (1 Å = 0.1 nm). The interior of this lumen is polar and negatively charged, consistent with the cation selectivity of PA_{63} channels. Domains 1′ and 2 pack against one another to form the heptamer, whereas domains 3 and 4 lie on the outside of the ring. Neither monomeric PA_{83} nor the water-soluble PA_{63} heptamer shows a region of hydrophobicity that might mediate insertion into a bilayer. For this reason, the structure of the water-soluble PA_{63} heptamer likely represents a "prepore" state.

The crystal structures of native PA and the PA_{63} prepore reveal the presence of a disordered, amphipathic loop (D2L2) that has alternating hydrophilic and hydrophobic residues reminiscent of the Gly-rich loop of the alpha-hemolysin from *S. aureus* (Fig. 4A). This loop in PA_{63}, which connects strands $2\beta2$ and $2\beta3$ within domain 2, projects outward from the side of this domain within the water-soluble heptamer (33). A significant conformational rearrangement would be

A)

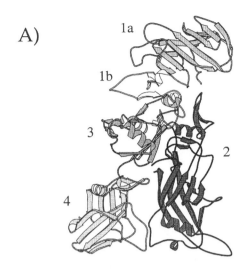

B)

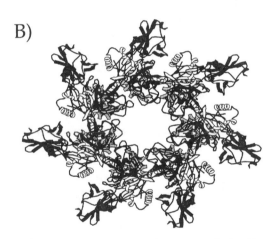

FIGURE 3 (A) X-ray crystal structure of PA$_{83}$. Domains are labeled as indicated (B) X-ray crystal structure of the PA$_{63}$ prepore, axial view. Domain 1b is indicated in black, 2 in light gray beneath domain 1b, 3 in white, and 4, protruding out from the heptamer, in dark gray.

the 24 residues of this loop. In this method, individual residues are replaced with cysteine and tested for accessibility to the positively charged bilayer-impermeant reagent methanethiosulfonate ethyltrimethylammonium (MTS-ET), which specifically reacts with water-accessible sulfhydryls. PA is ideally suited to this method, in that the native protein is devoid of cysteine. Should the cysteine of interest line the ion-conducting pathway, derivatization with MTS-ET would introduce a positive charge within the cation-selective channel and likely result in inhibition of channel conductance. Our results, described below, provide strong evidence in favor of the proposed model of membrane penetration by these loops in a β structure.

MACROSCOPIC CHANNEL EXPERIMENTS

A series of 24 mutations was generated that replaced each D2L2 residue individually with cysteine. The mutant proteins were purified to 90% homogeneity and proteolytically activated in vitro with trypsin, which cleaves PA into its 20-kDa and 63-kDa fragments. Each activated mutant was added to painted diphytanoylphosphatidylcholine planar membranes at pH 6.6. Once the current had plateaued, MTS-ET was added to the *trans* chamber (that opposite the chamber to which PA was added), and the resulting effect on macroscopic current (the collective effect of hundreds to thousands of channels within the membrane) was observed. At certain positions, an immediate and large inhibition of conductance was observed, whereas at others no inhibition was detected, even after several minutes. Figure 5 shows a typical trace of a MTS-ET-reactive mutant. Addition of 38 μM MTS-ET to channels formed by the N306C mutant inhibited macroscopic current nearly sixfold within seconds. Subsequent addition of 4 mM dithiothreitol (DTT) to these channels caused a reversal of inhibition (data not shown). At the concentrations used in these experiments, MTS-ET and DTT showed no effect on wild-type channels.

needed for this loop to participate in barrel formation, but a plausible mechanism for such a rearrangement has been proposed (Fig. 4B) (33).

To determine whether D2L2 forms a transmembrane barrel similar to that of the alpha-hemolysin, we employed the substituted-cysteine accessibility method (1) to

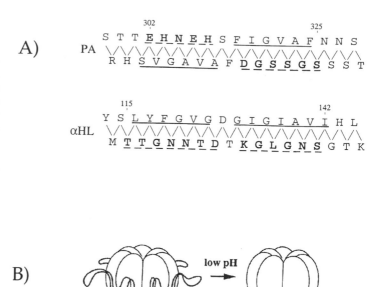

FIGURE 4 (A) Amphipathic sequences of the D2L2 loop of PA (after Petosa et al., 1997) and the Gly-rich loop of alpha-hemolysin (αHL). Residues that form the hydrophobic face of the β-barrel in alpha-hemolysin or have been proposed to form the hydrophobic face of the PA$_{63}$ pore are underscored with a solid line. Residues that form the hydrophilic face in alpha-hemolysin or have been proposed to form the hydrophilic face of the PA$_{63}$ pore are underscored with a dotted line. (B) Proposed model for pore formation by PA$_{63}$ (after Petosa et al., 1997). Following a low-pH trigger, the D2L2 loops move to the base of the heptamer and combine to form a 14-stranded transmembrane β-barrel.

Figure 6 shows the maximal inhibition of macroscopic current attained by each mutant within the first 3 min following MTS-ET addition. Within each of two stretches (E302C-A311C and I316C-S325C), alternating positions displayed an inhibition of current following the addition of MTS-ET. All hydrophilic positions within these stretches were responsive to MTS-ET, whereas all hydrophobic positions displayed little to no MTS-ET effect. The only exceptions were positions A307C and I316C, which showed a weak effect in some experiments. These stretches were bridged by a region of consecutive MTS-ET–responsive residues, from S312C to D315C. Although the absence of an MTS-ET effect does not prove that the unresponsive residues face the membrane, the pattern of MTS-ET sensitivity is consistent with the model of each D2L2 loop inserting into the membrane as two antiparallel β-strands, with alternating hydrophobic and hydrophilic amino acids facing the membrane and the ion-conducting channel, respectively. The stretch of consecutive MTS-ET–responsive residues likely represents the turn region connecting the β-strands at the far side of the membrane.

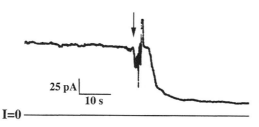

FIGURE 5 Effect of MTS-ET on N306C-induced macroscopic conductance. The current record (with the voltage held at +20 mV) begins 7 min after addition of trypsin-nicked PA N306C to a final concentration of 1.1 nM. At the arrow, MTS-ET was added *trans* to a concentration of 38 μM. After the initial artifactual increase in conductance due to the addition, the current is seen to decrease sixfold within seconds.

SINGLE-CHANNEL MEASUREMENTS

If the proposed model of channel formation is correct, single-channel measurements of MTS-ET–responsive mutants might permit one to resolve individual reactions between MTS-ET and each of the seven single cysteine residues within the heptameric pore. We have

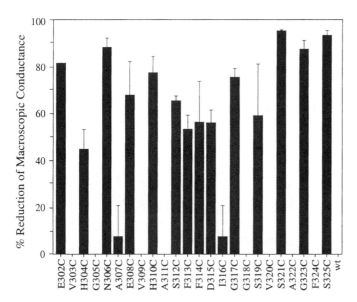

FIGURE 6 Reduction of conductance produced by *trans* MTS-ET as a function of location of Cys mutants within the D2L2 loop. Percentage reduction was calculated as $[1 - (I_{PA+MTS}/I_{PA})] \times 100$, where I_{PA} was the current immediately before MTS addition, and I_{PA+MTS} was the lowest current observed within 3 min following addition of MTS-ET. Values are reported as the mean ± standard error of 2 to 4 experiments. For A307C and I316C, MTS-ET–induced reduction in current was only seen in some experiments. Note the alternating pattern of reduction in conductance, except for the consecutive MTS-ET–responsive residues 312–315.

observed multiple MTS-ET reactions within single channels formed by N306C and H304C (the only two mutants tested). In a typical experiment, trypsin-activated mutant PA was added to a diphytanoylphosphatidylcholine membrane separating chambers of identical salt solutions (0.1 M KCl) at pH 6.6, and a single channel generally opened within 2 to 30 min. The conductance of the N306C and H304C channels was the same as that of wild-type channels (4) (~100 pS at an applied voltage of 50 mV). MTS-ET was then added to the *trans* compartment, the solutions were stirred briefly, and the effect on conductance was observed. With single N306C channels, stepwise jumps to lower conductance states were seen following addition of MTS-ET, consistent with multiple reactions within a multimeric channel (Fig. 7A). Furthermore, addition of DTT to channels of low conductance state reversed the MTS-ET effect: multiple stepwise increases in channel conductance, consistent with DTT-mediated reduction of the disulfide between the cysteines and MTS-ET, were seen until original channel conductance was regained (Fig. 7B). Similar effects were seen when MTS-ET was added to single channels formed by H304C.

We have been able to resolve at least five MTS-ET reactions per channel but do not believe this reflects the absolute number of monomers composing the channel. Each successive MTS-ET derivatization lowers conductance by introducing greater electrostatic repulsion and steric constraints within the channel, likely preventing complete channel derivatization within the duration of a normal single-channel experiment. Nonetheless, the observation of multiple-step conductance changes upon addition of MTS-ET to these single channels implies that the channel has an oligomeric structure.

CONCLUSION

We have identified the channel-lining residues of PA_{63} by observing the response to MTS-ET of channels containing cysteine substitutions within D2L2. The pattern of MTS-ET inhibition supports the model of insertion of each D2L2 as an antiparallel β-hairpin, with alternating hydrophobic and hydrophilic residues lining the membrane and aqueous pore, respectively (Fig. 8). Single-channel experiments showing multiple stepwise conductance changes following addition of MTS-ET confirm that the PA_{63} channel is oligomeric. Put

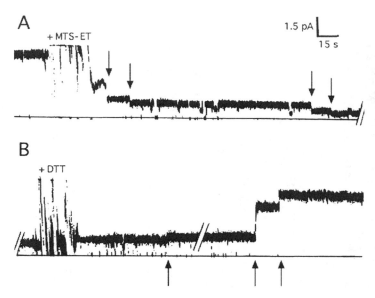

FIGURE 7 (A) Effect of MTS-ET on conductance of a single N306C channel. The trace begins after a single channel has opened with a conductance of 90 pS (at a holding potential of +50 mV). MTS-ET was then added to a concentration of 8 μM *trans*, and the current record was briefly obscured during stirring. One or more reactions occurred during stirring, since after the stirring was stopped, the conductance of the channel was about half that before MTS-ET addition. The arrows indicate stepwise decreases in single-channel conductance consistent with the reaction of MTS-ET with cysteines within the channel. (B) DTT reverses the MTS-ET effect. The trace begins 5 min after the final MTS-ET reaction was observed in panel A. DTT was added *trans* to a concentration of 1.2 mM, and the single-channel conductance immediately increased during stirring. The arrows indicate further stepwise increases in single-channel conductance, consistent with reduction of the mixed disulfides formed upon reaction of the cysteines with MTS-ET. At higher time resolution, the transition at the second arrow appears to be composed of 2 to 4 stepwise increases in conductance. (The last break in the record is 90 s.)

together, these results support the model of pore formation of PA_{63} as a transmembrane β-barrel formed from β-hairpins contributed by each PA_{63} protomer.

UNRESOLVED QUESTIONS AND FUTURE RESEARCH

Anthrax Toxin

Two major questions arise from the identification of D2L2 as the channel-forming motif of anthrax protective antigen: how can the D2L2 loops assemble into the transmembrane β-barrel, and what is the role of this channel in translocation of EF and LF? The orientation of the D2L2 strands within the water-soluble prepore poses a geometrical obstacle to their insertion into the membrane. Within the X-ray crystal structure of the PA63 prepore, the D2L2 loops are located midway up the surface of the globular domains, removed from the membrane surface. For the D2L2 loops to reach the membrane, a significant conformational change must take place, and this change will likely necessitate unfolding of the β-strands connecting D2L2 to the ordered globular domains. At low pH, the titration of

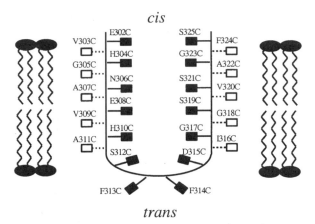

FIGURE 8 Model for the orientation of D2L2 within the membrane. The filled boxes indicate residues that are responsive to MTS-ET, on the basis of reduction of channel conductance. The open boxes indicate residues that show little or no effect upon MTS-ET addition. The pattern is consistent with each D2L2 contributing two antiparallel β-strands to make a 14-stranded β-barrel.

histidines in the vicinity of D2L2 may induce the necessary conformational change. Future experiments will investigate the role of the nearby histidines in pore formation. Future experiments will also extend electrophysiology experiments upon residues within the β-strands connecting D2L2, to define further the pore surface farther *cis* and to define the topology of the surface linking the β-barrel to the remainder of the globular domains.

The mechanism of membrane traversal is not well understood for any intracellularly acting toxin. For those that form pores, the actual pores may function as aqueous conduits for translocation or may instead form as byproducts of an insertion event that initiates translocation via another route. Translocation along any route presumably requires some degree of unfolding of the translocating moiety, either to enable it to fit through an aqueous pore or to expose hydrophobic regions that would contact the lipid upon membrane traversal. The dimensions of the anthrax toxin pore, determined experimentally through permeation studies (12 Å) (4) or estimated structurally from a structural model of the β-barrel pore (15 Å) (C. Petosa, personal communication), could accommodate translocation of an α-helix (10 to 12 Å anhydrous diameter) or an unfolded polypeptide (14). Assuming the conformation of the globular heptamer remains similar following pore formation, the narrowest diameter of the globular pore lumen (20 Å) would not pose additional restrictions upon translocation (33). On the other hand, EF and LF have been shown to insert into membranes at low pH even in the absence of PA (17). Thus, translocation conceivably may not require passage through an aqueous pore, but may proceed directly through the lipid or in contact with the lipid along a hydrophilic cleft formed by PA_{63}.

Although the involvement of the PA_{63} channel in translocation remains unclear, the identification of channel-lining residues may allow the design of future experiments to probe the role of the channel in the translocation process. For instance, by derivatizing channel-lining residues with bulky groups and blocking conductance from the interior of the channel, one may be able to ascertain whether or not channel conductance is required for the translocation event. Additionally, the isolation of intermediates in anthrax toxin translocation may facilitate fluorescence and cross-linking experiments that could identify the pathway traveled by the translocating moiety. In particular, placing cross-linking or fluorescent probes on residues lining the interior or exterior of the channel may differentiate, via cross-linking or transfer of fluorescence energy, whether or not derivatized residues on the translocating chain pass nearby the PA_{63} residue of interest. It has been shown that the existence of disulfide bonds within the translocating moiety or binding of a high-affinity inhibitor to induce tight folding of the translocation moiety prevents translocation in the anthrax toxin system (J. Wesche, J. Elliott, P. Falnes, S. Olsnes, and R. J. Collier, unpublished results). These species may represent translocation intermediates, and further experimentation will be needed to determine their utility in delineating the path of translocation.

Other Pore-Foming Toxins

Assembly of transmembrane β-barrels may serve as a common mechanism of membrane penetration by bacterial toxins. For instance, features of the water-soluble X-ray crystal structures of three other toxins suggest that membrane insertion will involve β structures. One is the pore-forming toxin aerolysin from *Aeromonas hydrophila*. This toxin of primarily β structure is secreted as a dimer that is activated by proteolysis to form a heptameric membrane-inserted pore (39, 41, 44). Formation of the stable heptamer has been shown to precede insertion into the membrane (38). The X-ray crystal structure of the pro-aerolysin dimer has been combined with low-resolution reconstructions of the channel to create a model of the membrane-inserted form in which the channel is composed of a β-barrel (30). As with PA_{63} and alpha-hemolysin, only a small part of each monomer would penetrate the membrane.

Another toxin, δ-endotoxin CytB from *Bacillus thuringiensis*, kills insects by forming a pore in the plasma membrane of midgut cells. This toxin is also secreted as a dimer in solution, and evidence supports the formation of an oligomeric channel within membranes (22, 27). The X-ray crystal structure of the water-soluble monomer shows that two layers of helical hairpins wrap around a five-stranded β-sheet (23). The orientation of these helical hairpins is such that they are able to move relative to the sheet without unraveling it. The three inner β-strands are 36 Å long, and their amphipathic nature has led to a model of transmembrane structure in which three strands from each protomer combine to form a β-barrel of 12 to 18 strands.

Finally, the water-soluble X-ray crystal structure of the thiol-activated cytolysin perfringolysin O (PFO) from *Clostridium perfringens* reveals a primarily β structure thought to undergo a novel means of membrane penetration (34). This toxin forms large multimeric pores (>150 Å) within membranes. A hydrophobic dagger within domain 4 has been proposed to initiate membrane insertion. The receptor, cholesterol, would then shield one face of the domain, while the opposite face is thought to form a continuous β-sheet with the same domain on other monomers. Proof for these models of membrane insertion awaits further biochemical and structural evidence.

Sequence homologies suggest that the family of β-barrel–inserting toxins may be even larger. The alpha-toxin from *Clostridium septicum* displays significant homologies to aerolysin and is also presumed to form a membrane-inserted β-barrel (2). Both VIP1 from *B. thuringiensis* and iota 1b from *C. perfringens* display significant homologies to PA and, in particular, contain two stretches of amphipathic residues similar to that of the D2L2 loop (32, 33, 42). In addition, protein subunits that make up the oligomeric pore-forming gamma-hemolysin and leukocidin F toxins of *S. aureus* display regions of homology to alpha-hemolysin (13). Besides homologies within internal regions suggesting similar folding organization, these subunits also contain Gly-rich regions that correspond to the Gly-rich, membrane-spanning regions of alpha-hemolysin, suggesting these homologs may also be capable of forming transmembrane β-barrel pores.

ACKNOWLEDGMENTS

We thank Can Cui for establishing PA cloning conditions, Jianmin Zhao for construction and purification of the H304C and G305C mutants, and Carlo Petosa and Bob Liddington for their work in solving the X-ray crystal structures of PA and PA63. Figures 1 and 4–8 are reprinted from *Biochemistry* (Benson et al., 1998), and Figure 3 is reprinted from *Nature* (Petosa et al., 1997), with permission.

REVIEWS AND KEY PAPERS

Benson, E. L., P. D. Huynh, A. Finkelstein, and R. J. Collier. 1998. Identification of residues lining the anthrax protective antigen channel. *Biochemistry* **37:**3941–3948.

Lesieur, C., B. Vescey-Semjen, L. Abrami, M. Fivaz, and F. G. van der Goot. 1997. Membrane insertion: the strategies of toxins. *Mol. Membr. Biol.* **14:**45–64.

Petosa, C., R. J. Collier, K. R. Klimpel, S. H. Leppla, and R. C. Liddington. 1997. Crystal structure of the anthrax toxin protective antigen. *Nature* **385:**833–838.

Song, L., M. R. Hobaugh, C. Shustak, S. Cheley, H. Bayley, and J. E. Gouaux. 1996. Structure of staphylococcal alpha-hemolysin, a heptameric transmembrane pore. *Science* **274:**1859–1866.

REFERENCES

1. **Akabas, M. H., D. A. Stauffer, M. Xu, and A. Karlin.** 1992. Acetycholine receptor channel structure probed in cysteine-substitution mutants. *Science* **258:**307–310.
2. **Ballard, J., J. Crabtree, B. A. Roe, and R. K. Tweten.** 1995. The primary structure of *Clostridium septicum* alpha-toxin exhibits similarity with that of *Aeromonas hydrophila* aerolysin. *Infect. Immun.* **63:**340–344.
3. **Blaustein, R. O., T. M. Koehler, R. J. Collier, and A. Finkelstein.** 1989. Anthrax toxin: channel-forming activity of protective antigen in planar phospholipid bilayers. *Proc. Natl. Acad. Sci. USA* **86:**2209–2213.
4. **Blaustein, R. O., E. J. Lea, and A. Finkelstein.** 1990. Voltage-dependent block of anthrax toxin channels in planar phospholipid bilayer membranes by symmetric tetraalkylammonium ions. Single-channel analysis. *J. Gen. Physiol.* **96:**921–942.
5. **Choe, S., M. J. Bennett, G. Fujii, P. M. Curmi, K. A. Kantardjieff, R. J. Collier, and D. Eisenberg.** 1992. The crystal structure of diphtheria toxin. *Nature* **357:**216–222.
6. **Cramer, W. A., Y. L. Zhang, S. Schendell, A. R. Merrill, H. Y. Song, C. V. Stauffacher, and F. S. Cohen.** 1992. Dynamic properties of the colicin E1 ion channel. *FEMS Microbiol. Immunol.* **5:**71–81.
7. **Duesbery, N. S., C. P. Webb, S. H. Leppla, V. M. Gordon, K. R. Klimpel, T. D. Copeland, N. G. Ahn, M. K. Oskarsson, K. Fukasawa, K. D. Paull, and G. F. Van de Woude.** 1998. Proteolytic inactivation of MAP-kinase-kinase by anthrax lethal factor. *Science* **280:**734–737.

8. **Elkins, P., A. Bunker, W. A. Cramer, and C. V. Stauffacher.** 1997. The crystal of the channel-forming domain of colicin E1. *Structure* **5:**443–458.
9. **Escuyer, V., and R. J. Collier.** 1991. Anthrax protective antigen interacts with a specific receptor on the surface of CHO-K1 cells. *Infect. Immun.* **59:**3381–3386.
10. **Friedlander, A. M.** 1986. Macrophages are sensitive to anthrax lethal toxin through an acid-dependent process. *J. Biol. Chem.* **261:**7123–7126.
11. **Gill, D. M.** 1978. Seven toxic peptides that cross cell membranes. *In* J. Jeljaszewicz and T. Wadstrom (ed.) *Bacterial Toxins and Cell Membranes*, p. 291–322. Academic Press, New York.
12. **Gordon, V. M., S. H. Leppla, and E. L. Hewlett.** 1988. Inhibitors of receptor-mediated endocytosis block the entry of *Bacillus anthracis* adenylate cyclase toxin but not that of *Bordetella pertussis* adenylate cyclase toxin. *Infect. Immun.* **56:**1066–1069.
13. **Gouaux, E., M. Hobaugh, and L. Song.** 1997. α-hemolysin, γ-hemolysin, and leukocidin from *Staphylococcus aureus*. Distant in sequence but similar in structure. *Protein Sci.* **6:**2631–2635.
14. **Hamman, B. D., J.-C. Chen, E. E. Johnson, and A. E. Johnson.** 1997. The aqueous pore through the translocon has a diameter of 40–60 Å during cotranslational protein translocation at the ER membrane. *Cell* **89:**535–544.
15. **Hanna, P. C., D. Acosta, and R. J. Collier.** 1993. On the role of macrophages in anthrax. *Proc. Natl. Acad. Sci. USA* **90:**10198–10201.
16. **Klimpel, K. R., S. S. Molloy, G. Thomas, and S. H. Leppla.** 1992. Anthrax toxin protective antigen is activated by a cell surface protease with the sequence specificity and catalytic properties of furin. *Proc. Natl. Acad. Sci. USA* **89:**10277–10281.
17. **Kochi, S. K., I. Martin, G. Schiavo, M. Mock, and V. Cabiaux.** 1994. The effects of pH on the interaction of anthrax toxin lethal and edema factors with phospholipid vesicles. *Biochemistry* **33:**2604–2609.
18. **Kochi, S. K., G. Schiavo, M. Mock, and C. Montecucco.** 1994. Zinc content of the *Bacillus anthracis* lethal factor. *FEMS Microbiol. Lett.* **124:**343–348.
19. **Koehler, T. M., and R. J. Collier.** 1991. Anthrax toxin protective antigen: low-pH-induced hydrophobicity and channel formation in liposomes. *Mol. Microbiol.* **5:**1501–1506.
20. **Leppla, S. H.** 1982. Anthrax toxin edema factor: a bacterial adenylate cyclase that increases cyclic AMP concentrations of eukaryotic cells. *Proc. Natl. Acad. Sci. USA* **79:**3162–3166.

21. Leppla, S. H., A. M. Friedlander, and E. M. Cora. 1988. Proteolytic activation of anthrax toxin bound to cellular receptors. *In* F. J. Ferenbach, J. E. Alouf, W. Goebel, J. Jeljaszewicz, D. Jurgen, and R. Rappouli (ed.) *Bacterial Protein Toxins.* Gustav Fischer, Stuttgart.

22. Lesieur, C., B. Vescey-Semjen, L. Abrami, M. Fivaz, and F. G. van der Goot. 1997. Membrane insertion: the strategies of toxins. *Mol. Membr. Biol.* **14**:45–64.

23. Li, J., P. A. Koni, and D. J. Ellar. 1996. Structure of the mosquitocidal d-endotoxin CytB from *Bacillus thuringiensis sp. kyushuensis* and implications for membrane pore formation. *J. Mol. Biol.* **257**:129–152.

24. Li, J. D., J. Carroll, and D. J. Ellar. 1991. Crystal structure of insecticidal delta-endotoxin from *Bacillus thuringiensis* at 2.5 Å resolution. *Nature* **353**:815–-821.

25. Little, S. F., J. M. Novak, J. R. Lowe, S. H. Leppla, Y. Singh, K. R. Klimpel, B. C. Lidgerding, and A. M. Friedlander. 1996. Characterization of lethal factor binding and cell receptor binding domains of protective antigen of *Bacillus anthracis* using monoclonal antibodies. *Microbiology* **142**:707–715.

26. London, E. 1992. Diphtheria toxin: membrane interaction and membrane translocation. *Biochim. Biophys. Acta* **1113**:25–51.

27. Maddrell, S. H., N. J. Lane, J. B. Harrison, J. A. Overton, and R. B. Moreton. 1988. The initial stages in the action of an insecticidal delta endotoxin of *Bacillus thuringiensis var. israelensis* on the epithelial cells of the malphigian tubules of the insect *Rhodnius prolixus. J. Cell. Sci.* **90**:131–144.

28. Milne, J. C., and R. J. Collier. 1993. pH-dependent permeabilization of the plasma membrane of mammalian cells by anthrax protective antigen. *Mol. Microbiol.* **10**:647–653.

29. Milne, J. C., D. Furlong, P. C. Hanna, J. S. Wall, and R. J. Collier. 1994. Anthrax protective antigen forms oligomers during intoxication of mammalian cells. *J. Biol. Chem.* **269**:20607–20612.

30. Parker, M. W., J. T. Buckley, J. P. Postma, A. D. Tucker, K. Leonard, F. Pattus, and D. Tsernoglou. 1994. Structure of the *Aeromonas* toxin proaerolysin in its water-soluble and membrane-channel states. *Nature* **367**:292–295.

31. Parker, M. W., F. Pattus, A. D. Tucker, and D. Tsernoglou. 1989. Structure of the membrane-pore-forming fragment of colicin A. *Nature* **337**:93–96.

32. Perelle, S., M. Gibert, P. Boquet, and M. R. Popoff. 1993. Characterization of *Clostridium perfringens* iota-toxin genes and expression in *Escherichia coli. Infect. Immun.* **61**:5147–5156.

33. Petosa, C., R. J. Collier, K. R. Klimpel, S. H. Leppla, and R. C. Liddington. 1997. Crystal structure of the anthrax toxin protective antigen. *Nature* **385**:833–838.

34. Rossjohn, J., S. C. Feil, W. J. McKinstry, R. K. Tweten, and M. W. Parker. 1997. Structure of a cholesterol-binding, thiol-activated cytolysin and a model of its membrane form. *Cell* **89**:685–692.

35. Schendel, S. L., and W. A. Cramer. 1994. On the nature of the unfolded intermediate in the *in vitro* transition of the colicin E1 channel domain from the aqueous to the membrane phase. *Protein Sci* **3**:2272–2279.

36. Singh, Y., K. R. Klimpel, C. P. Quinn, V. K. Chaudhary, and S. H. Leppla. 1991. The carboxyl-terminal end of protective antigen is required for receptor binding and anthrax toxin activity. *J. Biol. Chem.* **266**:15493–15497.

37. Song, L., M. R. Hobaugh, C. Shustak, S. Cheley, H. Bayley, and J. E. Gouaux. 1996. Structure of staphylococcal alpha-hemolysin, a heptameric transmembrane pore. *Science* **274**: 1859–1866.

38. van der Goot, F. G., J. Ausio, K. R. Wong, F. Pattus, and J. T. Buckley. 1993. Dimerization stabilizes the pore-forming toxin aerolysin in solution. *J. Biol. Chem.* **268**:18272–18279.

39. van der Goot, F. G., J. Lakey, F. Pattus, C. M. Kay, O. Sorokine, A. Van Dorsselaer, and J. T. Buckley. 1992. Spectroscopic study of the activation and oligomerization of the channel-forming toxin aerolysin: identification of the site of proteolytic activation. *Biochemistry* **31**: 8566–8570.

40. van der Goot, F. G., F. Pattus, K. Wong, and J. T. Buckley. 1993. Oligomerization of the channel-forming toxin aerolysin precedes insertion into lipid bilayers. *Biochemistry* **32**:2636–2642.

41. van der Goot, G., J. M. Gonzalez-Manas, J. H. Lakey, and F. Pattus. 1991. A "molten-globule" membrane-insertion intermediate of the pore-forming domain of colicin A. *Nature* **354**: 408–410.

42. Warren, G., et al. 1996. Novel pesticidal proteins and strains. Patent application WO 96/10083. World Intellectual Property Organization.

43. Wiener, M., D. Freymann, P. Ghosh, and R. M. Stroud. 1997. Crystal structure of colicin 1a. *Nature* **385**:461–464.

44. Wilmsen, H. U., K. R. Leonard, W. Tichelaar, and J. T. Buckley. 1992. The aerolysin membrane channel is formed by heptamerization of the monomer. *EMBO J.* **11**:2457–2463.

ENVIRONMENTAL SIGNALS CONTROLLING GENE EXPRESSION

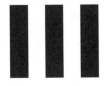

INTRODUCTION

David L. Gutnick

One of the major challenges to microbial populations in nature involves coping with drastic and often stressful changes in environmental conditions. To accomplish this, microbes have evolved a wide variety of functional and genetic strategies including sophisticated communication networks and regulatory systems at both cellular and intercellular levels. The versatility of the adaptation process clearly requires that the organisms maintain systems for sensing environmental signals and for transducing these signals into responses that may affect either the behavior of the individual cell or the population as a whole. Here we consider a number of genetic systems whose expression is affected by the sensing and transducing of various environmental signals. Microbial luminescence, the first model to be considered, represents a fascinating case of cell density-dependent gene expression regulated by a specific inducer from the class of homoserine lactone molecules. Derivatives of homoserine lactones enable the microbes to monitor their own population density, a process appropriately termed quorum sensing. Once induced, the actual luminescence system responds at the level of the individual cell to a variety of host factors, both specific, as well as global. The integration of such global processes forms the basis of the second presentation on luminescence. A third environmental signal is involved in controlling the response of the cell to oxygen stress induced by a variety of environmental insults such as chlorine pollution. In this presentation, the luminescence system is used primarily as a simple, quantitative, and sensitive gene reporter system for characterizing environmentally sensitive promoters whose expression reflects the presence of specific pollutants in the environment. Finally, one of the best-studied global responses in microbial physiology, the heat-shock response, is considered. This response leads to the induction of novel sigma factors governing the transcription initiation of specific regulons. Not only is the stress response system considered, but also its evolution and some unique aspects related to specific mRNA processing in organisms such as *Agrobacterium tumifaciens*. The models presented here are far from comprehensive, but they do serve to illustrate the versatility and efficiency with which microbes adapt genetically to adverse conditions of environmental stress.

David L. Gutnick, Department of Molecular Microbiology and Biotechnology, George S. Wise Faculty of Life Sciences, Tel Aviv University, Ramat Aviv 69978, Israel.

QUORUM SENSING IN GRAM-NEGATIVE BACTERIA: AN IMPORTANT SIGNALING MECHANISM IN SYMBIOSIS AND DISEASE

E. Peter Greenberg

9

This article represents an overview of the rapidly developing area of acylhomoserine lactone signaling and cell density-dependent control of gene expression in gram-negative bacteria. As is discussed, this type of bacterial cell-to-cell communication was first discovered in the context of microbial ecology, but it is now evident not only that acylhomoserine lactone signaling is relevant in plant and animal (including human) diseases, but the signaling pathway is an enticing target for the development of antivirulence therapies. Although it is not covered in this chapter, it has also become clear that bacterial cell-to-cell signaling and cell density-dependent gene expression is not always mediated by acylhomoserine lactones, and other signaling systems, while perhaps not as well understood at the mechanistic level, are important in the disease process. For example, recent evidence indicates that a novel cell-to-cell communication system is relevant to the pathogenesis of *Staphylococcus aureus* (2). It has become clear that the ability to communicate with one another and to organize into communal groups with char-

acteristics not exhibited by individual cells is prevalent in the bacterial world. Acylhomoserine lactone signaling is perhaps the best-studied communication mechanism, but even with this type of signaling, many important questions remain to be answered. It seems critically important that this emerging area of microbial cell-to-cell signaling continue its rapid expansion as a scientific endeavor.

OVERVIEW OF QUORUM SENSING IN GRAM-NEGATIVE BACTERIA

Over the past several years there has been an increasing appreciation among microbiologists that bacteria can perceive other bacteria and respond in some fashion. This capability is often important in the colonization of animal and plant hosts by symbiotic or pathogenic bacterial species. Although different bacterial groups have different mechanisms for monitoring their own abundance in a local environment, one mechanism that has emerged as common in many gram-negative bacteria is acylhomoserine lactone-mediated quorum sensing (for recent reviews see references 15 and 18).

The basic framework for quorum sensing was established in the early 1970s by Nealson et al. (35). They showed that the marine luminescent bacteria *Vibrio fischeri* and *Vibrio*

E. Peter Greenberg, Department of Microbiology, University of Iowa, Iowa City, Iowa 52242-1109.

Microbial Ecology and Infectious Disease, Edited by Eugene Rosenberg
©1999 American Society for Microbiology, Washington, D.C.

harveyi produce diffusible compounds, termed autoinducers, that accumulate in the medium during growth. These autoinducer signals can accumulate to sufficient concentrations only when there is a critical mass of cells in a confined environment. The signals from *V. fischeri* and *V. harveyi* do not cross-react. Thus, there is species specificity. *V. fischeri* is a specific symbiont in light organs of certain fish where it is found at very high density (10^{10} to 10^{11} cells/ml), and it also can be found free in seawater where it occurs at much lower densities (perhaps 5 cells/ml). Thus the autoinducer system allows *V. fischeri* to sense its presence in the light organ and express the luminescence system there, where it is required for the symbiosis, but not in seawater where luminescence, which is energetically expensive, would be frivolous.

This concept that bacteria produce pheromones and communicate with one another was not readily accepted by the scientific community in the 1970s. Evidence in favor of autoinduction began to build in the late 1970s and early 1980s, first with a careful chemostat study confirming that luminescence required high cell density (45). Next, the structure of the autoinducer signal was solved, *N*-3-(oxohexanoyl)homoserine lactone (13). This molecule was shown to move out of and into cells by passive diffusion (29). The genes for luminescence were cloned from *V. fischeri* into *Escherichia coli* (14). Fortunately, the genes for autoinduction are linked to the luminescence structural genes, and *E. coli* cells containing this *lux* gene cluster produce light in a cell density-dependent fashion (Fig. 1). Thus, quorum sensing could now be analyzed with the tools of *E. coli* genetics.

The regulatory region that enables autoinduction of luminescence consists of two genes, *luxR*, which encodes an autoinducer-responsive transcriptional activator, and *luxI*, which encodes a protein required for autoinducer synthesis (14). The region between *luxR* and *luxI* contains the regulated *lux* promoter elements. Of note, *luxI* is positively autoregulated so that basal levels of luminescence

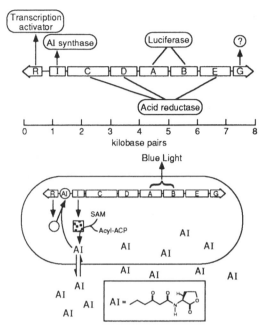

FIGURE 1   Quorum sensing in *Vibrio fischeri*. (Top) The *lux* gene cluster. The *luxR* gene encodes an autoinducer-dependent transcriptional activator of the *luxI-G* operon. The *luxI* product is the autoinducer synthase; *luxC, D,* and *E* form a complex responsible for generation of one of the substrates for the luciferase reaction, the long chain fatty aldehyde; *luxA* and *B* encode the two subunits of luciferase; and the function of *luxG* remains unknown. (Bottom) Cartoon of a *V. fischeri* cell producing the diffusible autoinducer signal. At low cell densities, the luminescence operon is transcribed at a basal level. At high cell densities, the autoinducer signal can reach a sufficient concentration and bind to the cellular LuxR protein, which will then activate transcription of the luminescence operon.

operon transcription lead to low rates of autoinducer production and quite high cell densities are necessary for activation of the luminescence genes. Once activation has occurred, the rate of autoinducer synthesis is more rapid, and the cell density must drop considerably before the rate of transcription of the luminescence operon returns to the basal level. Also, not surprisingly, autoinduction is just one of the regulatory systems that comes to bear on luminescence gene expression: *luxR* requires activation by cAMP and the cAMP receptor protein (12); iron can influence expression of luminescence (11, 27); FNR seems to exert an effect on *luxR* (28); and there appear to be other cellular regulatory elements that may exert effects on expression of the luminescence genes of *V. fischeri* (34).

As mentioned above, the *V. fischeri* autoinducer is free to diffuse out of and into cells. Thus the cellular concentration and the environmental concentration of this signal are equivalent (29). For this reason, the transcriptional activator, LuxR, which is located on the cytoplasmic side of the cell membrane (30), can respond to the environmental concentration of the autoinducer. The environmental concentration of the autoinducer increases with *V. fischeri* cell density (11).

A considerable amount is now known about LuxR and the regulatory DNA with which it interacts to activate expression of the luminescence operon (for a recent review see reference 48). LuxR is a 250-amino-acid polypeptide that consists of two domains and functions as a homomultimer (5–7, 24), likely a dimer, with σ^{70} RNA polymerase to activate *lux* gene expression (49, 50). It is a member of the LuxR superfamily of transcription factors, all of which contain somewhat similar H-T-H motifs in their DNA-binding regions (17). This family includes true LuxR homologs (see below) and also, MalT, GerE, NarL, and others. The N-terminal 160 amino acids or so constitute an autoinducer-binding, regulatory domain, which in the absence of sufficient autoinducer interferes with the C-terminal domain, the last 90 or so amino acids; binds to RNA polymerase, and the *lux* regulatory DNA; and activates transcription of the luminescence operon (Fig. 2). There is a 20-bp inverted repeat at about −40 from the start of transcription of the luminescence operon (Fig. 2), and this genetic element is required for autoinduction of luminescence (9). In vitro studies of LuxR have been difficult and slow, but such studies seem to indicate that LuxR and σ70-RNA polymerase are the only transcription factors required for activa-

tion of the *luxI* promoter and that these two factors bind synergistically to the promoter region (49, 50). Many autoinducer analogs with alterations in the acyl side chain can bind to LuxR, and some can serve weakly as autoinducers; it is perhaps more important to note that many can inhibit the activity of the natural autoinducer, presumably by competition for the autoinducer binding site (46).

More recently, we have begun to understand the mechanism by which the *luxI* gene directs the synthesis of the autoinducer signal (25, 26, 47). We now know that LuxI and LuxI homologs are autoinducer synthases that catalyze the formation of an amide bond between two substrates, a 6-carbon fatty acyl-ACP and *S*-adenosylmethionine (Fig. 3). Although it has been suggested that the acyl group forms a covalent bond with an active-site cysteine in LuxI, recent studies of cysteine substitution mutants indicate that this is not the case (26). Through studies of LuxI mutants and mutant forms of a related protein from *Pseudomonas aeruginosa*, RhlI (38), we have developed a view of the protein that indicates that the active site in which amide bond formation is catalyzed is roughly in the region of residues 25 to 104, and a region in the C terminus may be involved in selection of the appropriate acyl-ACP from those existing in the cellular pools (Fig. 3).

DISCOVERY OF LuxR-LuxI–TYPE QUORUM-SENSING SYSTEMS IN OTHER BACTERIA

Within the last 10 years, several groups made key discoveries that led to our current view that quorum sensing is common to many gram-negative bacterial species. First, LuxR homologs were discovered in *P. aeruginosa* (19) and *Agrobacterium tumefaciens* (41), and several bacterial species were shown to produce *N*-3-(oxohexanoyl)homoserine lactone (1). Then it was found that the *A. tumefaciens* and *P. aeruginosa* autoinducers are analogs of the *V. fischeri* autoinducer. For *A. tumefaciens*, the autoinducer is *N*-3-(oxooctanoyl) homoserine lactone (55), and *P. aeruginosa* has

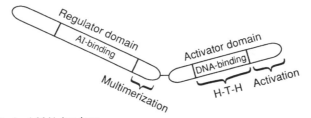

V. fischeri MJ1 lux box   A C C T G T A G G A T C G T A C A G G T
lux box-like consensus sequence   R N S T G V A X G A T N X T R C A S R T

FIGURE 2 Elements of autoinducible *lux* gene expression. (Top) Key regions of LuxR, the activator of luminescence gene transcription. The polypeptide consists of two domains. There is a C-terminal helix-turn-helix (H-T-H)-containing activator domain extending from about residue 160 to the C-terminal residue, 250. This domain interacts with the transcription initiation complex. The region from residue 230 to 250 is thought to be required for transcriptional activation but not for DNA binding. An N-terminal regulatory domain extends to about residue 160. A region of this domain is involved with autoinducer binding, residues 79 to 127, and a region is involved in multimer formation, about 120 to 160. In the absence of autoinducer, the regulatory domain interferes with activity of the activator domain. (Bottom) The *lux* box from *V. fischeri* strain MJ1 and a consensus sequence for *lux* box-like elements found in promoter regions of acylhomoserine-regulated genes from other bacterial species. The 20-bp *lux* box is centered at about −40 from the start of *luxI* transcription. Consensus sequence abbreviations: N, A, T, C, or G; R, A or G; S, C or G; Y, T or C; X, N or a gap in the sequence.

at least two quorum-sensing systems, one that uses *N*-3-(oxododecanoyl)homoserine lactone (39) and one that uses *N*-butyrylhomoserine lactone (32, 36, 37, 40, 54). The genes responsible for autoinducer production were sequenced, and their products are homologous to LuxI. Thus, the two systems have been termed *lasI-lasR* and *rhlI-rhlR*.

There are now over 15 LuxI homologs and 15 LuxR homologs in the protein sequence data bases. Furthermore, *lux* box-like sequences can be found in the promoter regions of many of the genes regulated by LuxR homologs in bacteria other than *V. fischeri*. The LuxI homologs direct the synthesis of acylhomoserine lactones with saturated or unsaturated acyl chains of 4 to 14 carbons, with either a hydroxyl group, a carbonyl group, or a hydrogen on the third carbon from the amide bond. The constant is the homoserine lactone; the acyl group provides signal specificity. Different LuxI homologs produce different

autoinducers, and the cognate LuxR homologs respond best to the appropriate autoinducer (for example see reference 46). Table 1 provides a partial list of bacteria known to produce acylhomoserine lactones.

What does autoinduction control in different bacteria? As discussed, *V. fischeri* uses quorum sensing to regulate transcription of the luminescence genes so that they are expressed in the light organ symbiosis. *A. tumefaciens* controls conjugal transfer genes by quorum sensing (16, 41). This is thought to ensure that this bacterial species possesses its catabolic Ti plasmid when present at high density in a crown gall tumor. *P. aeruginosa* is an opportunistic human pathogen, and quorum sensing is used to regulate expression of a battery of extracellular virulence genes including enzymes and exotoxins (for a recent review see reference 15). Autoinduction of extracellular enzymes is a common theme. One can envision that at low density, production of extra-

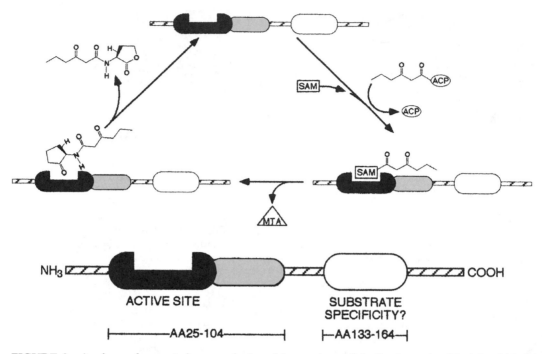

NH₃ ████ ACTIVE SITE ████ SUBSTRATE SPECIFICITY? ████ COOH

ACTIVE SITE

├────────AA25-104────────┤ ├─AA133-164─┤

FIGURE 3 A scheme for autoinducer synthesis and key regions of the LuxI protein. (Top) LuxI binds an acyl-ACP and SAM. The acyl group is transferred from the bound ACP, forming an amide bond with the SAM. Acyl-SAM is converted to acylhomoserine lactone with release of 5′-methylthioadenosine (MTA) and release of the acylhomoserine lactone. (Bottom) LuxI is 193 amino acids in length. A region extending from about residue 25 to somewhere between residue 70 and 104 appears to represent the active site for amide bond formation. There is limited evidence to suggest that a region between residue 133 and 164 is involved in selection of the appropriate acyl-ACP from the cellular pools.

cellular enzymes would be of no value. The enzymes would diffuse away from the cell, convert relatively little substrate to product, and because the environmental concentration of the product would not change appreciably, the bacterial cells would not benefit. When the bacteria have achieved a high enough density, production of an extracellular enzyme could have an impact on the environment. What about exotoxins? Here the analogy is to an invading army. The bacterial pathogen first masses the troops, but it does not reveal its weapons until they can be deployed in sufficient quantity to overwhelm the opposition. By not producing exotoxins at low cell densities and waiting until the host defenses can be overwhelmed, *P. aeruginosa* deprives the host of the chance to respond immunologi-

cally. In fact, *P. aeruginosa* quorum-sensing mutants are capable of initial colonization in a mouse lung model, but the progression of the disease is impaired, and unlike infection with wild type, infection with the quorum-sensing mutants does not lead to death (52). Another easily understood example of LuxR–LuxI-type quorum sensing is control, not only of extracellular enzymes in *Erwinia carotovora,* but also of carbepenem antibiotic synthesis (1, 42). The significance of some quorum-sensing systems is more difficult to picture; for example, the autoinduction of a set of genes in *Rhizobium leguminosarum* that is expressed just prior to root hair penetration together with the expression of functions that lead to stationary phase (23). A general theme that has emerged is that the bacteria that exhibit this type of cell

TABLE 1 Partial list of bacteria that produce acylhomoserine lactone signals

Vibrio fischeri

Vibrio harveyi

Pseudomonas aeruginosa

Agrobacterium tumefaciens

Erwinia carotovora

Erwinia herbicola

Erwinia stewartii

Chromobacterium violaceum

Rhizobium leguminosarum

Vibrio anguillarum

Pseudomonas aureofaciens

Pseudomonas solanacearum

Rhizobium meliloti

Aeromonas hydrophila

Aeromonas salmonicida

Burkholderia cepacia

Citrobacter freundii

Enterobacter agglomerans

Obseumbacterium sp.

Proteus mirabilis

Rhodobacter sphaeroides

Serratia liquefaciens

Yersinia enterocolitica

Hafnia sp.

Pseudomonas fluorescens

density-dependent gene regulation experience a plant or animal host association as part of their lifestyle. However, there are recently described examples that might provide an exception to this rule. For example, the photosynthetic bacterium *Rhodobacter sphaeroides* has a quorum-sensing system, and although one cannot rule out an involvement with a eukaryotic host, such an association has not been described (44).

Although the divergently transcribed *luxI* and *luxR* genes in *V. fischeri* are linked to each other and to the genes they regulate (Fig. 1), this is not always the case. In fact every sort of arrangement imaginable has been reported. The *R* and *I* genes can regulate unlinked genes and in some cases are not even linked to each other. There can be multiple LuxR and LuxI

homologs in a single bacterium, for example *P. aeruginosa* (32, 36, 37). There is now some evidence that *Burkholderia cepacia*, an opportunistic pathogen that can colonize lungs of cystic fibrosis patients, may sense and respond to the density of another bacterial species infecting the cystic fibrotic lung, *P. aeruginosa* (33). It appears that the elements of the LuxR-LuxI system evolved in gram-negative bacteria early or have moved from species to species by gene transfer and that each species has adapted these elements to its own needs.

RECENTLY DISCOVERED ROLES FOR ACYLHOMOSERINE LACTONE SIGNALING IN BIOFILM DIFFERENTIATION AND DISPERSAL FROM COMMUNITY STRUCTURES

Biofilms of mixed bacterial communities and of individual species such as *P. aeruginosa* form thick layers consisting of differentiated mushroom-shaped and pillarlike structures that consist primarily of an extracellular polysaccharide matrix in which the bacterial cells are embedded. The development of a biofilm involves several steps. First, individual bacteria must adhere to a surface. They must then proliferate, and at an appropriate time, there must be differentiation or morphogenesis into a mature, structured biofilm. This, taken together with the knowledge that *P. aeruginosa* produces extracellular signals involved in cell-to-cell communication and cell density-dependent expression of many secreted virulence factors, suggests that cell-to-cell signaling could be involved in the differentiation of *P. aeruginosa* into the mature biofilm form. Because quorum sensing requires a sufficient density of bacteria, we would not expect *P. aeruginosa* quorum-sensing signals to be involved in the initial attachment stage of biofilm formation. However, quorum sensing may be involved in biofilm differentiation.

The wild-type *P. aeruginosa* forms structured biofilms with stalked mushroom-shaped aggregates approximately 120 μm thick, with water-filled spaces in between. Biofilm bacteria are hundreds of times more resistant to antibiotics than are bacteria growing in broth culture. This makes biofilms of organisms like *P. aeruginosa* clinically relevant (8). One signal generator mutant, a *lasI* mutant, but not the other, a *rhlI* mutant, produces thin, unstructured biofilms about 10 to 20 μm thick. These thin biofilms are sensitive to environmental challenges that do not affect the wild-type biofilms. These challenges result in dispersal of the bacteria from the glass surface to which they are attached (8). When the biofilms of the *lasI* mutant are provided with 3-oxodo-decanoylhomoserine lactone, the LasI-generated signal, they appear identical to the wild type.

Control of biofilm differentiation and integrity by quorum sensing has important implications in medicine. *P. aeruginosa* can colonize devices such as catheters, and it colonizes the lungs of most cystic fibrosis patients (22, 43). Because of their innate resistance to antibiotics and other biocides, biofilms in these environments are difficult if not impossible to eradicate. Bacterial biofilms also present other problems of significant economic importance in both industry and medicine. The connection between biofilm and a quorum-sensing signal suggests that inhibition of these cell-to-cell signals could aid in the treatment of biofilms.

At least for *P. aeruginosa*, quorum-sensing signals are required for conversion to a mature biofilm. Are there signals for dispersal of biofilm cells back into the planktonic community? This is an area that merits intensive investigation. Although much more study is required, the case of quorum sensing in *R. sphaeroides* (44) brings evidence to bear on this question. Recently, we found that *R. sphaeroides* contains *luxI-luxR* homologs called *cerI-cerR*. The *cerI* gene directs synthesis of the quorum-sensing signal 7,8-*cis*-tetradecenoyl-homoserine lactone. In a broth medium, the wild type grows as individual cells in suspension. However, a *cerI* mutant grown under identical conditions occurs as a single large mucilaginous clump. Addition of the signal 7,8-*cis*-tetradecenoylhomoserine lactone to a

clumped mutant causes cells to disperse from the clump and grow as the wild type grows. The ecological significance of this observation is unknown, but it does provide some evidence that there may be acylhomoserine lactone signals involved in dispersal of biofilms. In fact, the gene designation *cer* is for community escape response (44).

A CASE OF CONVERGENT EVOLUTION

Understanding autoinduction of luminescence in *V. harveyi* has come more slowly than understanding of autoinduction in *V. fischeri*. This is in large part because the *V. harveyi* system is more complicated. There are two signaling systems that can function independently of each other (3). One of the systems involves an acylhomoserine lactone, N-(3-hydroxy-butyryl)homoserine lactone (4). The structure of the signal for the other system remains unknown, and it does not appear to be an acylhomoserine lactone (51). LuxR homologs have not been identified in *V. harveyi*. Rather, the signal sensors are complex proteins with sequence similarities to both components of two-component regulatory proteins. Two genes, *luxL* and *luxM*, are required for synthesis of N-(3-hydroxybutyryl)homoserine lactone (3). Neither of these genes encodes a protein that shows similarity to the *V. fischeri* LuxI protein or any of its homologs. It was surprising when Kuo et al. (31) discovered that *V. fischeri luxI* mutants produce octanoyl-homoserine lactone, which serves as a very poor substitute for the LuxI-produced 3-oxohexanoylhomoserine lactone in luminescence gene activation. The gene required for octanoylhomoserine lactone synthesis was cloned and sequenced, and although its product is not a LuxI homolog, there is a 38% sequence identity of its amino-terminal region and the *V. harveyi* LuxM. This suggests that there is a second family of acylhomoserine lactone-synthesizing enzymes (20). The mechanism of acylhomoserine lactone synthesis by this family has not yet been investigated.

UNANSWERED QUESTIONS

LuxR–LuxI-type quorum sensing plays a role not only in the curious light organ relationship between *V. fischeri* and its marine animal hosts but also in the virulence of certain human and plant pathogens. The research field is young, and there are many important areas to investigate. It is clear that LuxI and LuxR homologs of pathogens are targets for development of novel antimicrobial factors. We need to know more about how they function, and inhibitors need to be identified. With respect to inhibitors, at least one marine algal species produces a furanone compound that can inhibit autoinduction (21). This may explain why luminescent marine bacteria, which can be isolated from a variety of marine habitats, are not found on the surface of algae. We know little about quorum sensing in natural environments and in the biofilms in which bacteria often grow. Is communication between bacterial species in complex natural environments common or important? Why do bacteria have multiple quorum-sensing systems, and how many can be found in an individual strain? What is the significance of the "second family" of autoinducer synthetic enzymes? Finally, one might expect that with the intimate associations known to exist between mutualistic and pathogenic quorum-sensing bacteria and their plant and animal hosts, the hosts may have evolved systems that can sense and respond to acylhomoserine lactone signals. It has been reported that one of the *P. aeruginosa* autoinducers stimulates epithelial cell production of interleukin-8 (10). Other acylhomoserine lactones also appear to affect production of immunomodulators and cytokines (53), and we have shown that at concentrations as low as 5 nM, butyrylhomoserine lactone, which is produced by *P. aeruginosa*, stimulates mouse spleen cells to produce gamma interferon. In general, host detection and response to autoinducers is as yet an untapped avenue of investigation.

REVIEWS AND KEY PAPERS

Bassler, B. L. and M. R. Silverman. 1995. Intercellular communication in marine Vibrio species: density-dependent regulation of the expression of bioluminescence, p. 431–435. *In* J. A. Hoch and T. J. Silhavy (ed.), *Two-Component Signal Transduction.* American Society for Microbiology, Washington, D.C.

Davies, D. G., M. R. Parsek, J. A. Pearson, B. H. Iglewski, J. W. Costerton, and E. P. Greenberg. 1998. The involvement of cell-to-cell signals in the development of a bacterial bio film. *Science* **280:**295–298.

Engebrecht, J., K. H. Nealson, and M. Silverman. 1983. Bacterial bioluminescence: isolation and genetic analysis of the functions from *Vibrio fischeri. Cell* **32:**773–781.

Fuqua, C., and E. P. Greenberg. 1998. Self perception in bacteria: quorum sensing with acylated homoserine lactones. *Curr. Opin. Microbiol.* **1:**183–189.

Fuqua, W. C., S. C. Winans, and E. P. Greenberg. 1994. Quorum sensing in bacteria: the LuxR-LuxI family of cell density-responsive transcriptional regulators. *J. Bacteriol.* **176:**269–275.

Fuqua, W. C., S. C. Winans, and E. P. Greenberg. 1996. Census and consensus in bacterial ecosystems: the LuxR-LuxI family of quorum-sensing transcriptional regulators. *Annu. Rev. Microbiol.* **50:**727–751.

Gilson, L., A. Kuo, and P. V. Dunlap. 1995. AinS and a new family of antoinducer synthesis proteins. *J. Bacteriol.* **177:**6946–6951.

Greenberg, E. P. 1997. Quorum sensing in gram-negative bacteria. *ASM News* **63:**371–377.

Kaiser, D., and R. Losick. 1997. How and why bacteria talk to each other. *Sci. Am.* **276:**68–73.

Latifi, A., M. Foglino, K. Tanaka, P. Williams, and A. Lazdunski. 1996. A hierarchical quorum-sensing cascade in *Pseudomonas aeruginosa* links the transcriptional activators LasR and RhlR to expression of the stationary-phase sigma factor RpoS. *Mol. Microbiol.* **21:**1137–1146.

Pesci, E. C., and B. H. Iglewski. 1997. The chain of command in *Pseudomonas* quorum sensing. *Trends Microbiol.* **5:**132–135.

Pesci, E. C., J. P. Pearson, P. C. Seed, and B. H. Iglewski. 1997. Regulation of *las* and *rhl* quorum sensing systems in *Pseudomonas aeruginosa. J. Bacteriol.* **179:**3127–3132.

Ruby, E. G. 1996. Lessons from cooperative bacterial-animal associations: the *Vibrio fischeri-Euprymna scolopes* light organ. *Annu. Rev. Microbiol.* **50:**591–624.

Salmond, G. P. C., B. W. Bycroft, G. S. A. B. Stewart, and P. Williams. 1995. The bacterial "enigma": cracking the code of cell-cell communication. *Mol. Microbiol.* **16:**615–624.

Sitnikov, D. M., J. B. Schineller, and T. O. Baldwin. 1995. Transcriptional regulation of bioluminescence genes from *Vibrio fischeri. Mol. Microbiol.* **17:**801–812.

REFERENCES

1. **Bainton, N. J., P. Stead, S. R. Chhabra, B. W. Bycroft, G. P. C. Salmond, G. S. A. B. Stewart, and P. Williams.** 1992. A general role for the *lux* autoinducer in bacterial cell signalling: control of antibiotic synthesis in *Erwinia. Gene* **116:**87–91.
2. **Balaban, N., T. Goldkorn, R. T. Nhan, L. B. Dang, S. Scott, R. M. Ridgley, A. Rasooly, S. C. Wright, J. W. Larrick, R. Rasooly, and J. R. Carlson.** 1998. Autoinducer of virulence as a target for vaccine and therapy against *Staphylococcus aureus. Science* **280:**438–441.
3. **Bassler, B. L., and M. R. Silverman.** 1995. Intercellular communication in marine Vibrio species: density-dependent regulation of the expression of bioluminescence, p. 431–435. *In* J. A. Hoch and T. J. Silhavy (ed.), *Two-Component Signal Transduction.* American Society for Microbiology, Washington, D.C.
4. **Cao, J., and E. A. Meighen.** 1993. Biosynthesis and stereochemistry of the autoinducer controlling luminescence in *Vibrio harveyi. J. Bacteriol.* **175:**3856–3862.
5. **Choi, S. H., and E. P. Greenberg.** 1991. The C-terminal region of the Vibrio fischeri LuxR protein contains an inducer-independent lux gene activating domain. *Proc. Natl. Acad. Sci. USA* **88:**11115–11119.
6. **Choi, S. H., and E. P. Greenberg.** 1992. Genetic dissection of the DNA binding and luminescence gene activation by the *Vibrio fischeri* LuxR protein. *J. Bacteriol.* **174:**4064–4069.
7. **Choi, S. H., and E. P. Greenberg.** 1992. Genetic evidence for multimerization of LuxR, the transcriptional activator of Vibrio fischeri luminescence. *Mol. Mar. Biol. Biotech.* **1:**408–413.
8. **Davies, D. G., M. R. Parsek, J. A. Pearson, B. H. Iglewski, J. W. Costerton, and E. P. Greenberg.** 1998. The involvement of cell-to-cell signals in the development of a bacterial biofilm. *Science* **280:**295–298.
9. **Devine, J. H., G. S. Shadel, and T. O. Baldwin.** 1989. Identification of the operator of the *lux* regulon from *Vibrio fischeri* ATCC7744. *Proc. Natl. Acad. Sci. USA* **86:**5688–5692.
10. **DiMango, E., H. J. Zar, R. Bryan, and A. Prince.** 1995. Diverse *Pseudomonas aeruginosa* gene products stimulate respiratory epithelial cells to produce interleukin-8. *J. Clin. Invest.* **96:**2204–2210.
11. **Dunlap, P. V.** 1992. Mechanism for iron control of the *Vibrio fischeri* luminescence system: involvement of cyclic AMP and cyclic AMP receptor protein and modulation of DNA level *J. Biolumin. Chemilumin.* **7:**203–214.
12. **Dunlap, P. V., and E. P. Greenberg.** 1988. Analysis of the mechanism of *Vibrio fischeri* luminescence gene regulation by cyclic AMP and cyclic AMP receptor protein in *Escherichia coli. J. Bacteriol.* **170:**4040–4046.
13. **Eberhard, A., A. L. Burlingame, C. Eberhard, G. L. Kenyon, K. H. Nealson, and N. J. Oppenheimer.** 1981. Structural identification of autoinducer of *Photobacterium fischeri* luciferase. *Biochemistry* **20:**2444–2449.
14. **Engerbrecht, J., K. H. Nealson, and M. Silverman.** 1983. Bacterial bioluminescence: isolation and genetic analysis of the functions from *Vibrio fischeri. Cell* **32:**773–781.
15. **Fuqua, C., and E. P. Greenberg.** 1998. Self perception in bacteria: quorum sensing with acylated homoserine lactone. *Curr. Opin. Microbiol.* **1:**183–189.
16. **Fuqua, W. C., and S. C. Winans.** 1994. A LuxR-LuxI type regulatory system activates *Agrobacterium* Ti plasmid conjugal transfer in the presence of a plant tumor metabolite. *J. Bacteriol.* **176:**2796–2806.
17. **Fuqua, W. C., S. C. Winans, and E. P. Greenberg.** 1994. Quorum sensing in bacteria: the LuxR-LuxI family of cell density-responsive transcriptional regulators. *J. Bacteriol.* **176:**269–275.
18. **Fuqua, W. C., S. C. Winans, and E. P. Greenberg.** 1996. Census and consensus in bacterial ecosystems: the LuxR-LuxI family of quorum-sensing transcriptional regulators. *Annu. Rev. Microbiol.* **50:**727–751.
19. **Gambello, M. J., and B. H. Iglewski.** 1991. Cloning and characterization of the *Pseudomonas aeruginosa lasR* gene, a transcriptional activator of elastase expression. *J. Bacteriol.* **173:**3000–3009.
20. **Gilson, L., A. Kuo, and P. V. Dunlap.** 1995. AinS and a new family of autoinducer synthesis proteins. *J. Bacteriol.* **177:**6946–6951.
21. **Givskov, M. R. deNys, M. Manefield, L. Gram, R. Maximilien, L. Eberl, P. D. Steinberg, and S. Kjelleberg.** 1996. Eukaryotic interference with homoserine lactone-mediated prokaryotic signalling. *J. Bacteriol.* **178:**6618–6622.
22. **Govan, J. R. W., and V. Deretic.** 1996. Microbial pathogenesis in cystic fibrosis: mucoid *Pseudomonas aeruginosa* and *Burkholderia cepacia. Microbiol. Rev.* **60:**539–574.
23. **Gray, K. M., J. P. Pearson, J. A. Downie, B. E. A. Boboye, and E. P. Greenberg.** 1996.

Cell-to-cell signaling in the symbiotic nitrogen-fixing bacterium *Rhizobium leguminosarum*: auto-induction of a stationary phase and rhizosphere-expressed genes. *J. Bacteriol.* **178**:372–376.

24. **Hanzelka, B. L., and E. P. Greenberg.** 1995. Evidence that the N-terminal region of the *Vibrio fischeri* LuxR protein constitutes an autoinducer-binding domain. *J. Bacteriol.* **177**:815–817.

25. **Hanzelka, B. L., and E. P. Greenberg.** 1996. Quorum sensing in *Vibrio fischeri*: evidence that S-adenosylmethionine is the amino acid substrate for autoinducer systhesis. *J. Bacteriol.* **178**:5291–5294.

26. **Hanzelka, B. L., A. M. Stevens, M. R. Parsek, T. J. Crone, and E. P. Greenberg.** 1997. Mutational analysis of the *Vibrio fischeri* LuxI polypeptide: critical regions of an autoinducer synthase. *J. Bacteriol.* **179**:4882–4887.

27. **Haygood, M. G., and K. H. Nealson.** 1985. Mechanisms of iron regulation of luminescence in *Vibrio fischeri*. *J. Bacteriol.* **162**:209–216.

28. **Jekosch, K., and U. K. Winkler.** 1996. Anaerobic expression of the *Photobacterium fischeri* regulon requires the FNR protein which acts upon the left operon, p. 93–96. *In* J. W. Hastings, L. J. Kricka, and P. E. Stanley (ed.), *Proceedings of the 9th International Symposium on Bioluminescence and Chemiluminescence.*

29. **Kaplan, H. B., and E. P. Greenberg.** 1985. Diffusion of autoinducer is involved in regulation of the *Vibrio fischeri* luminescence system. *J. Bacteriol.* **163**:1210–1214.

30. **Kolibachuk, D., and E. P. Greenberg.** 1993. The *Vibrio fischeri* luminescence gene activator LuxR is a membrane-associated protein. *J. Bacteriol.* **175**:7307–7312.

31. **Kuo, A., N. V. Blough, and P. V. Dunlap.** 1994. Multiple N-acyl-L-homoserine lactone autoinducers of luminescence in the marine symbiotic bacterium *Vibrio fischeri*. *J. Bacteriol.* **176**:7558–7565.

32. **Latifi, A., K. M. Winson, M. Foglino, B. W. Bycroft, G. S. A. B. Stewart, A. Lazdunski, and P. Williams.** 1995. Multiple homologues of LuxR and LuxI control expression of virulence determinants and secondary metabolites through quorum sensing in *Pseudomonas aeruginosa* PAO1. *Mol. Microbiol.* **17**:333–344.

33. **McKenney, D., K. E. Brown, and D. G. Allison.** 1995. Influence of *Pseudonomas aeruginosa* exoproducts on virulence factor production in *Burkholderia cepacia*: evidence of interspecies communication. *J. Bacteriol.* **177**:6989–6992.

34. **Nealson, K. H., and J. W. Hastings.** 1979. Bacterial bioluminescence: its control and ecological significance. *Microbiol. Rev.* **43**:496–518.

35. **Nealson, K. H., T. Platt, and J. W. Hastings.** 1970. Cellular control of the synthesis and activity of the bacterial luminescence system. *J. Bacteriol.* **104**:313–322.

36. **Ochsner, U. A., A. K. Koch, A. Fiechter, and J. Reiser.** 1994. Isolation and characterization of a regulatory gene affecting rhamnolipid biosurfactant synthesis in *Pseudomonas aeruginosa*. *J. Bacteriol.* **176**:2044–2054.

37. **Ochsner, U. A., and J. Reiser.** 1995. Autoinducer-mediated regulation of rhamnolipid biosurfactant synthesis in *Pseudomonas aeruginosa*. *Proc. Natl. Acad. Sci. USA* **92**:6424–6428.

38. **Parsek, M. R., A. L. Schaefer, and E. P. Greenberg.** 1997. Analysis of random and site-directed mutations in *rhlI*, a *Pseudomonas aeruginosa* gene encoding an acylhomoserine lactone synthase. *Mol. Microbiol.* **26**:301–310.

39. **Pearson, J. P., K. M. Gray, L. Passador, K. D. Tucker, A. Eberhard, B. H. Iglewski, and E. P. Greenberg.** 1994. Structure of the autoinducer required for expression of *Pseudomonas aeruginosa* virulence genes. *Proc. Natl. Acad. Sci. USA* **91**:197–201.

40. **Pearson, J. P., L. Passador, B. H. Iglewski, and E. P. Greenberg.** 1995. A second N-acylhomoserine lactone signal produced by *Pseudomonas aeruginosa*. *Proc. Natl. Acad. Sci. USA* **92**:1490–1494.

41. **Piper, K. R., S. B. v. Bodman, and S. K. Farrand.** 1993. Conjugation factor of *Agrobacterium tumefaciens* regulates Ti plasmid transfer by autoinduction. *Nature* **362**:448–450.

42. **Pirhonnen, M., D. Flego, R. Heikiheimo, and E. T. Palva.** 1993. A small diffusible signal molecule is responsible for the global control of virulence and exoenzyme production in the plant pathogen *Erwinia carotovora*. *EMBO J.* **12**:2467–2476.

43. **Pollack, M. (ed.).** 1990. *Pseudomonas aeruginosa*. Churchill Livingstone, Ltd., Edinburgh.

44. **Puskas, A., E. P. Greenberg, S. Kaplan, and A. L. Schaefer.** 1997. A quorum sensing system in the free-living photosynthetic bacterium *Rhodobacter sphaeroides*. *J. Bacteriol.* **179**:7530–7537.

45. **Rosson, R. A., and K. H. Nealson.** 1981. Autoinduction of bacterial luminescence in a carbon limited chemostat. *Arch. Microbiol.* **159**:160–167.

46. **Schaefer, A. L., B. L. Hanzelka, A. Eberhard, and E. P. Greenberg.** 1996. Quorum sensing in *Vibrio fischeri*: autoinducer-LuxR interactions with autoinducer analogs. *J. Bacteriol.* **178**:2897–2901.

47. **Schaefer, A. L., D. L. Val, B. L. Hanzelka, J. E. Cronan, Jr., and E. P. Greenberg.** 1996. Generation of cell-to-cell signals in quorum sensing: acyl homoserine lactone synthase activity of

a purified *Vibrio fischeri* LuxI protein. *Proc. Natl. Acad. Sci. USA* **93**:9505–9509.

48. **Sitnikov, D. M., J. B. Schineller, and T. O. Baldwin.** 1995. Transcriptional regulation of bioluminescence genes from *Vibrio fischeri*. *Mol. Microbiol.* **17**:801–812.

49. **Stevens, A. M., K. M. Dolan, and E. P. Greenberg.** 1994. Synergistic binding of the *Vibrio fischeri* LuxR transcriptional activator domain and RNA polymerase to the *lux* promoter region. *Proc. Natl. Acad. Sci. USA* **91**:12619–12623.

50. **Stevens, A. M., and E. P. Greenberg.** 1997. Quorum sensing in *Vibrio fischeri*: essential elements for activation of the luminescence genes. *J. Bacteriol.* **179**:557–562.

51. **Surette, M. G., and B. L. Bassler.** 1998. Quorum sensing in *Escherichia coli* and *Salmonella typhimurium*. *Proc. Natl. Acad. Sci. USA* **95**:7046–7050.

52. **Tang, H. B., E. Dimango, R. Bryan, M. J. Gambello, B. H. Iglewski, J. B. Goldberg, and A. Prince.** 1996. Contribution of specific *Pseudomonas aeruginosa* virulence factors to pathogenesis of pneumonia in a neonatal mouse model of infection. *Infect. Immun.* **64**:37–43.

53. **Telford, G., D. Wheeler, P. Williams, P. T. Tompkins, P. Appleby, H. Sewell, G. S. Stewart, B. W. Bycroft, and D. I. Pritchard.** 1998. The *Pseudomonas aeruginosa* quorum-sensing signal molecule N-(3-oxododecanoyl)-L-homoserine lactone has immunomodulatory activity. *Infect. Immun.* **66**:36–42.

54. **Winson, M. K., M. Camara, A. Latifi, M. Foglino, S. R. Chhabra, M. Daykin, M. Bally, V. Chapon, G. P. C. Salmond, B. W. Bycroft, A. Lazdunski, G. S. A. B. Stewart, and P. Williams.** 1995. Multiple N-acyl-L-homoserine lactone signal molecules regulate production of virulence determinants and secondary metabolites in *Pseudomonas aeruginosa*. *Proc. Natl. Acad. Sci. USA* **92**:9427–9431.

55. **Zhang, L., P. J. Murphy, A. Kerr, and M. E. Tate.** 1993. *Agrobacterium* conjugation and gene regulation by N-acyl-L-homoserine lactones. *Nature* **362**:446–448.

INVOLVEMENT OF HOST FACTORS IN REGULATING THE *lux* SYSTEM OF *VIBRIO FISCHERI*

S. Ulitzur

10

The regulatory mechanism of the *Vibrio fischeri* *lux* system has been extensively studied during the past 10 years (see review references 22, 27, 30). The *lux* system of *V. fischeri* is encoded by two adjacent operons that are divergently transcribed. The right operon consists of seven genes (*luxICDABEG*) that encode the enzymes required for synthesis of the autoinducer (*luxI*) and the alpha (*luxA*) and beta (*luxB*) subunits of the luciferase enzyme. The *luxC*, *luxD*, and *luxE* genes encode the enzymes required for the luciferase substrate, a long-chain aldehyde. The role of *luxG* is unknown. The left operon constitutes a single gene encoding the regulatory protein LuxR (14, 28).

Luminous bacteria growing in complex or minimal media undergo induction of the *lux* system only for a brief period during late exponential growth phase. This phenomenon, termed "autoinduction," is attributed to accumulation of a cell product (autoinducer) in the growth medium (24). The autoinducer formed by *V. fischeri* was first identified by Eberhard et al. (13) as *N*-3-(oxohexanoyl)-L-homoserine lactone. More recently, Kuo et al.

(18), have shown that *V. fischeri* produces three chemically distinct autoinducers; the two new autoinducers were identified as *N*-hexanoyl-L-homoserine lactone and *N*-octanoyl-L-homoserine lactone.

Several lines of evidence indicate that growth conditions and the genetic background of the bacteria harboring the *lux* system strongly affect the timing of the onset of the *lux* system and the level of the developed luminescence. As a conceptual contrast to the situation with shaken broth culture, which is generally induced after attaining a cell density of about 5×10^7 to 10×10^8 cells/ml, Barak and Ulitzur (3) have shown that when a single bacterium of *V. fischeri* was cultivated on 1 ml of solid complex medium, induction occurred after only five or six generations. At this stage, the concentration of the luminous bacteria was only 50 to 100 cells/ml, although the population density in microcolonies was very high. To address the question of whether the early induction was due to nutrient limitation, *V. fischeri* cells were grown in artificial seawater containing low concentrations of nutrients (100 μg of tryptone and 50 μg of yeast extract per ml). Under these conditions, induction of the *lux* system took place at a cell density of about 10^6 cells/ml. At this stage of growth, the concentration of the autoinducer

S. *Ulitzur*, Department of Food Engineering and Biotechnology, Technion, Haifa 32000, Israel.

Microbial Ecology and Infectious Disease, Edited by Eugene Rosenberg
©1999 American Society for Microbiology, Washington, D.C.

in the growth medium was below 0.1 pg/ml, while under normal growth conditions, in the presence of a 50-fold higher nutrient content, induction of these cells occurred at a cell density of about 10^8 cells/ml, upon accumulation of about 150 pg of autoinducer in 1 ml of growth medium. Nutrient-depleted cells exhibited a thousand times higher sensitivity to exogenous autoinducer than nutrient-repleted cells (1). Moreover, addition of a low concentration of nutrients during the course of induction of the *lux* system of *V. fischeri* culture resulted in a transient inhibition of luminescence. Other chemophysical factors such as heat shock, oxygen tension (31), and high osmotic pressure (33) also altered the timing of the onset of luminescence and its level.

These and other observations indicated that the regulation of the *lux* system is more complex than previously assumed and that in addition to the autoinducer and the regulatory protein, other factors that do not belong to the *lux* system play a key role in the expression of the *lux* system of *V. fischeri*. Our studies in the last decade have revealed the key role of different groups of regulons, including the RecA and LexA proteins, σ^{32}, GroESL and Lon protease, as well as RpoS (σ^S) and H-NS in controlling the *lux* system of *V. fischeri*. The involvement of these proteins in controlling the formation and expression of *V. fischeri lux* system is described below.

ROLE OF cAMP AND CRP
The development of luminescence in *V. fischeri* and in recombinant *Escherichia coli* carrying the *lux* system of this strain is temporarily inhibited by growth in the presence of glucose. Mutants of transformed *E. coli* strains missing the gene for cyclic AMP (cAMP) or for cAMP-binding protein (CRP) are very dim. A consensus sequence for the binding of CRP has been located in the center of the intergenomic region between *luxR* and *luxI* (9–11). These studies demonstrated that CRP and cAMP activate transcription from the *luxR* promoter but inhibit expression of the right operon containing the *lux* structural

genes. However, if both operons were present, luminescence was stimulated by CRP and cAMP. High levels of LuxR, when supplied in *trans*, override the requirement for cAMP and CRP.

ROLE OF RecA AND LexA PROTEINS
The onset of induction of young cultures of *V. fischeri lux* system is greatly advanced by different DNA synthesis inhibitors, such as mitomycin C; gyrase inhibitors, such as nalidixic acid or novobiocin; as well as by DNA intercalating agents, such as ethidium bromide and proflavine (37). We (31) suggested that LexA inhibits the transcription of the *V. fischeri lux* system by occupying the LuxR DNA-binding site in the intergenomic region between *luxR* and *luxI*. The existence of sequence similarity between the consensus *E. coli* LexA binding site and the *V. fischeri lux* box (29) as well as the binding of *E. coli* LexA at this site (26) was in agreement with this assumption. Consistent with an involvement of LexA and RecA in luminescence, we (29) showed that *lux* plasmid-carrying *E. coli* mutant strains were either defective in *recA* or produced LexA resistant to RecA protease activity, emitted low-level luminescence, and were relatively insensitive to mitomycin C. Conversely, a *lux* plasmid-containing *E. coli* strain producing LexA with weak DNA binding, exhibited higher luminescence and higher sensitivity to mitomycin C than the *lexA*[+] control strain. Since high, but not low, concentrations of autoinducer overcome a mutation in *recA*, we proposed that a LexA-like protein acts as a weak repressor of the *lux* system, thus avoiding premature induction of the *lux* system.

In addition to their effect on the SOS system, some of the DNA synthesis inhibitors act indirectly on DNA topology, thereby affecting the expression of the *lux* system. We drew this conclusion (32) on the basis of our recent finding that the H-NS protein represses transcription of the *luxRI* and *luxC* genes of the *V. fischeri lux* system (see below). Regions upstream of these genes are especially enriched in poly(dA) and poly(dT) clusters characteristic of curved DNA, a preferred site for H-NS binding. H-NS binding to these DNA stretches results in changes in DNA topology that are assumed to interfere with the activity of RNA polymerase. The presence of gyrase inhibitors such as novobiocin or nalidixic acid resulted in DNA relaxation, thus enabling transcription of H-NS–repressed genes.

Taken together, the activity of DNA synthesis inhibitors in advancing the induction of the *lux* system may be due to two independent mechanisms. Activation of RecA protease and the consequent cleavage of LexA protein may relieve the inhibitory effect of LexA on the transcription of the *luxI* upstream promoter. Gyrase inhibitors may also act as DNA-relaxation agents that relieve the inhibitory effect of H-NS on the two promoters located upstream and downstream of the *luxI* gene (see below).

ROLE OF GroESL, HtpR, AND LonA

As discussed above, the onset of induction of the *lux* system of *V. fischeri* is not solely dependent on the concentration of the autoinducer in the growth medium. As we have shown (1), the major factor that governs the onset of autoinduction is the level of active LuxR protein in the cell. LuxR is a labile protein that tends to denature at temperatures above 30°C and consequently to undergo proteolytic degradation by LonA protease. An *E. coli lonA* mutant harboring the whole *lux* system of *V. fischeri* initiated luminescence earlier and at higher levels than wild-type cells (unpublished observation). Our earlier studies (31) revealed that mutants of *E. coli* defective in HtpR (σ^{32}) that carried the whole *lux* system of *V. fischeri* were very dim throughout the growth cycle. For some time, this observation has not received special attention, since addition of high concentrations of the autoinducer fully restored wild-type levels of luminescence in these mutant cells. It was eventually shown (1, 8) that σ^{32} does not act directly as a sigma factor but rather through GroESL proteins, which are controlled by

σ^{32}. The capacity of the LuxR to form a stable complex with the autoinducer is highly dependent on the presence of GroESL. In the presence of the *plac*-controlled *groESL* gene, LuxR binds the autoinducer at a very low concentration ($K_d = 7 \times 10^{-8}$ M), indicating that the β-GroESL chaperonin-mediated folding is necessary for stabilization of the native and active form of LuxR (2).

Limited availability of GroESL and competition among various GroESL-demanding proteins in the cell could contribute to cessation of LuxR–mediated *lux* operon expression. This effect is more pronounced when the stability of LuxR is more dependent on GroESL. Under these circumstances, (e.g., growth temperature above 30°C), the development of luminescence is largely dependent on the availability of GroESL. Thus, the development of light in *E. coli* cells carrying the whole *lux* system of *V. fischeri* is completely inhibited in the copresence of either *plac*-controlled *luxAB*-, *luxA*-, or *luxB*-carrying genes (34). As expected, luminescence in these cells can be fully recovered by introducing either *ptac*-controlled *groESL* genes or the *plac luxR*-controlled gene into these dim cells (unpublished observation). The activity of other GroESL-demanding proteins is also affected by the presence of *luxAB* genes. We have shown (unpublished observation) that the susceptibility to ampicillin of *E. coli* cells carrying a pBR322 plasmid was largely increased when *plac*-controlled *luxAB* genes were subcloned into this plasmid. Similarly, the lytic activity of T4 bacteriophage (which requires GroESL for propagation) is reduced in the presence of *luxAB* genes (unpublished observation).

ROLE OF RpoS AND H-NS PROTEINS

The involvement of RpoS (σ^S) and H-NS proteins in the regulation of bacterial bioluminescence has only recently been discovered (32). σ^S is the principal regulator of numerous stationary-phase genes in *E. coli* (11). Out of the many factors that are involved in the regulatory activity of RpoS, special attention has been given to H-NS (4). H-NS protein is a neutral homodimeric protein composed of 138 amino acids, which shows high affinity for double-stranded DNA, with preference to curved DNA. *hns* mutants show pleiotropic phenotypes, and many genes, including *drdX*, *bglY*, *osmZ*, *pilG*, and *virR*, were shown to be allelic to *hns* (4). The *lux* genes of all luminous bacteria show a typical base composition that characterizes curved DNA. The upstream regions of *luxR* of *V. fischeri* and the *luxC* genes of all species contain DNA fragments showing over 80% AT stretches, while other structural genes are also highly enriched with A tracts.

Self-expression in *E. coli* of the luminescence systems from light–emitting bacteria was observed only with the *V. fischeri lux* operons. *E. coli* MC4100 cells harboring the *lux* systems of *Vibrio harveyi*, *Photobacterium leiognathi*, *Photobacterium phosphoreum*, or *Xenorabdus luminescens* expressed them at very low levels. In contrast, *E. coli* MC4100 *hns* cells harboring the *lux* systems of the latter luminous bacteria developed high levels of in vivo luminescence (32). In this mutant background, the luminescence of the cloned *V. fischeri lux* system was constitutive, regardless the presence of either a *luxI* or *luxR* deletion. The *V. fischeri lux-CDABE* genes under *plac* control were dim in MC4100 *rpoS* mutant cells but emitted strong light in MC4100 *hns* or *hns rpoS* double mutant strains. The question of whether both the left and the right operons of the *V. fischeri lux* system are controlled by H-NS was recently addressed by us (29a) with the aid of plasmids harboring the *lacZ* gene fused with *luxR* or *luxI*. In the MC4100 *hns rpoS* background, *luxR* and *luxI* genes were transcribed very early and actively, as judged by β-galactosidase activity. The β-galactosidase activity in the wild-type cells was 20 to 40 times lower and occurred mainly during the second half of the growth cycle. Hence, we concluded that H-NS inhibits the transcription of three promoters of the *lux* system of *V. fischeri*: the left operon that codes for LuxR protein and two promoters located upstream and downstream of the *luxI* gene.

More recently (29b), we showed that transcription of *luxCDABE* genes in wild-type cells of *E. coli* is activated by LuxR in the absence of the autoinducer. The copresence of the *ptac*-controlled *luxR* gene in a *trans* position to a plasmid carrying the *luxCDABE* genes resulted in 100,000 times higher luminescence. In the absence of the autoinducer, the presence of the *luxR* gene under its own regulated control resulted in about a 150-fold increase in luminescence from the *luxC* upstream promoter.

Taken together, it seems that LuxR initiates transcription of the *V. fischeri lux* system cloned in *E. coli* from two promoters, located upstream and downstream of the *luxI* gene. Only the activation of the first site requires the presence of the autoinducer; the second site is fully activated by the LuxR protein in the absence of the autoinducer.

We assumed that transcription of the *luxI* gene in *V. fischeri* is negatively controlled by H-NS and is positively controlled by LuxR with the autoinducer. It appears that when both LuxR and the autoinducer are in optimal concentrations, they relieve H-NS repression. The 5′ end of LuxR is highly enriched with poly(dA·dT) stretches, suggesting potential H-NS DNA-binding sites. A possible H-NS binding site in the LuxR gene was shown by Davine et al. (6) and Choi and Greenberg (5). The latter showed that deletion of the fragment between 30 and 60 bp from the first codon of the *luxR* gene dramatically increased transcription of both operons of the *V. fischeri lux* system, independently of the presence of either the autoinducer or LuxR.

The involvement of H-NS and σ^S in the regulation of the *V. fischeri lux* system may explain some phenomena associated with bacterial bioluminescence. There is increasing evidence that the regulation of gene expression is affected by DNA supercoiling and that DNA topology varies in response to environmental signals such as osmolarity, temperature, or anaerobic conditions (16). Ulitzur and

Kuhn (31) showed that induction of the *lux* system in marine bacteria, as well as the cloned *lux* system, responds very rapidly to anaerobiosis. Ulitzur and Osman (33) have shown that addition of different salts, at concentrations of 0.3 to 0.4 M, or sugars at concentrations of 0.5 to 0.7 M to LB medium resulted in rapid induction of luminescence in recombinant *E. coli* harboring the whole *lux* system of *V. fischeri*. Moreover, *E. coli* cells that grew in high osmotic medium showed high luminescence at 37°C (a temperature at which wild-type cells are dark) and, like *hns*-deficient *E. coli* cells, did not respond to externally added inducer. Similarly, Mechthild et al. (21) showed that under hyperosmotic conditions, the accumulated K^+ ions in *E. coli* cells released DNA-bound H-NS and thus relieved its repression.

The rate of H-NS synthesis during the log and stationary phases of growth is a controversial matter. Dersch et al. (7) have suggested that more *hns* transcription occurs in the stationary phase than in the log phase, while Free and Dormain (15) recently showed that *hns* transcription occurs only during periods of DNA synthesis. According to these authors, the H-NS:DNA ratio is constant at all stages of growth, and the level of *hns* mRNA declines at the onset of the stationary phase. The two periods of H-NS synthesis may correlate well with the two periods of arrested *lux* system expression. After inoculation of luminescent cultures into fresh medium, de novo synthesis of the *lux* system is arrested, and in vivo luminescence declines. During the mid- to late-log phase of growth, the *lux* system undergoes an intense period of induction and then is once again arrested as cells enter the stationary phase.

LuxR is a well-studied member of the UhpA/FixJ family of prokaryotic transcriptional activators that share homology throughout their entire protein sequence (see E. P. Greenberg's chapter in this book). It is not surprising, therefore, that like LuxR, these genes are enriched with stretches of dA and dT. In most cases, these genes are induced in late-log phase upon accumulation of homoserine lactone derivatives in the growth medium. At this stage of growth, the H-NS content in the cells reaches its maximal level. It seems that the role of LuxR is to relieve H-NS repression, thereby inducing the formation of proteins essential for cell survival in the stationary phase.

Relief of H-NS repression by LuxR and the autoinducer raises the interesting possibility that other H-NS–repressed genes in *E. coli* might also be relieved by LuxR and the autoinducer and that other members of the UphA/FixJ proteins and their corresponding autoinducer(s) act as general H-NS–relieving agents in prokaryotic cells.

Kassen et al. (17) showed that many commonly used *E. coli* K-12 strains carry an amber mutation in the *rpoS* gene. Expression of the functional σ^S in these cells depends on the presence of amber suppressors. *E. coli* MC4100, which is *rpoS⁺* and *sup⁰*, emits high luminescence, while *E. coli rpoS⁻* strains are very dim (32). The appearance of *rpoS* missense mutants is often observed in old stationary-phase *E. coli* cultures (38). Similarly, old stationary cultures of luminous bacteria show a high percentage occurrence of pleothrophic dim mutants, known as K variants (24). K-variant strains regain wild-type levels of luminescence upon starvation (31) or in the presence of gyrase inhibitors and DNA intercalators (35, 37). The possibility that the K variants are naturally occurring *rpoS* mutants, that are subjected to stronger H-NS inhibition is supported by the findings of Free and Dorman (15). These authors showed that de novo synthesis of H-NS is arrested shortly after the synthesis of DNA is blocked and that starvation for amino acids activates the stringent control and consequently results in accumlation of ppGpp and activation of *rpoS* promoter (20).

There is increasing evidence that the regulation of gene expression is affected by DNA supercoiling and that DNA topology varies in response to environmental signals such as osmolarity, temperature, or anaerobic conditions

(16). The induction of the *lux* system in marine bacteria and that of the cloned *lux* system responds very rapidly to anaerobiosis (33). As mentioned above, high osmotic pressure also greatly increased luminescence in marine and cloned luminous bacteria.

ROLE OF Fnr PROTEIN

The *lux* system of *V. fischeri* and other luminous species is expressed under both aerobic and anaerobic conditions to about the same extant (19). Studies with *E. coli* carrying the *V. fischeri lux* system revealed that fumarate-nitrate reductase (Fnr) protein is required for expression of the *lux* system under anaerobic conditions. An Fnr DNA binding site was identified in the region adjacent to the CRP-binding site (23).

ROLE OF Lrp PROTEIN

Very recently, we have shown (in preparation) that yet another host factor is involved in regulation of the *V. fischeri lux* system in *E. coli*. The leucine-responsive regulatory protein (Lrp) affects the transcription of a large number of genes, increasing the expression of some and decreasing that of others (25). At some promoters, Lrp action is greatly modified by the presence of L-leucine in the growth medium, whereas at others, leucine has little or no effect. Lrp is a small basic, DNA-binding protein, consisting of two identical 18,800-Da subunits, which is highly abundant in *E. coli* cells (3,000 molecules per cell). The Lrp binds DNA at a large number of sites with varying affinity. Promoter regions that show higher affinity to Lrp seem be more affected. Wang and Calvo's (36) analysis of the six Lrp binding sites upstream of the *E. coli ilvH* operon revealed that those with strongest affinity for Lrp have a symmetric of putative consensus sequence of AGAATTTATTCT (24). The role of Lrp protein in regulating the *lux* system of *V. fischeri* has not yet been described. Our preliminary studies showed that a typical core of consensus Lrp DNA binding site (TTTATTCT) is located in the *luxC* gene of *P. leiognathi*, and a nine-nucleotide stretch (AATTTTATT) of the putative long consensus sequence is located at the end of the *luxR* gene of *V. fischeri*. We found that *E. coli* W3110 cells carrying the whole *lux* system of *V. fischeri* became very dim in the presence of a *plac*-controlled *lrp* gene, regardless of the presence of externally added autoinducer, and that leucine inhibited the development of light in *lux*-carrying *E. coli* cells as well as in different luminous marine bacteria. The possibility that leucine-bound Lrp, like H-NS, binds to the promoter site(s) of the *lux* system is under study.

SUMMARY

LuxR may be viewed as the only ultimate and indispensable transcriptional factor required for the activation of *V. fischeri lux* system (see Fig. 1). Our recent studies (submitted) have shown that the presence of the autoinducer is required only for the activation of the *luxI* upstream promoter. LuxR-mediated transcription from the newly discovered *luxC* upstream promoter is independent of the autoinducer. A plausible scenario is that binding of the autoinducer to the folded LuxR results in configurational changes that expose the LuxR DNA binding domain to the *luxI* upstream promoter, while binding of LuxR to the *luxC* upstream promoter is independent of the autoinducer but requires a much higher concentration of active LuxR protein. It seems that the LuxR-RNA polymerase complex is able to initiate transcription of the *lux* system in the presence of H-NS. In the absence of H-NS, neither LuxR nor the autoinducer is required for luminescence development of the *V. fischeri lux* system in recombinant *E. coli* cells (32).

Other regulatory factors, including cAMP, CRP, and GroESL, as well as RecA that is associated with the formation or activity of the LuxR protein, may greatly influence the onset of induction and the level of developed luminescence of the *lux* system. RpoS seems to act mainly at the level of H-NS repression,

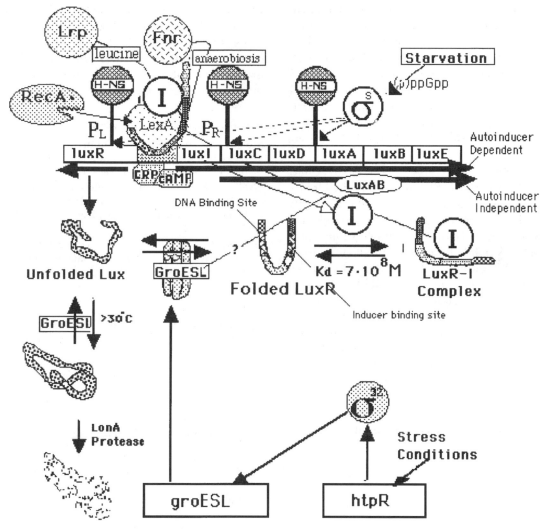

FIGURE 1 Involvement of host factors in the regulatory circuitry of the *V. fischeri lux* system.

since *E. coli rpoS* mutants carrying the whole *lux* system of *V. fischeri* are very dim (while the *hns rpoS* double-mutant strain is very bright). The relationship between the activity of host factors and the critical concentration of autoinducer required for induction of the *lux* system is very complex. A relatively high concentration of autoinducer (>30 ng/ml) overcomes the ultimate requirement for GroESL or RpoS. On the other hand, high activity of GroESL proteins diminishes by

hundredfolds the critical concentration of autoinducer required for induction of the *lux* system (1).

OPEN QUESTIONS AND FUTURE PERSPECTIVES

Studies describing the role of different host factors in regulating the *V. fischeri lux* system were mainly performed on *E. coli* transformed with recombinant plasmids containing the *V. fischeri lux* genes. This raises the question of whether some of the observed phenomena were due to abnormal levels of the *lux* system components and/or regulatory elements. Similarly, some results may be attributed to possible differences in the composition of *E. coli* and *V. fischeri* cellular milieus. The recently introduced possibility of genetically manipulating *V. fischeri* (30) may allow direct confirmation of the role of host factors in *lux*-system regulation.

Luminescence, like other extracellular products made by the members of the UphA/FixJ family, requires a certain critical intensity level to exert its ecological or physiological impact. As a single bacterial cell cannot produce enough light, or other products by itself, a collaborative and coordinated attempt should simultaneously be made by all members of the bacterial community. This goal may be achieved with the help of the diffusible autoinducer(s) that acts as a quorum sensing message that ensures accumulation of a critical mass of the formed product. It seems, however, that the critical concentration of the autoinducer required for triggering the *lux* system is highly dependent on the physiological state of the bacterial community. Under stress conditions, when the activities of the GroESL and RpoS proteins are high and/or when the activities of the H-NS and Lrp are low, the requirement for the autoinducer is hundreds of times lower than under optimal growth conditions. Moreover, in the absence of H-NS, both autoinducer and LuxR protein are not required for luminescence development. Thus, control of the complex regulatory system of *V. fischeri lux* system is a summation of multiple cross-acting regulatory elements and is not just a result of "accumulation of the autoinducer in the medium," as current dogma would suggest. According to our model, induction of bacterial bioluminescence may also occur under nonconfined conditions, such as those existing in the open sea. We found (unpublished observations) that typical bacterial luminescence is associated with particulate marine organic matter. Development of luminescence in particulate or-

ganic matter in the sea may attract fish that in turn carry bacteria to their desired nutritional niche, the fish gut. Indeed, a very high percentage of luminous bacteria can be found in marine fish gut flora (unpublished observation).

REVIEWS AND KEY PAPERS

Meighen, E. A., and P. V. Dunlap. 1993. Physiology biochemical and genetic control of bacterial bioluminescence. *Adv. Microbiol. Physiol.* **34:**1–67.

Sitnikov, D. M., J. B. Schineller, and T. O. Baldwin. 1995. Transcriptional regulation of bioluminescence genes from *Vibrio fischeri. Mol. Microbiol.* **17:**901–912.

Ulitzur, S., and P. Dunlap. 1995. Regulatory circuitry controlling luminescence autoinduction in *Vibrio fischeri. Photobiol. Photochem.* **62:**625–632.

REFERENCES

1. **Adar, Y., M. Siman, and S. Ulitzur.** 1992. Formation of the LuxR protein in the *Vibrio fischeri lux* system is controlled by HtpR through the GroESL proteins. *J. Bacteriol.* **174:**7138–7143.

2. **Adar, Y., and S. Ulitzur.** 1993. GroESL proteins facilitate binding of externally added inducer by LuxR protein containing *E. coli* cells. *J. Biolumin. Chemilumin.* **8:**261–266.

3. **Barak, M., and S. Ulitzur.** 1981. The induction of the bacterial luminescence system on solid media. *Curr. Microbiol.* **4:**597–601.

4. **Barth, M., C. Marschall, A. Muffler, D. Fischer, and R. Hengge-Aronis.** 1995. Role for the histone-like protein H-NS in growth phase-dependent and osmotic regulation of σ^S and many σ^S dependent genes in *Escherichia coli. J Bacteriol.* **177:**3455–3464.

5. **Choi, S. M., and E. P. Greenberg.** 1991. The C terminal region of *V. fischeri* LuxR protein contains an inducer-independent *lux* gene activating domain. *Proc. Natl. Acad. Sci. USA* **88:**11115–11119.

6. **Davine, J. H., G. S. Shadal, and T. O. Baldwin.** 1989. Identification of the operon of the operator of the *lux* regulon from the *V. fischeri* strain ATCC 7744. *Proc. Natl. Acad. Sci. USA* **86:**5689–5692.

7. **Dersch, P., K. Schmidt, and E. Bremer.** 1993. Synthesis of the *Escherichia coli* K-12 nucleoid-associated DNA-binding protein H-NS is subjected to growth-phase control and autoregulation. *Mol. Microbiol.* **8:**875–889.

8. **Dolan, K. M., and E. P. Greenberg.** 1992. Evidence that GroESL, not σ^{32}, is involved in

transcription regulation of the *Vibrio fischeri* luminescence genes in *Escherichia coli*. *J. Bacteriol.* **174:**5132–5135.

9. **Dunlap, P. V.** 1989. Regulation of luminescence by cAMP in *cya*-like and *crp*-like mutants of *Vibrio fischeri*. *J. Bacteriol.* **171:**1199–1202.

10. **Dunlap, P. V., and E. P. Greenberg.** 1985. Control of *Vibrio fischeri* luminescence gene expression in *Escherichia coli* by cAMP and cAMP receptor protein. *J. Bacteriol.* **164:**45–50.

11. **Dunlap, P. V., and E. P. Greenberg.** 1988. Control of *Vibrio fischeri lux* gene transcription by cAMP receptor protein-LuxR regulatory circuit. *J. Bacteriol.* **170:**4040–4046.

12. **Dunlap, P. V., and A. Kuo.** 1992. Cell density dependent modulation of the *Vibrio fischeri* luminescence system in the absence of autoinducer and LuxR protein *J. Bacteriol.* **174:**2440–2448.

13. **Eberhard, A., A. Burlingame, C. Eberhard, G. Kenyon, K. H. Nealson, and N. J. Oppenheimer.** 1981. Structural identification of autoinducer of *Photobacterium fischeri* luciferase. *Biochemistry* **20:**2444–2449.

14. **Engebrecht J., K. Nealson, and M. Silverman.** 1984. Identification of gene and gene products necessary for bacterial bioluminescence *Proc. Natl. Acad. Sci. USA* **81:**4154–4158

15. **Free, A., and C. Dorman.** 1995. Coupling of *Escherichia coli hns* mRNA levels to DNA synthesis by autoregulation: implications for growth phase control. *Mol. Microbiol.* **18:**101–113.

16. **Hulton, C. S. J., A. Seirafi, J. C. D. Hinton, J. M. Sidebortham, L. Waddell, G. D. Pavitt. T. Owen-Hughes, A. Spassky, H. Buc, and C. Higgins.** 1990. Histone like protein H1 (H-NS), DNA supercoiling, and gene expression in bacteria. *Cell* **63:**631–642.

17. **Kassen, I., P. Falkenberg, D. B. Styrvold, and A. R. Strom.** 1992. Molecular cloning and physical mapping of the *otsBA* genes, which encode the osmoregulatory trehalose pathway of *E. coli*: evidence that transcription is activated by KatF (AppR). *J. Bacteriol.* **174:**889–898.

18. **Kuo, A., N. V. Blough, and P. V. Greenberg.** 1994. Multiple *N*-acyl-homoserine lactone autoinducers of luminescence in the marine symbiotic bacterium *Vibrio fischeri*. *J. Bacteriol.* **176:**7558–7565.

19. **Levi, B.-Z., and S. Ulitzur.** 1983. Proflavin and norharman induce luciferase synthesis under anaerobiosis. *Arch. Mikrobiol.* **13:**281–284.

20. **Loewen, C. P., and R. Hengge-Aronis.** 1994. The role of the sigma factor σ^S (KatF) in bacterial global regulation. *Annu. Rev. Microbiol.* **48:**53–80.

21. **Mechthild, B., C. A. Marschall, D. Muffler, and R. Hengge-Aronis.** 1995. Role for the histone-like H-NS in growth phase-dependent and osmotic regulation of σ^S and many σ^S dependent genes in *Escherichia coli*. *J. Bacteriol.* **177:** 3455–3464.

22. **Meighen, E. A., and P. V. Dunlap.** 1993. Physiology biochemical and genetic control of bacterial bioluminescence. *Adv. Microbiol. Physiol.* **34:**1–67.

23. **Muller-Breitkreutz, K., and U. K. Winkler.** 1993. Anaerobic expression of *Vibrio fischeri lux* regulon in *E. coli* is Fnr-dependent. *J. Biolumin. Chemilumin.* **8:**108.

24. **Nealson, K. H., and J. W. Hastings.** 1992. The luminous bacteria, p. 625–639. *In* A. Balows, H. G. Truper, M. Dworkin, W. Harder, and W. K. H. Schleifer (ed.), *The Prokaryotes*, 2nd ed. Springer-Verlag, Berlin.

25. **Newman, E. B., R. T. Lin, and R. D'Ari.** 1996. The leucine/Lrp regulon, p. 1513–1525. *In* F. C. Neidhardt, R. Curtiss III, J. L. Ingraham, E. C. C. Lin, K. B. Low, Jr., B. Magasanik, W. S. Reznikoff, M. Riley, M. Schaechter, and H. E. Umbarger (ed.), *Escherichia coli and Salmonella*: *Cellular and Molecular Biology*, 2nd ed. American Society for Microbiology, Washington, D.C.

26. **Shadel, G. S., J. H. Devine, and T. O. Baldwin.** 1990. Control of the *lux* regulon of *Vibrio fischeri*. *J. Biolumin. Chemilumin.* **5:**99–106.

27. **Sitnikov, D. M., J. B. Schineller, and T. O. Baldwin.** 1995. Transcriptional regulation of bioluminescence genes from *Vibrio fischeri*. *Mol. Microbiol.* **17:**901–912.

28. **Stevens, A. M., K. M. Dolan, and E. P. Greenberg.** 1994. Synergistic binding of the *Vibrio fischeri* transcriptional activator domain and RNA polymerase to the *lux* promoter region. *Proc. Natl. Acad. Sci. USA* **91:**12619–12623.

29. **Ulitzur, S.** 1989. The regulatory control of the bacterial luminescence system: a new view. *J. Biolumin. Chemilumin.* **4:**317–325.

29a.**Ulitzur, S.** 1998. H-NS controls the transcription of three promoters of *Vibrio fischeri lux* cloned in *Escherichia coli*. *J. Biolumin. Chemilumin.* **13:**1–4.

29b.**Ulitzur, S.** 1998. LuxR controls the transcription of two promoters located upstream and downstream of *luxI* gene in *Vibrio fischeri lux* system. 10th International Symposium on Bioluminescence and Chemiluminescence, September 4–8, 1998, Bologna, Italy.

30. **Ulitzur, S., and P. Dunlap.** 1995. Regulatory circuitry controlling luminescence autoinduction in *Vibrio fischeri*. *Photobiol. Photochem.* **62:**625–632.

31. **Ulitzur, S., and J. Kuhn.** 1988. The transcription of bacterial luminescence is regulated by sigma 32. *J. Biolumin. Chemilumin.* **2:**81–93.

32. **Ulitzur, S., A. Matin, C. Fraley, and E. A. Meighen.** 1977. H-NS protein represses transcription of the *lux* systems of *Vibrio fischeri* and other luminous bacteria cloned into *Escherichia coli*. *Curr. Microbiol.* **35:**336–342.

33. **Ulitzur, S., and M. Osman.** 1994. The expression of the whole *lux* system of *Vibrio fischeri* in recombinant *Escherichia coli* at 37°C requires high ionic strength and the presence of either GroESL proteins or externally added inducer, p. 515–520. *In* A. K. Campbell, L. J. Kricka, and P. E. Stanley (ed.), *Bioluminescence and Chemiluminescence—Fundamentals and Applied Aspects*. John Wiley & Sons, Inc., New York.

34. **Ulitzur, S., M. Simaan, and J. Kuhn.** 1987. α-Subunit of bacterial luciferase inhibits the expression of the luminescence genes, p. 381–384. *In* J. Scholmerich, R. Andreesen, A. Kapp, M. Ernst, and W. G. Woods (ed.), *Bioluminescence and Chemiluminescence: New Perspectives*. John Wiley, Chichester.

35. **Ulitzur, S., and I. Weiser.** 1981. Acridine dyes and other DNA-intercalating agents induce luminescence in luminous bacteria and their dark variants. *Proc. Natl. Acad. Sci. USA* **78:**3338–3342.

36. **Wang, Q., and J. M. Calvo.** 1993. Lrp, a major regulatory protein of *Escherichia coli*, binds cooperatively to multiple sites and activates transcription of *ilv*H. *J. Mol. Biol.* **229:**306–318.

37. **Weiser, I., S. Ulitzur, and S. Yannai.** 1981. DNA damaging agents and DNA synthesis inhibitors induce luminescence in dark variants of luminous bacteria. *Mutat. Res.* **91:**443–450.

38. **Zambrano, M. M., D. Siegele, M. Almiron, A. Tormo, and R. Kolter.** 1993. Microbial competition: *Escherichia coli* mutants that take over stationary phase cultures. *Science* **259:**1757–1760.

DEATH BY DISINFECTION: MOLECULAR APPROACHES TO UNDERSTANDING BACTERIAL SENSITIVITY AND RESISTANCE TO FREE CHLORINE

Shimshon Belkin, Sam Dukan, Yves Levi, and Danièle Touati

Uncombined chlorine, in the form of unionized hypochlorous acid (HOCl), is an extremely potent bactericidal agent even at concentrations lower than 0.1 mg/liter (41). As a direct consequence, chlorination is the most widely used method for disinfection of water and wastewater. Nevertheless, the mechanism by which HOCl exerts its lethal effects on microorganisms has never been fully elucidated experimentally. Specific and general damage caused by exposure to free chlorine has been documented in many reports (4, 9, 12, 18, 19, 33, 34, 36, 38, 49, 50, 62, 63), but in most cases, it is difficult to differentiate between primary and secondary effects. Some of the more reactive hypochlorous acid targets seem to be membrane and protein associated (28, 52). They appear to be mostly protein amino and sulfhydryl groups (52), nonheme Fe/S clusters, cytochromes, and conjugated polyenes (31).

Recent data (24) indicate that the bactericidal effect of free chlorine may involve, at least in part, hydroxyl radicals generated by a Fenton-type reaction. It has also been shown that genes that are a part of *Escherichia coli*'s defenses against hydrogen peroxide are involved in free chlorine resistance, indicating a possible overlap in the defense circuits. A different set of experiments suggested a specific, *oxyR*-independent adaptive response to HOCl (24). This finding may be in agreement with an earlier observation (42) that starved bacteria exhibit increased resistance to disinfection, probably implicating, among others, the global regulatory circuit now known to be controlled by *rpoS* (37).

In contrast to bacterial responses to free chlorine, their ability to resist and to adapt to the presence of hydrogen peroxide has been extensively studied. In *E. coli*, a major regulatory circuit involved is the *oxyR* regulon (17, 35, 51). One of the genes positively regulated by the OxyR protein is *katG*, encoding the HPI catalase. Another catalase (HPII, *katE*) is regulated by *rpoS* (*katF*; 37); the latter circuit apparently functions in *katG* regulation as well (32). It has also been shown that hydrogen peroxide activates genes that are part of the heat shock (15, 44, 45, 57) and the SOS (61) responses.

Shimshon Belkin, Environmental Sciences, The Fredy & Nadine Herrmann Graduate School of Applied Science, The Hebrew University of Jerusalem, Jerusalem 91904, Israel. *Yves Levi*, Faculté de Pharmacie, Laboratoire Santé Publique—Environnement, Université Paris Sud, 5 rue J. B. Clément, 92296 Chatenay-Malabry Cedex, France. *Sam Dukan and Danièle Touati*, Institut Jacques Monod, CNRS-Universités Paris 7-Paris 6, 2 place Jussieu, 75251 Paris Cedex 05, France.

Microbial Ecology and Infectious Disease, Edited by Eugene Rosenberg
©1999 American Society for Microbiology, Washington, D.C.

Another major *E. coli* defense circuit in the fight against reactive oxygen species is *soxRS*, known to be activated by superoxide radicals (17, 35). Among the genes belonging to this regulon are *sodA*, coding for the Mn-superoxide dismutase (SOD) (53). Other global regulators involved, often with a considerable degree of overlap, are the *rpoH* (45), *rpoS* (37), *soxQ* (27), *fur*, *arcA*, *fnr* (16), and possibly other circuits.

To begin to decipher the mode of action of free chlorine, we have set out to examine the effects of this oxidant in several directions, two of which are described in this article.

First, we have attempted to identify the genes induced following a low-dosage HOCl exposure. Several genes, belonging to different regulatory systems known to be involved in the defenses against oxidative stress, were selected for this purpose. To monitor their induction in real time, we have used a set of plasmids on which the promoters of the studied genes were fused to the bioluminescence operon derived from the marine bacterium *Vibrio fischeri* (43). The parental plasmid used, pUCD615 (48), contained *luxCDABE* genes downstream from a multiple cloning site, into which promoters of the selected genes were inserted. Members of this set of plasmids have been previously described (6–8, 57–60), and the advantages of their uses as general and specific reporters for bacterial stress were documented.

Second, we have tried to study the involvement of O_2 in the damage inflicted by HOCl, especially in regard to the recovery process of injured cells. For this purpose, we have compared the survival of HOCl-treated aerobically and anaerobically grown *E. coli* cells, allowed to recover in the presence or absence of oxygen. To clarify the importance of oxygen in the recovery phase, the survival of mutants in different regulatory circuits was compared with that of the parental strains.

This chapter integrates results that were partly reported in more detail in a recent series of articles (22–24), along with others that have not been previously published (21). While at-tempting to summarize these data, it became all too apparent that the efforts to unravel some of the mystery surrounding a highly applied question relating to water disinfection may help to shed light on a similar phenomenon from a very remote field, highly relevant to the fight against infectious disease. The molecular mechanisms determining bacterial resistance and/or sensitivity to disinfection of drinking water must also be involved in the fight the same bacteria put up when challenged with the oxidative attack of macrophages; the tools used, as well as the results obtained in our studies of the former situation, may offer a most useful approach for addressing the latter.

EXPERIMENTAL APPROACH

To achieve the two goals described above, two complementary experimental approaches were used in the course of this study. First, we attempted to identify molecular defense systems that may be important in combating HOCl by exposing *E. coli* cells to *sublethal* HOCl concentrations, using *E. coli* strains containing different oxidative stress-responsive *lux* fusions. Second, we followed the recovery of culturability after *lethal* doses of HOCl to clarify the significance of oxygen and thus of antioxidative defenses in the recovery process. For that purpose, *E. coli* mutants defective in antioxidative defenses were compared.

Definition of "Lethal" and "Sublethal" Conditions

We have empirically defined "sublethal" as the conditions under which loss of culturability (colony formation on LB agar at 37°C) amounted to less than 50%. Since HOCl can be rapidly consumed by medium constituents as well as by the target cells themselves, the establishment of such conditions depends not only upon HOCl concentrations. At a cell density of 10^8/ml, in phosphate buffer (pH 7.0) at 26°C, HOCl concentrations up to 1 mg/liter conformed with that restriction (60 ± 20% survival at 1 mg/liter; 22). These were therefore the conditions used in the experiments described below in which activation of the different *lux*-fused defense circuits was monitored (Figs. 1–3 and Table 1). In the experiments described later in this article (Figs. 4 and 5), the conditions used were such that colony-forming ability of the wild-type strain was reduced by at least 99%.

Identification of Regulatory Circuits Activated by HOCl

Using the "sublethal" conditions described above, we attempted to identify the regulatory circuits activated upon exposure to HOCl. For this purpose, we have used plasmid-borne *lux* fusions, in which luminescence was driven by promoters of regulons known to be responsive to oxidative stress (Table 1). The *E. coli* genes thus tested were the heat shock gene *grpE*, *micF* (controlled by the redox regulon *soxRS*), *katG* (under *oxyR* control), *recA* (SOS), and the "universal stress protein" *uspA* (47).

As also indicated in Table 1, under our experimental conditions, only two of the five circuits were clearly activated within the first 2 h: the *rpoH*-controlled heat shock response, represented by *grpE*, and the *soxRS*-regulated "superoxide response," exemplified by *micF*. Figure 1 presents the kinetics of both responses, and Fig. 2 the dependency on HOCl concentration as well as on the designated regulatory circuit. Results similar to those obtained for *grpE* were obtained with two other *rpoH*-activated genes, *dnaK* and *lon* (22).

Induction of the heat shock system by free chlorine, demonstrated for the first time in this study, was not unexpected. Whether in response to a protein conformational change or as part of a more global effect, this system is readily activated by a variety of environmental insults. Induction of the *soxRS* circuit, however, was somewhat of a surprise, partly since the *soxRS* regulon was previously shown to be activated by one-electron reactions of either superoxide (17) or nitric oxide (46). Direct activation by hypochlorous acid, a two-electron redox agent, may be questionable, and an indirect induction pathway not involving superoxides seemed more likely. Indeed, the assumption that superoxides are not involved in this process was supported by the fact that the degree of activation of *micF′*::*lux* was not affected by a double superoxide dismutase (*sodA*, *sodB*) mutation (Fig. 3). More-circuitous support for the same suggestion was presented by the lack of *katG′*::*lux* induction by HOCl (Table 1): it had previously been shown that *oxyR* is induced by superoxides (6), apparently due to SOD-dependent dismutation of the superoxide radicals to hydrogen peroxide. Lack of *oxyR* induction, therefore, suggests that HOCl treatment does not promote the immediate generation of superoxides.

A possible hypothesis to explain *soxRS* induction under these conditions may be that exposure to free chlorine limited the availability of compounds necessary to maintain SoxR in its reduced form, such as NADPH (40) or reduced flavodoxins or ferrodoxins. At least in vitro, plant and bacterial ferrodoxins were shown to be very sensitive to free chlorine (2). Whatever the true explanation, we are faced with the fact that exposure to hypochlorous acid, while it may not involve actual generation of superoxides, nevertheless activates the defense circuits against such radicals. As is shown below, this may be an important factor in the recovery process.

Colony-Forming Ability following HOCl Challenge

In the previous section, sublethal HOCl concentrations were used to identify defense circuits activated in the presence of free chlorine.

TABLE 1 HOCl activation of regulatory circuits involved in antioxidative defense

Circuit	Gene tested	Response
oxyR	*katG*	−
"Universal stress"	*uspA*	−
SOS	*recA*	−
soxRS	*micF*	+
rpoH (heat shock)	*grpE*	+

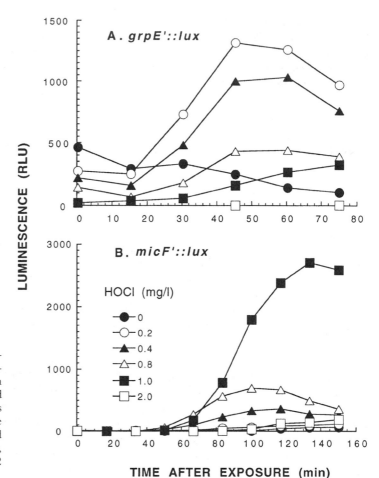

FIGURE 1 Luminescent responses of *grpE* (A) and *micF* promoter::*lux* fusions to a 20-min exposure to HOCl at the indicated concentrations. Luminescence values are arbitrary relative light units of the microtiter plate luminometer used (Lucy 1, Anthos Labtech, Salzburg, Austria). Adapted from reference 22 with permission.

Are these circuits the ones determining the survival of *E. coli* in response to higher doses of the oxidant? This question has not yet been fully addressed in regard to all of the regulons represented in Table 1. Thus, we have not yet tested whether heat shock mutations affect the sensitivity to HOCl treatment. Some of the results obtained so far, however, clearly corroborate those described above pertaining to other antioxidative response circuits. For instance, mutations in *oxyR* or in *recA* did not significantly affect survival, and a double catalase mutant (*katG katE*) did not exhibit a survival pattern significantly different from that of the wild type (24). Dramatic effects were observed, however, when the *recA* or *katG katE* mutants were further afflicted with

a *dps* mutation. The absence of this DNA-protecting protein (even by itself) increased HOCl lethality by several orders of magnitude (24).

In Fig. 4, a similar sensitivity pattern is exhibited by superoxide defenses. Whereas neither a *soxS* nor a double *sodA sodB* mutation significantly affected survival, the triple mutation had a striking effect. In spite of our earlier discussion concerning superoxides, therefore, it nevertheless seems that combating reactive oxygen species is important for surviving HOCl injury. It is possible, however, that this survival depends not only upon the type of damage inflicted by free chlorine; it is expected that a role will also be played by molecular adaptations that the cells have under-

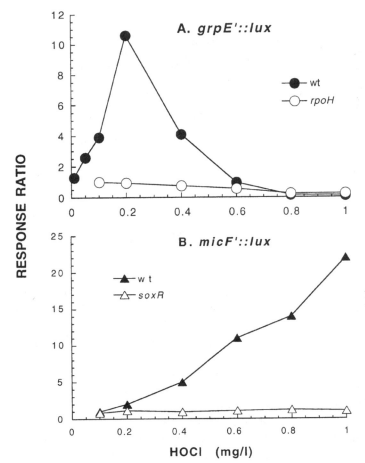

FIGURE 2 Dependency of the *grpE* (A) and *micF* (B) responses on HOCl concentration and on the intactness of the regulatory circuit. Values depict the ratios of the luminescence in the treated sample to that in the untreated control. Adapted from reference 22 with permission.

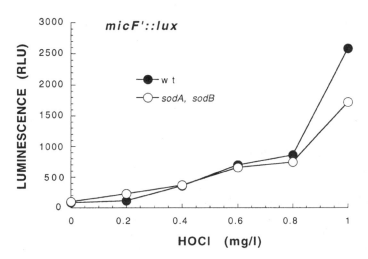

FIGURE 3 Superoxide dismutase mutations do not affect HOCl induction of *micF′::lux*. Adapted from reference 22 with permission.

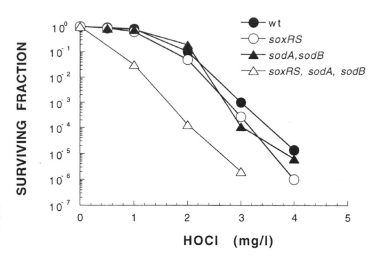

FIGURE 4 Survival of various *E. coli* mutants following a 20-min HOCl treatment at the designated concentrations. Initial cell density was 10^8 CFU/ml.

gone *before* treatment, as well as by conditions prevailing *after* it (i.e., during the recovery process). It was previously shown that H_2O_2 pretreatment promotes some HOCl resistance (24), and we have set out to find whether simple exposure to atmospheric concentrations of molecular oxygen also had a decisive influence. As demonstrated in Fig. 5, this was indeed the case, in two opposite manners: whereas aerobic growth before treatment had a beneficial adaptive influence (Fig. 5A), the presence of oxygen during the recovery period was deleterious (Fig. 5B). While the effect demonstrated in Fig. 5B may not appear dramatic, it was nevertheless clear and reproducible. In the presence of 4 mg of HOCl per liter, for instance, the ratio of anaerobic to aerobic survivors was 49 ± 14.3 (an average of four independent experiments) (21). The damaging effect of oxygen was more strongly manifested at the higher HOCl concentrations.

Following HOCl injury, therefore, the ability of some of the damaged cells to recover sufficiently to form a colony on a solid medium can be affected by the presence of oxygen. This is in good agreement with the results presented in Fig. 4, which highlighted the importance of superoxide defenses in the recovery phase. Indeed, direct superoxide assays indicated a fivefold increase in net cyto-plasmic radical production rates, from 0.24 to 1.19 nmol/min/mg of protein, following HOCl treatment that caused a 100-fold decrease in viability (21). This increase in steady-state superoxide levels is likely to be due to a decrease in the radical-scavenging capabilities of the culture, rather than to an increase in actual superoxide production rates. This assumption is supported by the observation that SOD activities were drastically reduced as a result of the same treatment, thus depleting the cells of essential protection at a time when it is sorely needed.

CONCLUSIONS

The results described in this chapter were obtained in the framework of a study aimed at understanding microbial responses in a very specific and highly stressed biotope, drinking water distribution systems after disinfection by free chlorine. The importance and practical aspects of the topic are obvious, since both sensitivity and resistance of bacteria to disinfection as well as the parameters governing subsequent regrowth have clear implications on drinking water quality.

Bacteria may face very similar challenges in a completely different environment, the vacuolar space of a phagocytic white blood cell, a macrophage. This mechanism for combating infectious agents uses strong oxidants, includ-

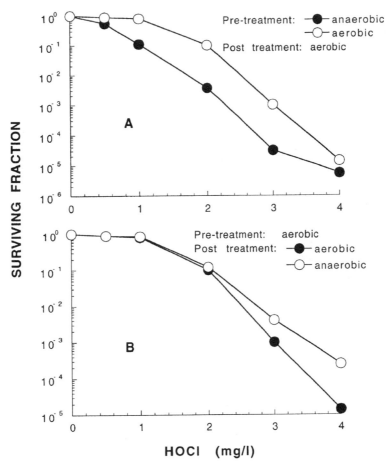

FIGURE 5 Aerobically grown cells are more resistant to HOCl treatment, but cells survive better anaerobically.

ing peroxides, superoxides, and even hypochlorous acid to "disinfect" the environment. As in the case of drinking water, the molecular mechanisms determining bacterial survival are far from being completely understood. Presently, intensive research efforts appear to be made in the medical direction, mostly because of the immediate implications of understanding microbial resistance to macrophage attack.

As a direct consequence of these research efforts, progress is continuously made in understanding the regulation of bacterial genes allowing survival in the hostile phagocyte milieu on the one hand and controlling the virulence to the host on the other hand. The bacterial functions involved in both of these aspects of infection are being defined, as are the genes responsible for these activities (1, 3, 5, 10, 11, 14, 20, 25, 26, 29, 30, 39, 54–56). An important trend in these studies is the increase in reported experimental attempts at in vivo identification of genes expressed and proteins synthesized following phagocytosis. One of the characteristics of the emerging pattern is that gene expression inside the macrophages differs from that in vitro experiments (1, 54), thereby reemphasizing the importance of in vivo analysis. Reporter gene technology has naturally found its uses in such studies (10, 14, 20, 25, 26, 30, 54–56). One of the exciting developments in this field is the use of *gfp* (the *Aequorea victoria* green fluorescent protein gene) (13) as a reporter in combination with fluorescence-activated cell sorting to select for genes preferentially expressed upon association with a host cell (55).

Investigations such as the one described here, though driven by completely different research targets, may nevertheless complement studies like those quoted above. In the search for answers to problems in water disinfection, they can also illuminate aspects of microbial sensitivity/resistance to macrophage attack. Furthermore, the approach used in our study—monitoring bacterial luminescence as a reporter on the activation of promoters of interest—can probably find immediate and fruitful uses in unraveling some of the mysteries surrounding life in a macrophage, possibly highlighting additional real-time quantitative and kinetic aspects.

REFERENCES

1. **Abshire, K. Z., and F. C. Neidhardt.** 1993. Analysis of proteins synthesized by *Salmonella typhimurium* during growth within a host macrophage. *J. Bacteriol.* **175:**3734–3743.
2. **Albrich, J. M., C. A. McCarthy, and J. K. Hurst.** 1981. Biological reactivity of hypochlorous acid: implications for microbicidal mechanisms of leukocyte myeloperoxidase. *Proc. Natl. Acad. Sci. USA* **78:**210–214.
3. **Barak, M., S. Ulitzur, and D. Merzbach.** 1983. Phagocytosis-induced mutagenesis in bacteria. *Mutat. Res.* **121:**7–16.
4. **Barrette, W. C., Jr., D. M. Hannum, W. D. Wheeler, and J. K. Hurst.** 1989. General mechanism for the bacterial toxicity of hypochlorous acid: abolition of ATP production. *Biochemistry* **28:**9172–9178.
5. **Baumler, A. J., J. G. Kusters, I. Stojiljkovic, and F. Heffron.** 1994. *Salmonella typhimurium* loci involved in survival within macrophages. *Infect. Immun.* **62:**1623–1630.
6. **Belkin, S., D. R. Smulski, A. C. Vollmer, T. K. Van Dyk, and R. A. LaRossa.** 1996. Oxidative stress detection with *Escherichia coli* bearing a *katG'::lux* fusion. *Appl. Environ. Microbiol.* **62:**2252–2256.
7. **Belkin, S., D. R. Smulski, S. Dadon, A. C. Vollmer, T. K. Van Dyk, and R. A. LaRossa.** 1997. A panel of stress-responsive lumi-

8. **Belkin, S., T. K. Van Dyk, A. C. Vollmer, D. R. Smulski, and R. A. LaRossa.** 1996. Monitoring sub-toxic environmental hazards by stress-responsive luminous bacteria. *Environ. Toxicol. Water Qual.* **11:**179–185.
9. **Bernarde, M. A., W. B. Snow, V. P. Olivieri, and B. Davidson.** 1967. Kinetics and mechanism of bacterial disinfection by chlorine dioxide. *Appl. Microbiol.* **15:**257–265.
10. **Buchmeier, N., S. Bossie, C. Y. Chen, F. C. Fang, D. G. Guiney, and S. J. Libby.** 1997. SlyA, a transcriptional regulator of *Salmonella typhimurium*, is required for resistance to oxidative stress and is expressed in the intracellular environment of macrophages. *Infect. Immun.* **65:**3725–3730.
11. **Buchmeier, N. A., and F. Heffron.** 1990. Induction of *Salmonella* stress proteins upon infection of macrophages. *Science* **248:**730–732.
12. **Camper, A. K., and G. A. McFeters.** 1979. Chlorine injury and the enumeration of waterborne coliform bacteria. *Appl. Environ. Microbiol.* **37:**633–641.
13. **Chalfie, M., Y. Tu, G. Euskirchen, W. W. Ward, and D. C. Prasher.** 1994. Green fluorescent protein as a marker for gene expression. *Science* **263:**802–805.
14. **Chen, C. Y., L. Eckmann, S. J. Libby, F. C. Fang, S. Okamoto, M. F. Kagnoff, J. Fierer, and D. G. Guiney.** 1996. Expression of *Salmonella typhimurium rpoS* and *rpoS*-dependent genes in the intracellular environment of eukaryotic cells. *Infect. Immun.* **64:**4739–4743.
15. **Christman, M. F., R. W. Morgan, F. S. Jacobson, and B. N. Ames.** 1985. Positive control of a regulon for defenses against oxidative stress and some heat shock proteins in *Salmonella typhimurium*. *Cell* **41:**753–762.
16. **Compan, I., and D. Touati.** 1993. Interaction of six global transcription regulators in expression of manganese superoxide dismutase in *Escherichia coli* K-12. *J. Bacteriol.* **175:**1687–1696.
17. **Demple, B.** 1991. Regulation of bacterial oxidative stress genes. *Annu. Rev. Genet.* **25:**315–337.
18. **Dennis, W. H., V. P. Olivieri, and C. W. Kruse.** 1979. The reaction of nucleotides with aqueous hypochlorous acid. *Water Res.* **13:**357–362.
19. **Dennis, W. H., V. P. Olivieri, and C. W. Kruse.** 1979. Mechanism of disinfection: incorporation of Cl-36 into f2 virus. *Water Res.* **13:**363–369.
20. **Dhandayuthapani, S., L. E. Via, C. A. Thomas, P. M. Horowitz, D. Deretic, and V.**

7. (continued) nous bacteria for toxicity detection. *Water Res.* **31:**3009–3016.

Deretic. 1995. Green fluorescent protein as a marker for gene expression and cell biology of mycobacterial interactions with macrophages. *Mol. Microbiol.* **17:**901–912.

21. **Dukan, S., S. Belkin, and D. Touati.** Unpublished.

22. **Dukan, S., S. Dadon, D. R. Smulski, and S. Belkin.** 1996. Hypochlorous acid activates the heat shock and *soxRS* systems of *Escherichia coli*. *Appl. Environ. Microbiol.* **62:**4003–4008.

23. **Dukan, S., Y. Levi, and D. Touati.** 1997. Recovery of culturability of an HOCl-stressed population of *Escherichia coli* after incubation in phosphate buffer: resuscitation or regrowth? *Appl. Environ. Microbiol.* **63:**4204–4209.

24. **Dukan, S., and D. Touati.** 1996. Hypochlorous acid stress in *Escherichia coli*: resistance, DNA damage, and comparison with hydrogen peroxide stress. *J. Bacteriol.* **178:**6145–6150.

25. **Francis, K. P., and M. P. Galllagher.** 1993. Light emission from a Mudlux transcriptional fusion in *Salmonella typhimurium* is stimulated by hydrogen peroxide and by interaction with the mouse macrophage cell line J774.2. *Infect. Immun.* **61:**640–649.

26. **Francis, K. P., P. D. Taylor, C. J. Inchley, and M. P. Galllagher.** 1997. Identification of the *ahp* operon of *Salmonella typhimurium* as a macrophage-induced locus. *J. Bacteriol.* **179:** 4046–4048.

27. **Greenberg, J. T., J. H. Chou, P. A. Monach, and B. Demple.** 1991. Activation of oxidative stress genes by mutations at the *soxQ/cfxB/marA* locus of *Escherichia coli*. *J. Bacteriol.* **173:**4433–4439.

28. **Hannum, D. M., W. C. Barrette, Jr., and J. K. Hurst.** 1995. Subunit sites of oxidative inactivation of *Escherichia coli* F1-ATPase by HOCl. *Biochem. Biophys. Res. Commun.* **212:**868–874.

29. **Hassett, D. J., and M. S. Cohen.** 1989. Bacterial adaptation to oxidative stress: implications for pathogenesis and interaction with phagocytic cells. *FASEB J.* **3:**2574–2582.

30. **Heithoff, D. M., C. P. Conner, P. C. Hanna, S. M. Julio, U. Hentschel, and M. J. Mahan.** 1997. Bacterial infection as assessed by *in vivo* gene expression. *Proc. Natl. Acad. Sci. USA* **94:**934–939.

31. **Hurst, J. K., W. C. Barrette, Jr., B. R. Michel, and H. Rosen.** 1991. Hypochlorous acid and myeloperoxidase catalyzed oxidation of iron sulfur clusters in bacterial respiratory dehydrogenases. *Eur. J. Biochem.* **202:**1275–1282.

32. **Ivanova, A., C. Miller, G. Glinski, and A. Eisenstark.** 1994. Role of *rpoS* (*katF*) in *oxyR*-independent regulation of hydroperoxidase I in *Escherichia coli*. *Mol. Microbiol.* **12:**571–578.

33. **Jacangelo, J. G., and V. P. Olivieri.** 1985. Aspects of the mode of action of monochloramine. *Water Chlorination* **5:**575–586.

34. **Jacangelo, J. G., and V. P. Olivieri.** 1987. Oxidation of sulfhydryl groups by monochloramine. *Water Res.* **21:**1339–1344.

35. **Jamieson, D. J., and G. Storz.** 1997. Transcriptional regulators of oxidative stress responses, p. 91–115. *In* J. G. Scandalios (ed.), *Oxidative Stress and the Molecular Biology of Antioxidant Defenses*. Cold Spring Harbor Laboratory Press, Plainview, N.Y.

36. **Knox, W. E., P. K. Stumpf, D. E. Green, and Y. H. Auerbach.** 1948. The inhibition of sulfhydryl enzymes as the basis of the bacterial action of chlorine. *J. Bacteriol.* **55:**451–458.

37. **Lange, R., and R. Hengge-Aronis.** 1991. Identification of a central regulator of stationary-phase gene expression in *Escherichia coli*. *Mol. Microbiol.* **5:**49–59.

38. **Larson, R. A., and A. L. Rockwell.** 1979. Chloroform and chlorophenol production by decarboxylation of natural acids during aqueous chlorination. *Environ. Sci. Technol.* **13:**325–329.

39. **Lee, C. A., B. D. Jones, and S. Falkow.** 1992. Identification of a *Salmonella typhimurium* invasion locus by selection for hyperinvasive mutants. *Proc. Natl. Acad. Sci. USA* **89:**1847–1851.

40. **Liochev, S. I., A. Hausladen, W. F. Beyer, and I. Fridovich.** 1994. NADPH:ferredoxin oxidoreductase acts as a paraquat diaphorase and is a member of the *sox* regulon. *Proc. Natl. Acad. Sci. USA* **91:**1328–1331.

41. **Ludovici, P. P., R. A. Phillips, and W. S. Jeter.** 1977. Comparative inactivation of bacteria and viruses in tertiary-treated wastewater by chlorination, p. 359–390. *In* J. D. Johnson (ed.), *Disinfection: Water and Wastewater*. Ann Arbor Science, Ann Arbor, Mich.

42. **Matin, A., and S. Harakeh.** 1990. Effect of starvation on bacterial resistance to disinfectants, p. 88–103. *In* G. A. McFeters (ed.), *Drinking Water Microbiology*. Springer-Verlag, New York.

43. **Meighen, E. M., and P. V. Dunlap.** 1993. Physiological, biochemical and genetic control of bacterial bioluminescence. *Adv. Microb. Physiol.* **34:**1–67.

44. **Morgan, R. W., M. F. Christman, F. S. Jacobson, G. Storz, and B. N. Ames.** 1986. Hydrogen peroxide inducible proteins in *Salmonella typhimurium* overlap with heat shock and other stress proteins. *Proc. Natl. Acad. Sci. USA* **83:**8059–8063.

45. **Neidhardt, F. C., and R. H. VanBogelen.** 1987. Heat shock response, p. 1334–1345. *In* F. C. Neidhardt, J. L. Ingraham, K. B. Low, B. Magasanik, M. Schaechter, and H. E. Umbarger

(ed.), *Escherichia coli and Salmonella typhimurium*: *Cellular and Molecular Biology*. American Society for Microbiology, Washington, D.C.

46. **Nunoshiba, T., T. deRojas-Walker, J. S. Wishnok, S. R. Tannenbaum, and B. Demple.** 1993. Activation by nitric oxide of an oxidative-stress response that defends *Escherichia coli* against activated macrophages. *Proc. Natl. Acad. Sci. USA* **90**:9993–9997.

47. **Nystrom, T., and F. C. Neidhardt.** 1994. Expression and role of the universal stress protein, UspA, of *Escherichia coli* during growth arrest. *Mol. Microbiol.* **11**:537–544.

48. **Rogowsky, P. M., T. J. Close, J. A. Chimera, J. J. Shaw, and C. I. Kado.** 1987. Regulation of the *vir* genes of *Agrobacterium tumefaciens* plasmid pTiC58. *J. Bacteriol.* **169**:5101–5112.

49. **Shih, K. L., and J. Lederberg.** 1976. Effects of chloramine on *Bacillus subtilis* deoxyribonucleic acid. *J. Bacteriol.* **125**:934–945.

50. **Sips, H. J., and M. N. Hamers.** 1981. Mechanism of the bacterial action of myeloperoxidase: increased permeability of the *Escherichia coli* cell envelope. *Infect. Immun.* **31**:11–16.

51. **Storz, G., L. A. Tartaglia, S. B. Farr, and B. N. Ames.** 1990. Bacterial defenses against oxidative stress. *Trends Genet.* **6**:363–368.

52. **Thomas, E. L.** 1979. Myeloperoxidase, hydrogen peroxide, chloride antimicrobial system: nitrogen chlorine derivatives of bacterial components in bacterial action against *Escherichia coli*. *Infect. Immun.* **23**: 522–531.

53. **Touati, D.** 1997. Superoxide dismutases in bacteria and pathogen protists, p. 447–493. *In* J. G. Scandalios (ed.), *Oxidative Stress and the Molecular Biology of Antioxidant Defenses*. Cold Spring Harbor Laboratory Press, Plainview, N.Y.

54. **Valdivia, R. H., and S. Falkow.** 1996. Bacterial genetics by flow cytometry: rapid isolation of *Salmonella typhimurium* acid-inducible promoters by differential fluorescence induction. *Mol. Microbiol.* **22**:367–378.

55. **Valdivia, R. H., and S. Falkow.** 1997. Fluorescence-based isolation of bacterial genes expressed within host cells. *Science* **277**:2007–2011.

56. **Valdivia, R. H., A. E. Hromockyj, D. Monack, L. Ramakrishanan, and S. Falkow.** 1996. Applications for green fluorescent protein (GFP) in the study of host-pathogen interactions. *Gene* **173**:47–52.

57. **Van Dyk, T. K., W. R. Majarian, K. B. Konstantinov, R. M. Young, P. S. Dhurjati, and R. A. LaRossa.** 1994. Rapid and sensitive pollutant detection by induction of heat shock gene-bioluminescence gene fusions. *Appl. Environ. Microbiol.* **60**:1414–1420.

58. **Van Dyk, T. K., T. R. Reed, A. C. Vollmer, and R. A. LaRossa.** 1995. Synergistic induction of the heat shock response in *Escherichia coli* by simultaneous treatment with chemical inducers. *J. Bacteriol.* **177**:6001–6004.

59. **Van Dyk, T. K., D. R. Smulski, T. R. Reed, S. Belkin, A. C. Vollmer, and R. A. LaRossa.** 1995. Responses to toxicants of an *Escherichia coli* strain carrying a *uspA'::lux* genetic fusion and an *E. coli* strain carrying a *grpE'::lux* fusion are similar. *Appl. Environ. Microbiol.* **61**: 4124–4127.

60. **Vollmer, A. C., S. Belkin, D. R. Smulski, T. K. Van Dyk, and R. A. LaRossa.** 1997. Detection of DNA damage by use of *Escherichia coli* carrying *recA'::lux*, *uvrA'::lux*, or *alkA'::lux* reporter plasmids. *Appl. Environ. Microbiol.* **63**: 2566–2571.

61. **Walker, G. C.** 1987. The SOS response of *Escherichia coli*, p. 1400–1416. *In* F. C. Neidhart, R. Curtis III, J. L. Ingraham, E. C. C. Lin, K. B. Low, B. Magasanik, W. S. Reznikoff, M. Riley, M. Schaechter and H. E. Umbarger (ed.) *Escherichia coli and Salmonella: Cellular and Molecular Biology*, 2nd ed. American Society for Microbiology, Washington, D.C.

62. **Wenkobachar, C., L. Iyengar and A. V. S. P. Rav.** 1975. Mechanism of disinfection. *Water Res.* **9**:119–124.

63. **Wenkobachar, C., L. Iyengar, and A. V. S. P. Rav.** 1977. Mechanism of disinfection: effect of chlorine on cell membrane function. *Water Res.* **11**:727–729.

CONTROL ELEMENTS IN THE REGULATION OF BACTERIAL HEAT SHOCK RESPONSE

Eliora Z. Ron, Gil Segal, Marc Robinson, and Dan Graur

12

The heat shock response is a global regulatory network found in all living cells. It involves the induction of many proteins—called heat shock proteins, or Hsps—in response to elevation of temperature (56). Many of the heat shock proteins, such as chaperones and proteases, are important for overcoming changes that involve protein denaturation. The same proteins are also induced by other environmental changes, such as the addition of ethanol, heavy metals, high osmolarity, pollutants, starvation, or interaction with eukaryotic hosts (5, 26, 51, 76, 77). Therefore, the heat shock response can be considered a general stress response. In bacteria, the heat shock response is essential for adaptation to elevated temperatures and to stressful environmental conditions. Induction of this response improves thermotolerance, salt tolerance, and tolerance to heavy metals (29, 37, 38, 58, 78). Moreover, in several bacterial species, heat shock proteins have been shown to play an important role in pathogenesis (31, 36, 39, 44, 66, 67). For example, virulence of *Listeria mono-* *cytogenes* involves the heat shock protein lysteriolysin (7, 32, 35, 47, 73), and heat shock proteins are required for binding of *Salmonella typhimurium* to mucosal cells (19) and for survival within macrophages (3). Heat shock response was also implicated in pathogenesis of *Helicobacter pylori* (17), *Mycobacterium leprae*, *Mycobacterium tuberculosis* (48), *Legionella pneumophila* (21, 45), *Chlamydia trachomatis* (9) and *Brucella abortus* (18). Recent results indicated that heat shock proteins are also essential for stationary phase (51) and for differentiation of myxobacteria and *Bacillus subtilis* (16, 80). These findings indicate that the heat shock response is a central control system that is vital for all aspects of bacterial life. Moreover, the heat shock response is critical for bacterial adaptation to changes in the environment, whether as free living organisms or in association with eukaryotic hosts, and is therefore one of the major links between microbial ecology and microbial pathogenesis.

The heat shock response controls the expression of more than 15 genes, possibly as many as 26 genes (12, 56), that code for chaperones, proteases, and regulatory proteins. The induced proteins are similar in all organisms, and several of them are highly conserved in evolution. Two of these proteins, Hsp70 (the product of the bacterial *dnaK* gene) and the

Eliora Z. Ron and Gil Segal, Department of Molecular Microbiology and Biotechnology, *and Marc Robinson and Dan Graur*, Department of Zoology, George S. Wise Faculty of Life Sciences, Tel Aviv University, Tel Aviv, Israel 69978.

Microbial Ecology and Infectious Disease, Edited by Eugene Rosenberg
©1999 American Society for Microbiology, Washington, D.C.

Hsp10+Hsp60 complex (products of the *groESL* operon), show about 40% homology in amino acids from bacteria to mammals (8, 25). These proteins act as chaperones, maintaining the correct folding of cellular proteins. Because these chaperone proteins are physiologically important, are produced in very high levels under all conditions, and constitute major bacterial antigens, they have been extensively studied in many organisms, including a large number of bacterial species. Therefore, more data are available about the *groE* and *dnaK* genes and on the Hsp60 and Hsp70 proteins than about any other heat shock gene or protein, and the models concerning the heat shock response and its regulation are largely based on these data. The present review is also based mainly on results obtained from studies of the genes and products of the *groE* and *dnaK* operons, the major shock operons. Our understanding of the heat shock response and its control still lacks experimental results from other heat shock genes and operons.

In bacteria, an additional regulatory system exists that is activated by high temperatures. The best-studied gene activated by this system is *htrA*, whose product is essential for bacterial growth only at elevated temperatures (41, 42, 57). This system is activated by σ^E, a second heat shock sigma factor encoded by the *rpoE* gene (20, 28, 59, 62). This gene is also important for pathogenesis and was shown to control mucoidy in cystic fibrosis isolates of *Pseudomonas aeruginosa* (66). This system is much more limited in the number of genes that are involved and the stresses it responds to. The two heat-induced systems are connected in more than one way.

TRANSCRIPTIONAL ACTIVATION OF SPECIFIC HEAT-SHOCK PROMOTERS BY AN ALTERNATIVE SIGMA FACTOR (HEAT-SHOCK SIGMA FACTOR, RpoH, OR σ^{32})

The first and most extensive studies on bacterial heat shock response were performed in *Escherichia coli*. The heat-shock genes in *E. coli* K-12 have specific heat shock promoters, rec-

ognized by the heat shock sigma factor (σ^{32}, the product of the *rpoH* gene) that acts as a transcriptional activator (6, 13, 14, 46, 74). Although the *rpoH* gene is transcriptionally activated when the temperature is elevated, the major control of its expression is posttranscriptional, regulated at several levels including proteolysis (34, 46, 54, 83). In *E. coli*, σ^{32} has a short half-life and is degraded by a specific protease, the product of the *hflB* (*ftsH*) gene (23, 27, 34, 75). Damaged proteins produced upon a shift to a higher temperature, or exposure to other conditions that bring about protein denaturation initiate a cascade of events that brings about stabilization of σ^{32} and preferential expression of heat shock genes (10, 11, 22, 24, 33, 34, 37).

In *E. coli*, transcriptional activation of heat shock genes by σ^{32} is the only known control of the major heat shock operons. In the last few years, it became clear that the regulation of heat shock genes in other bacteria is more complex. For example, in gram-positive bacteria, there are at least three regulons of heat-shock genes, only one of which is activated by a specific heat shock sigma factor, σ^B (26).

TRANSCRIPTIONAL ACTIVATION BY RELEASE OF REPRESSION INVOLVING AN INVERTED REPEAT (IR, CIRCE) AND A REPRESSOR PROTEIN (PRODUCT OF THE *hrcA* GENE)

In most bacterial species there exists another transcriptional control system that regulates expression of one or more of the heat shock genes. This transcriptional control is mediated by an inverted repeat located at the upstream regulatory region of heat shock operons. This inverted repeat (IR)—also called CIRCE (controlling IR of chaperone expression)—acts as a binding site for a protein repressor, Orf39 (or OrfA, in *B. subtilis*), the product of the *hrcA* gene. Deletion of the IR results in constitutive expression of the operon (2, 26, 30, 50, 61, 65, 68, 71, 72, 81, 82, 85).

The IR is highly conserved, as demonstrated in Table 1. So far it was found only in

TABLE 1 The conserved inverted repeat in *groE* operons

Mycobacterium tuberculosis	cTAGCACTC-N9-GAGTGCTAg
Staphylococcus aureus	TTAGCACTC-N9-aAGTGCTAA
Bacillus subtilis	TTAGCACTC-N9-GAGTGCTAA
Chlamydia pneumoniae	TTAGCACT t-N9-GAGTGCTAA
Brucella abortus	TTAGCACTC-N9-GAGTGCTAA
Bordetella pertussis	TTAGCACTC-N9-GAGTGCTAA

the upstream region of *groE*, *dnaK* and *dnaJ* operons or genes, all of them coding for the major chaperones. However, as mentioned above, these major chaperones are highly significant in bacterial physiology and pathogenicity and constitute dominant antigens, and therefore, sequence data are available from bacteria belonging to most phylogenetic groups. Since not much is known about other heat shock genes, it is still impossible to determine if the IR is unique to operons coding for chaperones.

The bacteria that use the IR as a control element can be divided into two groups, with respect to the types of regulatory systems. The first regulatory system has been demonstrated in several gram-positive bacteria of the low-G+C group. In these bacteria all the operons coding for chaperones are transcribed by the vegetative sigma factor—σ^{70} or σ^{A}—and the IR regulates this transcription.

The second regulatory system has been demonstrated in bacteria belonging to the α-purple proteobacteria: *Agrobacterium tumefaciens*, *Bradyrhizobium japonicum*, and *Caulobacter crescentus*. In these bacteria, the heat shock operons contain a specific heat shock promoter that is unique and differs from the vegetative promoter and from the heat shock promoter of *E. coli* (69). This promoter is recognized by a heat shock sigma factor (σ^{32}-like factor) that activates the genes (49, 55, 69). Several, but not all, of the heat shock operons contain the conserved IR in addition and respond to the Orf39 repressor (1, 68). From the available data, it appears that in bacteria that control heat shock transcription by a combination of a heat shock sigma factor and a repressor-

binding IR, the latter is not present in *dnaK* operons. In these bacteria, the IR element is present in the *groE* operon or in at least one of the *groE* operons in bacteria that have more than one such operon (49, 72). The significance of this finding is not yet understood.

TRANSCRIPTIONAL ACTIVATION OF HEAT SHOCK GENES IN THE ALPHA SUBDIVISION OF PROTEOBACTERIA (α-PURPLE PROTEOBACTERIA)

The alpha subdivision of proteobacteria, α-purple proteobacteria, contains a large group of well-studied bacteria. These include bacteria of industrial importance, such as *Zymomonas* and *Acetobacter*, and bacteria with unusual cell cycles, such as *Caulobacter*. To this subdivision belong several groups of nitrogen fixers, such as *Rhodospirillum* and *Azospirillum*, as well as the plant symbionts *Rhizobium* and *Bradyrhizobium*. This subdivision also contains important human pathogens, such as *Brucella* and *Rickettsia* and plant pathogens such as *Agrobacterium tumefaciens*.

The heat shock operons of α-purple proteobacteria are activated by a σ^{32}-like transcription factor that recognizes heat shock promoters. This heat shock promoter was identified by comparing nine sequences of known heat shock operons from bacteria belonging to the α-purple proteobacteria (69). These operons include six *groESL* operons from *B. abortus*, *A. tumefaciens*, *C. crescentus*, *B. japonicum*, *Rhizobium meliloti*, and *Zymomonas mobilis* and three *dnaK* operons from *A. tumefaciens*, *C. crescentus*, and *Brucella bovis*. From these data, a consensus promoter sequence could be deduced. This putative consensus promoter is different from both the vegetative and the heat shock promoter consensus sequences of *E. coli* (Table 2).

The identification of a unique heat shock promoter is compatible with the finding that the heat-shock activator (σ^{32}-like factor) of the α-purple proteobacteria differs from its homolog of the γ-purple proteobacteria in several aspects, including the sites responsible for promoter recognition (Table 2) (53, 54, 69). The promoter-recognition domain of the vegetative sigma factor (σ^{70}) is quite similar between the two groups, as expected from the similarity of the vegetative promoters.

Transcriptional activation of the *dnaK* operons of the α-purple proteobacteria is presumably carried out by the heat shock sigma factor, since no other control element has been identified in any of them. The situation is different in the *groE* operons, specifically in those that contain the CIRCE element. The roles of each of the control elements in the regulation of *groE* transcription was studied in *A. tumefaciens*, a plant pathogen that belongs to the group of α-purple bacteria. Introduction of mutations and deletions that decreased the stability of the putative "stem" formed by the IR resulted in increased transcription of the operon under non–heat-shock conditions but did not decrease the level of heat shock

activation (71). This situation differs from that in the gram-positive bacteria, in which the IR actually controls heat shock activation.

We therefore assume that in bacteria that have a complex heat shock control consisting of an alternative sigma factor and a regulatory IR (e.g., α-purple bacteria), the heat shock sigma factor is responsible for heat shock activation of the operon, and the IR control system is involved in maintaining a low level of expression under non–heat-shock conditions.

STABILIZATION OF TRANSCRIPTS OF HEAT SHOCK GENES

The two control mechanisms described above act at the level of transcription. Two additional regulatory elements of the heat shock response are posttranscriptional. The finding that the IR can be transcribed raised the possibility that it is also active at the mRNA level. Evidence for this activity was obtained in *B. subtilis* and *A. tumefaciens* (71, 81). In *A. tumefaciens*, the half-life of the *groEL* transcript increased twofold when deletions were introduced into the IR. The deletions were found to increase the half-life of the transcript under non–heat-shock conditions (71). These results indicate that when it is transcribed, the IR functions at the level of the RNA as well as at the level of the DNA. In both situations, it

TABLE 2 Putative heat-shock promoters and promoter recognition domains of σ^{32} and σ^{70} in α-purple and γ-purple proteobacteria

Putative promoters			
α-Purple proteobacteria heat shock promoter	CTTG	⟨17/18⟩	CYTAT-T
γ-Purple proteobacteria heat shock promoter	TCTC-CCTTGAA	⟨13/14⟩	CCCAT-AT
γ-Purple proteobacteria vegetative promoter	TTGACA	⟨17⟩	TATAAT

Promoter recognition domains		
	2.4	4.2
α-Purple proteob. σ^{32}	IKA**SIQ**EYILR**SWSL**VK**M**GTT	YGVS**R**ERVRQ**IEK**R**AMKKLR
γ-Purple proteob. σ^{32}	IKA**EIH**EYVLR**NWRI**VK**V**ATT	YGVS**A**ERVRQ**LEK**N**AMKKLR
	* * * * **	* * *
α-Purple proteob. σ^{70}	IRQAITRSIADQARTIRIPVHM	F**S**VTRERIRQIEAKALRNV**K**
γ-Purple proteob. σ^{70}	IRQAITRSIADQARTIRIPVHM	F**D**VTRERIRQIEAKALRNV**R**
		* *

decreases the expression of the operon under non–heat-shock conditions.

PROCESSING OF TRANSCRIPTS OF HEAT SHOCK GENES TO FACILITATE DIFFERENTIAL EXPRESSION

An additional posttranscriptional control mechanism was demonstrated in *A. tumefaciens* and involves specific cleavage of the *groESL* operon transcript between the *groES* and the *groEL* genes (70). The resulting *groES* transcript is rapidly degraded, while the *groEL* transcript is stable. The outcome of this cleavage is differential expression of the two genes of the operon. This mRNA processing is temperature dependent and is probably the first example of controlled processing of transcripts in bacteria.

The result of this process is that GroEL is produced at higher levels than GroES. The physiological significance of this is not yet understood. However, many bacteria have molecular mechanisms that result in more GroEL than GroES. This is achieved by having more genes coding for GroEL than for GroES or having several *groE* operons, not all of which contain the *groES* gene (1, 15, 72).

PHYLOGENETIC ASPECTS

An interesting question is how and when the various control systems evolved. For a comprehensive understanding, more data are needed. For example, the genes coding for alternative sigma factors have been cloned and sequenced from only a few bacteria, all belonging to the α-purple bacteria and γ-purple bacteria (4, 52, 53, 60, 63, 79). In addition, it appears that the IR was lost in many *dnaK* operons, but in many cases the upstream sequences available are too short to be certain that this structure is indeed absent. Nevertheless, several interesting conclusions can be drawn from available information, especially from data on the *groE* operons.

Figure 1 shows a phylogenetic tree based on the nonsynonymous substitutions of *groE*. The phylogenetic relationships obtained are the same as these obtained from sequences of the small RNA subunit. The data indicate that the control system involving the repressor-binding IR (CIRCE) is probably the ancient control mechanism and was lost in evolution only twice—once in the $\gamma 2/\gamma 3$-purple bacteria and once in *H. pylori*, of the δ-purple bacteria. It should be noted that in *Campylobacter jejuni*, also of the δ-subdivision of proteobacteria, the IR of the *groE* operon was retained.

UNRESOLVED PROBLEMS AND OPEN QUESTIONS

The most important unresolved problem concerning the heat shock response is what triggers this response at the molecular level. It remains to be determined if—or how—temperature elevation or other environmental stresses affect the regulatory IR, its repressor, or the interaction of the two components. It may be even more difficult to explain the triggering of the σ^{32}-dependent cascade of events. It has been assumed that the transcriptional activator σ^{32} (RpoH) is stabilized at high temperatures, concurrently with the increased level of denatured proteins and decreased availability of the major chaperones. However, studies of mutants with the *rpoH* gene deleted indicate that the heat shock response is already active at temperatures as low as 22°C (84). Clearly, this range of temperatures is too low to support the assumption that only temperature-denatured proteins trigger the heat shock response.

Other questions have to do with the fact that so far most of the information has been obtained on very few heat shock genes and proteins. Additional information is required before comprehensive models can be constructed. For example, one interesting control element is the temperature-dependent cleavage of the *groESL* transcript of *A. tumefaciens* resulting in differential expression of the two genes. Is this mechanism unique to *A. tumefaciens* or to the *groESL* operon? Are there additional controlled transcript-cleavage mechanisms in other bacteria or other operons?

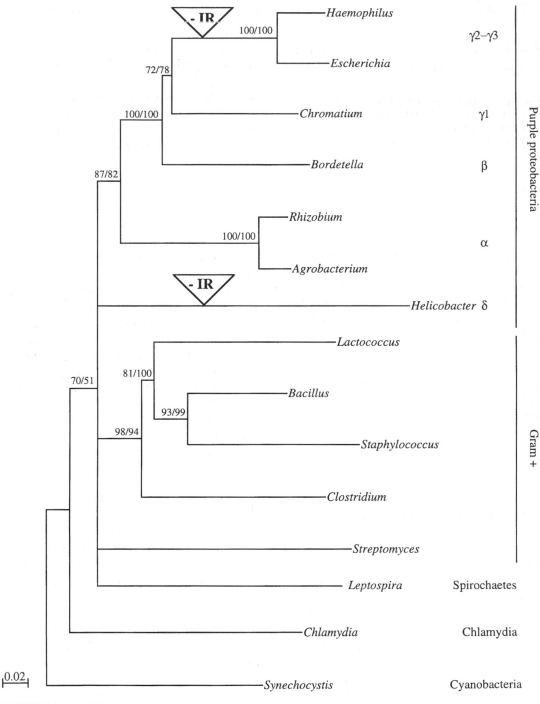

FIGURE 1 *groES/groEL* phylogeny obtained by neighbor-joining (64) with the Ka distance of Li (40). Shown above nodes are the bootstrap values (in %) obtained with 1,000 repetitions for concatenated genes *groES+ groEL* (left of slash) as well as bootstrap values for the same nodes with 16S rRNA sequences (neighbor-joining with the LogDet distance [43]), right of slash. Nodes supported by bootstrap values smaller than 50% with *groE* sequences are resolved differently by *groE* and by 16S rRNA sequences and are indicated as unresolved. Bootstrap values for 16S rRNA sequences are indicated for analysis with complete sequences only (1271 sites), the bootstrap value for the branch leading to *Haemophilus* and *Escherichia* is based on 861 aligned basepairs. Arrows indicate losses of the inverted repeat in *groE*. The scale bar represents 0.02 nonsynonymous substitutions per site.

What is the physiological/molecular reason for the differential expression of these two genes that code for proteins that are presumably working together in complexes? There is no obvious physiological explanation for the excess of GroEL over GroES, yet, as discussed above, such an excess is achieved by several different mechanisms in bacteria.

So far there are extensive experiments on *E. coli*, which uses only σ^{32} activation of heat shock promoters, and on *B. subtilis*, which has at least three regulons for heat shock response genes and in which the operons coding for Hsp60 and Hsp70 are transcribed by the vegetative sigma factor and activated by CIRCE. Many bacterial groups appear to combine the two control elements; the *dnaK* and *groE* operons appear to be activated by an alternative heat shock sigma factor but there is also an IR control element that represses the heat shock genes (or only the *groESL* operon?) in non-heat-shock conditions. Very little information is available about the control of operons other than *groE* and *dnaK* in these organisms.

Several phylogenetic questions are still unresolved, mainly because sequences are available only from a limited number of bacteria. Did the control start with a CIRCE element in all heat shock operons, to be replaced later by σ^{32} activation? When did the alternative heat shock sigma factor emerge? What are the advantages of having each of the control elements involved in the heat shock response?

ACKNOWLEDGMENTS

This work was supported in part by a grant from the Israel Academy of Science and by the Manja and Morris Leigh Chair for Biophysics and Biotechnology.

REVIEWS AND KEY PAPERS

Bukau, B. 1993. Regulation of the *Escherichia coli* heat-shock response. *Mol. Microbiol.* **9**:671–680.

Craig, E. A., B. D. Gambill, and R. J. Nelson. 1993. Heat shock proteins: molecular chaperones of protein biogenesis. *Microbiol. Rev.* **57**:402–414.

Gottesman, S. 1996. Proteases and their targets in *Escherichia coli*. *Annu. Rev. Genet.* **30**:465–506.

Mager, W. H., and A. J. De Kruijff. 1995. Stress-induced transcriptional activation. *Microbiol. Rev.* **59**:506–531.

Segal, R., and E. Z. Ron. 1996. Regulation and organization of the *groE* and *dnaK* operons in eubacteria. *FEMS Microbiol. Lett.* **138**:1–10.

Yura, T., H. Nagai, and H. Mori. 1993. Regulation of the heat-shock response in bacteria. *Annu. Rev. Microbiol.* **47**:321–350.

REFERENCES

1. Babst, M., H. Hennecke, and H. M. Fischer. 1996. Two different mechanisms are involved in the heat-shock regulation of chaperonin gene expression in *Bradyrhizobium japonicum*. *Mol. Microbiol.* **19**:827–839.

2. Bahl, H., H. Muller, S. Behrens, H. Joseph, and F. Narberhaus. 1995. Expression of heat shock genes in *Clostridium acetobutylicum*. *FEMS Microbiol. Rev.* **17**:341–348.

3. Baumler, A. J., J. G. Kusters, I. Stojiljkovic, and F. Heffron. 1994. *Salmonella typhimurium* loci involved in survival within macrophages. *Infect. Immun.* **62**:1623–1630.

4. Benvenisti, L., S. Koby, A. Rutman, H. Giladi, T. Yura, and A. B. Oppenheim. 1995. Cloning and primary sequence of the *rpoH* gene from *Pseudomonas aeruginosa*. *Gene* **155**:73–76.

5. Blom, A., W. Harder, and A. Matin. 1992. Unique and overlapping pollutant stress proteins of *Escherichia coli*. *Appl. Environ. Microbiol.* **58**:331–334.

6. Bloom, M., S. Skelly, R. VanBogelen, F. Neidhardt, N. Brot, and H. Weissbach. 1986. *In vitro* effect of the *Escherichia coli* heat shock regulatory protein on expression of heat shock genes. *J. Bacteriol.* **166**:380–384.

7. Bohne, J., Z. Sokolovic, and W. Goebel. 1994. Transcriptional regulation of *prfA* and PrfA-regulated virulence genes in *Listeria monocytogenes*. *Mol. Microbiol.* **11**:1141–1150.

8. Boorstein, W. R., T. Ziegelhoffer, and E. A. Craig. 1994. Molecular evolution of the HSP70 multigene family. *J. Mol. Evol.* **38**:1–17.

9. Brunham, R. C., and R. W. Peeling. 1994. *Chlamydia trachomatis* antigens: role in immunity and pathogenesis. *Infect. Agents Dis.* **3**:218–233.

10. Buchberger, A., H. Schroder, T. Hesterkamp, H. J. Schonfeld, and B. Bukau. 1996. Substrate shuttling between the DnaK and GroEL systems indicates a chaperone network promoting protein folding. *J. Mol. Biol.* **261**:328–333.

11. Bukau, B. 1993. Regulation of the *Escherichia coli* heat-shock response. *Mol. Microbiol.* **9**:671–680.

12. Chuang, S. E., and F. R. Blattner. 1993. Characterization of twenty-six new heat shock genes of *Escherichia coli*. *J. Bacteriol.* **175**:5242–5252.

13. **Cowing, D. W., J. C. Bardwell, E. A. Craig, C. Woolford, R. W. Hendrix, and C. A. Gross.** 1985. Consensus sequence for *Escherichia coli* heat shock gene promoters. *Proc. Natl. Acad. Sci. USA* **82**:2679–2683.

14. **Cowing, D. W., and C. A. Gross.** 1989. Interaction of *Escherichia coli* RNA polymerase holoenzyme containing sigma 32 with heat shock promoters. DNase I footprinting and methylation protection. *J. Mol. Biol.* **210**:513–520.

15. **de Leon, P., S. Marco, C. Isiegas, A. Marina, J. L. Carrascosa, and R. P. Mellado.** 1997. *Streptomyces lividans groES, groEL1* and *groEL2* genes. *Microbiology* **143**:3563–3571.

16. **Deuerling, E., A. Mogk, C. Richter, M. Purucker, and W. Schumann.** 1997. The *ftsH* gene of *Bacillus subtilis* is involved in major cellular processes such as sporulation, stress adaptation and secretion. *Mol. Microbiol.* **23**:921–933.

17. **Dunn, B. E., N. B. Vakil, B. G. Schneider, M. M. Miller, J. B. Zitzer, T. Peutz, and S. H. Phadnis.** 1997. Localization of *Helicobacter pylori* urease and heat shock protein in human gastric biopsies. *Infect. Immun.* **65**:1181–1188.

18. **Elzer, P. H., R. W. Phillips, M. E. Kovach, K. M. Peterson, and R. M. Roop, 2nd.** 1994. Characterization and genetic complementation of a *Brucella abortus* high-temperature-requirement A (*htrA*) deletion mutant. *Infect. Immun.* **62**:4135–4139.

19. **Ensgraber, M., and M. Loos.** 1992. A 66-kilodalton heat shock protein of *Salmonella typhimurium* is responsible for binding of the bacterium to intestinal mucus. *Infect. Immun.* **60**:3072–3078.

20. **Erickson, J. W., and C. A. Gross.** 1989. Identification of the sigma E subunit of *Escherichia coli* RNA polymerase: a second alternate sigma factor involved in high-temperature gene expression. *Genes Dev.* **3**:1462–1471.

21. **Fernandez, R. C., S. M. Logan, S. H. Lee, and P. S. Hoffman.** 1996. Elevated levels of *Legionella pneumophila* stress protein Hsp60 early in infection of human monocytes and L929 cells correlate with virulence. *Infect. Immun.* **64**:1968–1976.

22. **Gamer, J., G. Multhaup, T. Tomoyasu, J. S. McCarty, S. Rudiger, H. J. Schonfeld, C. Schirra, H. Bujard, and B. Bukau.** 1996. A cycle of binding and release of the DnaK, DnaJ and GrpE chaperones regulates activity of the *Escherichia coli* heat shock transcription factor sigma32. *EMBO J.* **15**:607–617.

23. **Gottesman, S.** 1996. Proteases and their targets in *Escherichia coli*. *Annu. Rev. Genet.* **30**:465–506.

24. **Grossman, A. D., D. B. Straus, W. A. Walter, and C. A. Gross.** 1987. Sigma 32 synthesis can regulate the synthesis of heat shock proteins in *Escherichia coli*. *Genes Dev.* **1**:179–184.

25. **Gupta, R. S.** 1995. Evolution of the chaperonin families (Hsp60, Hsp10 and Tcp-1) of proteins and the origin of eukaryotic cells [see comments]. *Mol. Microbiol.* **15**:1–11.

26. **Hecker, M., W. Schumann, and U. Volker.** 1996. Heat-shock and general stress response in *Bacillus subtilis*. *Mol. Microbiol.* **19**:417–428.

27. **Herman, C., D. Thevenet, R. D'Ari, and P. Bouloc.** 1995. Degradation of sigma 32, the heat shock regulator in *Escherichia coli*, is governed by HflB. *Proc. Natl. Acad. Sci. USA* **92**:3516–3520.

28. **Hiratsu, K., M. Amemura, H. Nashimoto, H. Shinagawa, and K. Makino.** 1995. The *rpoE* gene of *Escherichia coli*, which encodes sigma E, is essential for bacterial growth at high temperature. *J. Bacteriol.* **177**:2918–2922.

29. **Inbar, O., and E. Z. Ron.** 1993. Induction of cadmium tolerance in *Escherichia coli* K-12. *FEMS Lett.* **113**:197–200.

30. **Jayaraman, G. C., J. E. Penders, and R. A. Burne.** 1997. Transcriptional analysis of the *Streptococcus mutans hrcA, grpE* and *dnaK* genes and regulation of expression in response to heat shock and environmental acidification. *Mol. Microbiol.* **25**:329–341.

31. **Johnson, K., I. Charles, G. Dougan, D. Pickard, P. O'Gaora, G. Costa, T. Ali, I. Miller, and C. Hormaeche.** 1991. The role of a stress-response protein in *Salmonella typhimurium* virulence. *Mol. Microbiol.* **5**:401–407.

32. **Jones, S., and D. A. Portnoy.** 1994. Characterization of *Listeria monocytogenes* pathogenesis in a strain expressing perfringolysin O in place of listeriolysin O. *Infect. Immun.* **62**:5608–5613.

33. **Kandror, O., L. Busconi, M. Sherman, and A. L. Goldberg.** 1994. Rapid degradation of an abnormal protein in *Escherichia coli* involves the chaperones GroEL and GroES. *J. Biol. Chem.* **269**:23575–23582.

34. **Kanemori, M., K. Nishihara, H. Yanagi, and T. Yura.** 1997. Synergistic roles of HslVU and other ATP-dependent proteases in controlling in vivo turnover of sigma-32 and abnormal proteins in *Escherichia coli*. *J. Bacteriol.* **179**:7219–7225.

35. **Karunasagar, I., R. Lampidis, W. Goebel, and J. Kreft.** 1997. Complementation of *Listeria seeligeri* with the *plcA-prfA* genes from *Listeria monocytogenes* activates transcription of seeligerolysin and leads to bacterial escape from the phagosome of infected mammalian cells. *FEMS Microbiol. Lett.* **146**:303–310.

36. **Kaufmann, S. H.** 1992. Heat shock proteins in health and disease. *Int. J. Clin. Lab. Res.* **21**:221–226.

37. **Kusukawa, N., and T. Yura.** 1988. Heat shock protein GroE of *Escherichia coli*: key pro-

tective roles against thermal stress. *Genes Dev.* **2:** 874–882.

38. **LaRossa, R. A., and T. K. Van Dyk.** 1991. Physiological roles of the DnaK and GroE stress proteins: catalysts of protein folding or macromolecular sponges? *Mol. Microbiol.* **5:**529–534.

39. **Lathigra, R. B., P. D. Butcher, T. R. Garbe, and D. B. Young.** 1991. Heat shock proteins as virulence factors of pathogens. *Curr. Top. Microbiol. Immunol.* **167:**125–143.

40. **Li, W. H.** 1993. Unbiased estimation of the rates of synonymous and nonsynonymous substitution. *J. Mol. Evol.* **36:**96–99.

41. **Lipinska, B., O. Fayet, L. Baird, and C. Georgopoulos.** 1989. Identification, characterization, and mapping of the *Escherichia coli htrA* gene, whose product is essential for bacterial growth only at elevated temperatures. *J. Bacteriol.* **171:**1574–1584.

42. **Lipinska, B., S. Sharma, and C. Georgopoulos.** 1988. Sequence analysis and regulation of the *htrA* gene of *Escherichia coli*: a sigma 32-independent mechanism of heat-inducible transcription. *Nucleic Acids Res.* **16:**10053–10067.

43. **Lockhart, P. J., M. A. Steel, M. D. Hendy, and D. Penny.** 1994. Recovering evolutionary trees under a more realistic model of sequence evolution. *Mol. Biol. Evol.* **11:**605–612.

44. **Macario, A. J.** 1995. Heat-shock proteins and molecular chaperones: implications for pathogenesis, diagnostics, and therapeutics. *Int. J. Clin. Lab. Res.* **25:**59–70.

45. **Mauchline, W. S., B. W. James, R. B. Fitzgeorge, P. J. Dennis, and C. W. Keevil.** 1994. Growth temperature reversibly modulates the virulence of *Legionella pneumophila*. *Infect. Immun.* **62:**2995–2997.

46. **McCarty, J. S., S. Rudiger, H. J. Schonfeld, J. Schneider Mergener, K. Nakahigashi, T. Yura, and B. Bukau.** 1996. Regulatory region C of the *E. coli* heat shock transcription factor, sigma32, constitutes a DnaK binding site and is conserved among eubacteria. *J. Mol. Biol.* **256:** 829–837.

47. **McKay, D. B., and C. Y. Lu.** 1991. Listeriolysin as a virulence factor in *Listeria monocytogenes* infection of neonatal mice and murine decidual tissue. *Infect. Immun.* **59:**4286–4290.

48. **Meghji, S., P. A. White, S. P. Nair, K. Reddi, K. Heron, B. Henderson, A. Zaliani, G. Fossati, P. Mascagni, J. F. Hunt, M. M. Roberts, and A. R. Coates.** 1997. *Mycobacterium tuberculosis* chaperonin 10 stimulates bone resorption: a potential contributory factor in Pott's disease. *J. Exp. Med.* **186:**1241–1246.

49. **Minder, A. C., F. Narberhaus, M. Babst, H. Hennecke, and H. M. Fischer.** 1997. The *dnaKJ* operon belongs to the sigma32-dependent class of heat shock genes in *Bradyrhizobium japonicum*. *Mol. Gen. Genet.* **254:**195–206.

50. **Mogk, A., G. Homuth, C. Scholz, L. Kim, F. X. Schmid, and W. Schumann.** 1997. The GroE chaperonin machine is a major modulator of the CIRCE heat shock regulon of *Bacillus subtilis*. *EMBO J.* **16:**4579–4590.

51. **Muffler, A., M. Barth, C. Marschall, and R. Hengge Aronis.** 1997. Heat shock regulation of sigmaS turnover: a role for DnaK and relationship between stress responses mediated by sigmaS and sigma32 in *Escherichia coli*. *J. Bacteriol.* **179:**445–452.

52. **Naczynski, Z. M., C. Mueller, and A. M. Kropinski.** 1995. Cloning the gene for the heat shock response positive regulator (sigma 32 homolog) from *Pseudomonas aeruginosa*. *Can. J. Microbiol.* **41:**75–87.

53. **Nakahigashi, K., H. Yanagi, and T. Yura.** 1995. Isolation and sequence analysis of *rpoH* genes encoding sigma 32 homologs from gram negative bacteria: conserved mRNA and protein segments for heat shock regulation. *Nucleic Acids Res.* **23:**4383–4390.

54. **Nakahigashi, K., H. Yanagi, and T. Yura.** 1998. Regulatory conservation and divergence of sigma32 homologs from gram-negative bacteria: *Serratia marcescens*, *Proteus mirabilis*, *Pseudomonas aeruginosa*, and *Agrobacterium tumefaciens*. *J. Bacteriol.* **180:**2402–2408.

55. **Narberhaus, F., P. Krummenacher, H. M. Fischer, and H. Hennecke.** 1997. Three disparately regulated genes for sigma 32-like transcription factors in *Bradyrhizobium japonicum*. *Mol. Microbiol.* **24:**93–104.

56. **Neidhardt, F., and R. A. VanBogelen.** 1987. Heat shock response, p. 1334–1345. *In* F. C. Neidhardt, J. L. Ingraham, K.B. Low, Jr., B. Magasanik, M. Schaechter, and H. E. Umbarger (ed.), *Escherichia coli* and *Salmonella typhimurium*: *Cellular and Molecular Biology*, American Society for Microbiology, Washington, D.C.

57. **Pallen, M. J., and B. W. Wren.** 1997. The HtrA family of serine proteases. *Mol. Microbiol.* **26:**209–221.

58. **Qi, H., R. Menzel, and Y. C. Tse Dinh.** 1996. Effect of the deletion of the sigma 32-dependent promoter (P1) of the *Escherichia coli* topoisomerase I gene on thermotolerance. *Mol. Microbiol.* **21:**703–711.

59. **Raina, S., D. Missiakas, and C. Georgopoulos.** 1995. The *rpoE* gene encoding the sigma E (sigma 24) heat shock sigma factor of *Escherichia coli*. *EMBO J.* **14:**1043–1055.

60. **Reisenauer, A., C. D. Mohr, and L. Shapiro.** 1996. Regulation of a heat shock sigma32 hom-

olog in *Caulobacter crescentus*. *J. Bacteriol.* **178:** 1919–1927.

61. **Roberts, R. C., C. Toochinda, M. Avedissian, R. L. Baldini, S. L. Gomes, and L. Shapiro.** 1996. Identification of a *Caulobacter crescentus* operon encoding *hrcA*, involved in negatively regulating heat-inducible transcription, and the chaperone gene *grpE*. *J. Bacteriol.* **178:** 1829–1841.

62. **Rouviere, P. E., A. De Las Penas, J. Mecsas, C. Z. Lu, K. E. Rudd, and C. A. Gross.** 1995. *rpoE*, the gene encoding the second heat-shock sigma factor, sigma E, in *Escherichia coli*. *EMBO J.* **14:**1032–1042.

63. **Sahu, G. K., R. Chowdhury, and J. Das.** 1997. The *rpoH* gene encoding sigma 32 homolog of *Vibrio cholerae*. *Gene* **189:**203–207.

64. **Saitou, N., and M. Nei.** 1987. The neighbor-joining method: a new method for reconstructing phylogenetic trees. *Mol. Biol. Evol.* **4:**406–425.

65. **Schulz, A., and W. Schumann.** 1996. *hrcA*, the first gene of the *Bacillus subtilis dnaK* operon encodes a negative regulator of class I heat shock genes. *J. Bacteriol.* **178:**1088–1093.

66. **Schurr, M. J., and V. Deretic.** 1997. Microbial pathogenesis in cystic fibrosis: co-ordinate regulation of heat-shock response and conversion to mucoidy in *Pseudomonas aeruginosa*. *Mol. Microbiol.* **24:**411–420.

67. **Schurr, M. J., H. Yu, J. C. Boucher, N. S. Hibler, and V. Deretic.** 1995. Multiple promoters and induction by heat shock of the gene encoding the alternative sigma factor AlgU (sigma E) which controls mucoidy in cystic fibrosis isolates of *Pseudomonas aeruginosa*. *J. Bacteriol.* **177:** 5670–5679.

68. **Segal, G., and E. Z. Ron.** 1993. Heat shock transcription of the *groESL* operon of *Agrobacterium tumefaciens* may involve a hairpin-loop structure. *J. Bacteriol.* **175:**3083–3088.

69. **Segal, G., and E. Z. Ron.** 1995. The *dnaKJ* operon of *Agrobacterium tumefaciens*: transcriptional analysis and evidence for a new heat shock promoter. *J. Bacteriol.* **177:**5952–5958.

70. **Segal, G., and E. Z. Ron.** 1995. The *groESL* operon of *Agrobacterium tumefaciens*: evidence for heat shock-dependent mRNA cleavage. *J. Bacteriol.* **177:**750–757.

71. **Segal, G., and E. Z. Ron.** 1996. Heat shock activation of the *groESL* operon of *Agrobacterium tumefaciens* and the regulatory roles of the inverted repeat. *J. Bacteriol.* **178:**3634–3640.

72. **Segal, R., and E. Z. Ron.** 1996. Regulation and organization of the *groE* and *dnaK* operons in eubacteria. *FEMS Microbiol. Lett.* **138:**1–10.

73. **Sheehan, B., C. Kocks, S. Dramsi, E. Gouin, A. D. Klarsfeld, J. Mengaud, and P. Cossart.** 1994. Molecular and genetic determinants of the *Listeria monocytogenes* infectious process. *Curr. Top. Microbiol. Immunol.* **192:**187–216.

74. **Straus, D. B., W. A. Walter, and C. A. Gross.** 1987. The heat shock response of *E. coli* is regulated by changes in the concentration of sigma 32. *Nature* **329:**348–351.

75. **Tomoyasu, T., J. Gamer, B. Bukau, M. Kanemori, H. Mori, A. J. Rutman, A. B. Oppenheim, T. Yura, K. Yamanaka, H. Niki, S. Hiraga, and T. Ogura.** 1995. *Escherichia coli* FtsH is a membrane-bound, ATP-dependent protease which degrades the heat-shock transcription factor sigma 32. *EMBO J.* **14:**2551–2560.

76. **Van Bogelen, R., P. M. Kelley, and F. Neidhardt.** 1987. Differential induction of heat shock, SOS and oxidation stress regulons and accumulation of nucleotides in *Escherichia coli*. *J. Bacteriol.* **169:**26–32.

77. **Van Dyk, T. K., T. R. Reed, A. C. Vollmer, and R. A. LaRossa.** 1995. Synergistic induction of the heat shock response in *Escherichia coli* by simultaneous treatment with chemical inducers. *J. Bacteriol.* **177:**6001–6004.

78. **Volker, U., H. Mach, R. Schmid, and M. Hecker.** 1992. Stress proteins and cross-protecion by heat shock and salt stress in *Bacillus subtilis*. *J. Gen. Microbiol.* **138:**2125–2135.

79. **Wu, J., and A. Newton.** 1996. Isolation, identification, and transcriptional specificity of the heat shock sigma factor sigma32 from *Caulobacter crescentus*. *J. Bacteriol.* **178:**2094–2101.

80. **Yang, Z., Y. Geng, and W. Shi.** 1998. A DnaK homolog in *Myxococcus xanthus* is involved in social motility and fruiting body formation. *J. Bacteriol.* **180:**218–224.

81. **Yuan, G., and S. L. Wong.** 1995. Isolation and characterization of *Bacillus subtilis groE* regulatory mutants: evidence for *orf39* in the *dnaK* operon as a repressor gene in regulating the expression of both *groE* and *dnaK*. *J. Bacteriol.* **177:**6462–6468.

82. **Yuan, G., and S. L. Wong.** 1995. Regulation of *groE* expression in *Bacillus subtilis*: the involvement of the sigma A-like promoter and the roles of the inverted repeat sequence (CIRCE). *J. Bacteriol.* **177:**5427–5433.

83. **Yura, T.** 1996. Regulation and conservation of the heat-shock transcription factor sigma32. *Genes Cells* **1:**277–284.

84. **Zhou, Y. N., N. Kusukawa, J. W. Erickson, C. A. Gross, and T. Yura.** 1988. Isolation and characterization of *Escherichia coli* mutants that lack the heat shock sigma factor sigma 32. *J. Bacteriol.* **170:**3640–3649.

85. **Zuber, U., and W. Schumann.** 1994. CIRCE, a novel heat shock element involved in regulation of heat shock operon *dnaK* of *Bacillus subtilis*. *J. Bacteriol.* **176:**1359–1363.

ECOLOGY OF SPECIFIC HUMAN PATHOGENS

IV

INTRODUCTION

Itzhak Ofek

This section focuses on five human pathogens, four bacteria and a protozoan parasite, each of which has a different ecology. Each of these pathogens uses different strategies to occupy specific sites and niches. Chiang and Mekalanos review the present knowledge of the molecular aspects of *Vibrio cholerae* virulence. They present data indicating that pathogenic *V. cholerae* arose from nonpathogenic strains by acquiring mobile genetic elements encoding virulence factors. This type of horizontal gene transfer appears to be still occurring, resulting in new types of virulent *V. cholerae*.

Gil Segal and Howard Shuman discuss an intracellular bacterium, *Legionella pneumophila*, whose natural habitat is a freshwater unicellular protozoan. Occasionally, the organisms are inhaled in large quantities by humans exposed to ventilation of water systems and reach the alveolar macrophages of the lung, where they proliferate intracellularly. The identification of the genes required by the pathogens to multiply in both human macrophages and protozoa is now under intense research, and recent data on this issue are presented. A total of 20 or more genes appear to be essential for intracellular multiplication, and these so-called *icm* genes are located in two regions of the chromosome. In the years ahead, it is likely that the roles of the *icm* genes in the intracellular lifestyle of the pathogen will be defined. This may enable a better approach to the control of Legionnaires disease.

Trinad Chakraborty and colleagues describe *Listeria* spp., a foodborne intracellular bacterium that is now emerging as a major threat, especially in areas of increased consumption of food products that are stored for various periods of time under refrigeration. The search for ecologically specific gene expression is discussed because it may provide prophylactic measures to control the transition of the pathogenic *Listeria* spp. from the environment to the host.

Identification of the virulent genes of the protozoan parasite *Entamoeba histolytica* became feasible with new molecular biology techniques. This approach is discussed by David Mirelman and Serge Ankri. It is suggested that antisense inhibition of expression of the key virulent genes as well as specific inhibitors of cystein proteases may help control the virulence of the parasite.

Finally, Hervé Bercovier discusses the epidemiology of tuberculosis, emphasizing the resurgence of this disease in recent years in Asia and Africa as opposed to decline or no change in the Western developing countries. The promise of a new vaccine regimen for controlling this infection is encouraging.

Itzhak Ofek, Department of Human Microbiology, Sackler Faculty of Medicine, Tel Aviv University, Ramat Aviv 69978, Israel.

HORIZONTAL GENE TRANSFER IN THE EMERGENCE OF VIRULENT *VIBRIO CHOLERAE*

Su L. Chiang and John J. Mekalanos

13

Cholera is a potentially life-threatening diarrheal disease caused by the bacterium *Vibrio cholerae*. The disease is capable of killing its victims within hours of the onset of symptoms, and it spreads rapidly when introduced into previously unaffected areas. Reemergence of cholera in the Americas between 1991 and 1993 resulted in more than 820,000 reported cases of cholera, with almost 7,000 deaths (89), and mortality during an African epidemic in 1991 reached nearly 14,000 deaths out of approximately 153,000 reported cases (85). The disease is endemic in the Indian subcontinent, with the incidence in Asia and Africa estimated to exceed 5 million cases each year (33). The clinical severity and geographic spread of cholera have made it the focus of intensive study for decades and will certainly cause it to remain so until it no longer poses such a formidable threat to human health.

The origin of virulent *V. cholerae* has been the subject of much speculation (16, 48). Accounts of a severe diarrheal disease of high mortality occur in Sanskrit literature that is at least 1,000 years old, suggesting that the geographic origin of this disease was the Indian subcontinent. While the species *V. cholerae* exists throughout the world in aquatic environments, not all *V. cholerae* isolates are the same. Pathogenic strains are distinct in their genetic composition in that they possess, for example, genes encoding toxins and intestinal colonization factors that are lacking in most environmental isolates of *V. cholerae* (91). Furthermore, when pathogenic strains are found in water, they are usually only found in regions of the world with endemic or epidemic cholera. Phylogenetic analysis suggests that pathogenic strains are highly related to each other and can be divided into a series of clones that have spread globally (49, 96). Nonetheless, the level of relatedness between pathogenic and nonpathogenic strains is high enough to indicate the existence of a common ancestor for both these classes of *V. cholerae* (although depending upon which specific strains are being compared, such a common ancestral strain might have existed a thousand or more years ago). It is therefore likely that pathogenic *V. cholerae* arose from nonpathogenic environmental strains by acquiring mobile genetic elements encoding virulence factors. The clones that first acquired these virulence genes subsequently expanded and

Su L. Chiang and John J. Mekalanos, Department of Microbiology and Molecular Genetics and Shipley Institute of Medicine, Harvard Medical School, 200 Longwood Avenue, Boston, MA 02115.

Microbial Ecology and Infectious Disease, Edited by Eugene Rosenberg
©1999 American Society for Microbiology, Washington, D.C.

continue to evolve even today, resulting in the periodic emergence of distinctly new types of virulent *V. cholerae*. This chapter reviews our present knowledge of the molecular aspects of *V. cholerae* virulence and the genetic factors that have contributed to the emergence of this important human pathogen.

V. CHOLERAE: ECOLOGY AND EPIDEMIOLOGY

The bacterium *V. cholerae* is a gram-negative, nonsporulating, straight or curved rod. It possesses a single polar sheathed flagellum and is highly motile. A halophilic organism, it is found in estuarine or marine environments, and its growth in laboratory media is generally stimulated by the presence of 5 to 90 mM sodium, depending on actual culture conditions. Outside the human host, *V. cholerae* has been found free-living in water and also in association with plankton, most notably copepods, but present understanding of this aspect of *V. cholerae* ecology is rather limited (16, 17).

Although at least 151 serogroups of *V. cholerae* have been recognized, only the O1 and O139 serovars are known to cause epidemic cholera. The O1 serogroup is further divided into two biotypes, classical and El Tor, on the basis of the unique ability of El Tor strains to produce hemolysin and mannose-sensitive hemagglutinin (MSHA). In actuality, all but the earliest isolated El Tor strains are nonhemolytic, and MSHA production is the only reliable means of distinguishing between classical and El Tor strains. Of the six cholera pandemics since 1817, classical strains are known to be responsible for at least the fifth (1881–1896) and the sixth (1899–1923). The El Tor biotype is responsible for the seventh and current pandemic (1961–present), though this biotype had caused only sporadic outbreaks of cholera before rising to epidemic prominence in 1961. The O139 serovar appeared in India and Bangladesh in late 1992 and was the first non-O1 serovar found to cause epidemic cholera (1, 71). O139 strains are closely related to O1 El Tor strains but have a different O-antigen structure and are encapsulated (44, 97). Molecular characterization of the genes encoding O139 antigen biosynthesis suggests that an El Tor O1 may have acquired *rfb* genes from O22, O141, and other related non-O1 *V. cholerae* strains (7, 95). It was thought that the emergence of the O139 serovar might represent the beginning of a new pandemic, but these strains have not yet caused epidemics on other continents.

PATHOPHYSIOLOGY OF CHOLERA

In its most severe form, cholera is capable of causing death within 3 h after the onset of symptoms (35), which occurs 12 to 72 h after ingestion of *V. cholerae* (11). The distinctive feature of the disease is the profuse secretory diarrhea that results from the action of cholera toxin on cells of the intestinal epithelium. Fluid loss by this route can reach as much as 200 ml/kg of body weight per day, with total losses exceeding 100% of body weight over the course of several days. The concomitant loss of plasma solutes such as sodium, potassium, and chloride ions leads to electrolyte imbalances, acidosis, and ultimately death. However, effective treatment of cholera is both simple and relatively inexpensive, consisting of oral and/or intravenous rehydration therapy coupled with administration of antibiotics. With timely and appropriate intervention, a cholera patient can be discharged in 1 to 3 days (5).

Cholera typically begins with the ingestion of *V. cholerae* in contaminated food or water. A relatively large inoculum of 10^8 to 10^{11} organisms is required for successful infection, presumably because *V. cholerae* is acid sensitive and a great many vibrios therefore perish in the low-pH environment of the stomach (33, 56, 64). Those bacteria that reach the small intestine must penetrate the mucus gel covering the intestinal epithelium and colonize the epithelium itself. This process of colonization is as yet poorly characterized, but there is an absolute requirement for expression of the toxin-coregulated pilus (TCP), a filamentous appendage that is required for autoagglutination of bacterial cells in culture and that may play a similar role on the mucosal surface. Other factors implicated in colonization are discussed below, though the exact role of these is unclear.

The next step in the pathogenesis of the disease is the secretion by *V. cholerae* of cholera toxin, which consists of five identical B subunits and one A subunit. The B pentamer binds to GM_1 gangliosides on target cells, and the A subunit enters the target cell. Proteolytic cleavage and disulfide bond reduction of the A subunit subsequently release the A_1 and A_2 peptides into the cytoplasm of the target cell, where ADP-ribosylation of the regulatory protein $G_{s\alpha}$ by the A_1 peptide leads to constitutive activation of adenylate cyclase. This in turn increases levels of intracellular cyclic AMP (cAMP), which stimulates secretion of chloride, potassium, and bicarbonate ions into the gut lumen and inhibits active uptake of sodium. The resulting osmotic gradient causes water to move into the lumen in such enormous quantities that the absorptive capacity of the intestine is utterly insufficient to prevent net fluid loss (5, 47).

It has been postulated that the induction of diarrhea by cholera toxin aids in dissemination of vibrios back into the environment, from which they can be acquired by subsequent hosts. Some investigators have suggested that the sodium efflux induced by cholera toxin may provide more-favorable conditions for survival of *V. cholerae* in the intestine (4, 8), but this hypothesis remains largely untested. Proteases have also been implicated in dissemination, in that they may function to help *V. cholerae* detach from the epithelium and so pass more easily out of the intestine (29). However, the multifactorial nature of interactions among *V. cholerae*, human hosts, and the environment makes it difficult to investigate these theories.

V. CHOLERAE VIRULENCE FACTORS AND THEIR EXPRESSION

Cholera toxin expression is regulated by the ToxR and ToxT transcriptional activators in response to a variety of environmental signals (21, 67). ToxR is a 32-kDa transmembrane protein, the cytoplasmic domain of which is homologous to two-component response regulators (2, 62). ToxR has been shown to bind to sequences upstream of the cholera toxin genes (*ctxAB*) (62) and, possibly in conjunction with ToxS, to activate transcription of *ctxAB* (22, 60). ToxR also stimulates expression of the outer-membrane protein OmpU (61) and ToxT, an AraC-like protein that also modulates toxin expression. ToxT additionally controls expression of a number of genetic loci that are coordinately expressed with *ctxAB* (12, 39, 40), including the *acf* genes and the genes of the *tcp* operon (9, 23). cAMP and the cAMP receptor protein (CRP) provide negative regulation of toxin and TCP (80), and recently identified additional regulators of *toxT* expression include the TcpP and TcpH proteins, which act synergistically with ToxR and ToxS (10, 41).

TCP are generally thought to function as adhesins, although no host receptor for TCP has been identified. As assessed in the infant mouse model, TCP are the most important colonization factor identified thus far in classical, El Tor, and O139 strains (3, 52, 92, 93). TCP are required for successful colonization of the human intestine (38) and also serve as receptors for the cholera toxin phage (CTXφ) (98).

Biogenesis of TCP is apparently directly controlled by the *tcp* operon genes and the unlinked *tcpG* locus (42, 51, 65, 69). Several of the *tcp* operon genes have been analyzed in detail. The pilus subunit TcpA is a member of the type IV pilin family (77), which includes pilins from various pathogenic bacteria such as gonococci, meningococci, *Pseudomonas aeruginosa*, and enteropathogenic *Escherichia coli* (83). The *tcpI* gene may be involved in regulation of chemotaxis and motility (36), and *tcpJ* encodes a signal peptidase required for processing of the TcpA prepilin (50). TcpP and TcpH as stated above, activate expression of the ToxR regulon. The only other extensively characterized gene in this operon is the *toxT* gene, which lies toward the distal end of the operon and whose activity has been described above. *tcpG* encodes a periplasmic thiol:disulfide isomerase, and although a *tcpG* mutant assembles surface TCP, it has defects in the TCP-associated phenotypes of autoagglutination and colonization and furthermore displays defective secretion of cholera toxin and protease (69).

It was recently reported that a Tn*5* insertion in the *rfb* operon of *V. cholerae* 569B prevents translocation of TcpA, the structural subunit of TCP (43). The *rfb* genes are predicted to be involved in biosynthesis of the O-antigen component of lipopolysaccharide (LPS) (26, 82, 101). Since TCP are critical for colonization, the colonization defects observed in LPS mutants (14, 79, 97) could be simply due to interference with proper TCP expression. However, an *rfbB* insertion mutation in *V. cholerae* strain O395 caused no detectable defects in production of surface TCP, as assessed by immunoelectron microscopy and CTX phage transduction (S. C. and J. J. M., submitted). These data do not exclude the possibility that *rfb* mutations result in subtle changes in TCP structure or function, but it seems clear that *rfb* mutations do not always cause gross defects in TCP expression.

Several additional factors have been implicated in colonization, although none of these has been as well characterized as TCP. One of these is the MSHA, a type IV pilus (46) that apparently contributed strongly to colonization in a rabbit model (30). MSHA is readily expressed by El Tor strains (though not by classical strains), and it elicits an immunogenic response in humans (45, 84). Although MSHA was thought to aid in colonization by El Tor strains (66), it is not required for colonization of the infant mouse (93) and is evidently not critical for colonization of humans (87). This discrepancy is possibly due to some peculiarity of the rabbit model. Finally, although MSHA is apparently unnecessary for colonization of the host, it may be required for growth or survival outside the host.

The mannose-fucose-resistant hemagglutinin (MFRHA) is thought to be a cationic outer-membrane protein, and it also appears to play a role in colonization. An MFRHA mutant was constructed in classical strain 569B and found to be severely reduced in virulence as assessed by LD_{50} and infant mouse colonization assays (31). These data are highly intriguing, but unfortunately, no further information on MFRHA has been published. A recent hypothesis suggests that MFRHA genes are associated with an integron-like DNA structure and therefore may also have been acquired by horizontal transfer and subsequent chromosomal integration (15).

IrgA is an outer-membrane protein whose expression is highly induced under iron-limiting conditions. An *irgA* mutant demonstrates reduced colonization ability in the infant mouse model, and the LD_{50} for this strain is 100-fold greater than that for the wild-type parental strain (34). *irgA* and other iron-regulated genes are apparently important for in vivo growth in rabbit ileal loops (88), but the specific contribution of these genes to survival in the host remains unknown.

The accessory colonization factor genes (*acfABCD*) were identified in a screen for ToxR-regulated loci, and transposon insertions in these loci were found to substantially reduce colonization ability (70). It was subsequently determined that the *acf* cluster was physically adjacent to the *tcp* operon (25) and that the expression of *tcp* and *acf* genes is linked in several ways (9). Sequence analysis of the *acfB* gene suggests that it encodes an inner-membrane protein with homology to a variety of signal-transduction proteins, and *acfB* mutants display increased swarming on semisolid agar. Constitutive expression of AcfB resulted in decreased swarming (24).

The inverse correlation between motility and virulence was also observed in analyses of spontaneous and transposon-induced motility mutants (32). Nonmotile mutants displayed a ToxR-constitutive phenotype of toxin and TCP production under normally repressing laboratory conditions, while many hyperswarmer mutants showed decreased toxin and TCP production. Furthermore, certain hyperswarmer strains were defective in colonization of the infant mouse, but nonmotile mutants were generally competent for colonization. This ToxR-constitutive, colonization-competent phenotype was also observed in a flagellated, nonmotile strain created by insertional disruption of *motB* in a classical strain background. A nonmotile, nonflagellated *flaA* mutant similarly showed no impairment of colonization in infant mice, although this strain did not demonstrate any changes in toxin or TCP expression (54). Earlier work had indicated that loss of motility decreased colonization in the rabbit RITARD model but not in the infant mouse model (73).

It has been suggested that the inverse relationship between motility and the ToxR regulon reflects the changing needs of *V. cholerae* at different stages of infection (24, 32). Motility may be required for the bacterium to penetrate the mucus gel, but continued motility after reaching the intestinal epithelium might prevent efficient adhesion to host cells. Toxin and TCP, conversely, may be most beneficial to *V. cholerae* if they are expressed after bacterial attachment to host cells.

Signature-tagged transposon mutagenesis (STM) (37) was recently used to screen a large random bank of *V. cholerae* transposon insertion mutants for colonization-defective mutants (14). This screen resulted in identification of a number of genetic loci critical for colonization. Several of these were previously known to be involved in TCP biogenesis, confirming the ability of STM to detect colonization-defective mutants of *V. cholerae*. Purine and biotin biosynthesis were both found to be critical for colonization, indicating that these substances are limiting for growth in the infant mouse intestine. In accordance with previous observations (79, 97), mutations in LPS biosynthetic genes were also determined to cause severe colonization defects. Two STM-identified loci appear to encode phosphotransferases, and since mutations in these genes reduce production of both toxin and TCP, these putative phosphotransferases are apparently involved in control of the ToxR regulon. Other identified loci had no previously known function in pathogenesis, and one had no homology to any known genes.

Understanding the colonization process is vital not only because successful infection of the host cannot occur without it, but also because colonization may influence the safety of live, attenuated cholera vaccines. In clinical trials in human volunteers, several live vaccines were quite effective at inducing immunity to *V. cholerae* infection, but unfortunately, almost all caused mild diarrhea and other adverse reactions in a subset of vaccinees (48, 57, 86). Strains that colonize poorly were not reactogenic, but neither were they particularly immunogenic (38, 57). These results raised the possibility that reactogenicity was inextricably linked to colonization, which in turn appeared to be required for immunogenicity. It has, however, been noted that nonmotile, live-vaccine candidates not only induce strong immunogenic responses in human volunteers, but these strains apparently do not possess the reactogenicity problems that have plagued many otherwise acceptable live-vaccine strains (20, 53, 90).

MOBILE GENETIC ELEMENTS OF *V. CHOLERAE*

Several studies have characterized various aspects of genome plasticity in *V. cholerae*, particularly with respect to the role played by mobile genetic elements in the virulence of this organism. Such elements affect diverse characteristics of *V. cholerae*, including the ability to produce toxin and TCP, antibiotic resistance, and serogroup antigenicity. Only a brief description of this area of research is presented here, as it was recently reviewed extensively (75).

As noted above, the pathogenesis of *V. cholerae* depends almost exclusively on its ability to produce cholera toxin. The *ctxAB* genes are located within a region of the *V. cholerae* chromosome called the CTX genetic element (58, 68), and genes associated with this element were found to encode a site-specific re-combination system capable of mediating integration of the CTX element into the *V. cholerae* chromosome (68). It was subsequently discovered that the CTX element is in fact the genome of a filamentous bacteriophage, CTXφ, and that the receptor for this phage is TCP (98). This filamentous phage is quite un-usual in that it will form true lysogens. Adjacent to the structural genes for cholera toxin are two genes that were originally postulated to encode proteins with enterotoxic activity, *ace* (94) and *zot* (27). However, additional genetic analysis indicates that these genes are involved in morphogenesis of the CTXφ particles (98), bringing their roles as toxin genes into question.

As mentioned above, TCP are the functional receptors for CTXφ. Interestingly, the *tcp* operon is itself located on a chromosomal segment that is absent in most environmental strains of *V. cholerae* (91). Hybridization analysis suggests that this unique segment is approximately 35 kb in size and may be flanked by small direct repeats corresponding to the recombination site of a linked integrase (55). Thus, this chromosomal insert is apparently a pathogenicity island that encodes TCP and other ToxR-regulated virulence factors (e.g., accessory colonization factor) (25). The island also carries several regulatory genes, including the *toxT*, *tcpP*, and *tcpH* genes (9).

Codon usage by genes located on the TCP island differs from that of other *V. cholerae* genes, indicating that it may be derived from another bacterial species. It follows that the TCP pathogenicity island was acquired by *V. cholerae* via horizontal transmission, although how this transfer occurred remains unknown (25, 55). All toxinogenic *V. cholerae* strains possess the TCP pathogenicity island, sug-gesting that nontoxinogenic strains of *V. cholerae* are capable of acquiring the toxin genes only if they express TCP. Some nontoxino-genic strains contain the TCP pathogenicity island, while others do not (74). These obser-vations led to the hypothesis that pathogenic strains of *V. cholerae* may arise by acquiring

first the TCP pathogenicity island and then the toxin genes via infection by CTXφ (98). Since TCP expression occurs optimally in the gastrointestinal tract, the acquisition of CTXφ probably occurred within this host compart-ment in a manner that was modulated by host environmental signals (59, 98).

Since the discovery of CTXφ, several other filamentous phages of *V. cholerae* have been reported. Phage VSK (76) was isolated from an O139 serogroup strain. Like CTXφ, VSK is also capable of integrating into the genome, but so far no virulence factor has been shown to be encoded by this phage. Two other fil-amentous phages of *V. cholerae*, called fs1 and fs2 (78), have also not been implicated in vir-ulence thus far.

In contrast, another type of temperate phage, called kappa, may be involved in al-tering virulence in *V. cholerae* (72). Phage K139 is related to the kappa family of bacte-riophages previously described in El Tor O1 *V. cholerae* and present in classical strains in defective form. Phage K139 lysogens express a secreted protein known as Glo (for G protein-like open reading frame). Glo displays significant sequence similarity to a eukaryotic GTP-binding protein, and like many small eukaryotic G proteins, Glo displays a C-terminal CAAX box motif. This motif is rec-ognized in eukaryotic cells by enzymes that catalyze the isoprenylation of the cysteine res-idue within the CAAX motif (102). The sim-ilarity of Glo to GTP-binding proteins is especially interesting given that cholera toxin itself targets a GTP-binding protein ($G_{s\alpha}$) and requires a second GTP-binding protein (ARF) for optimal activity (28). Finally, genetic anal-ysis supports a role for Glo in virulence. Comparison of isogenic *V. cholerae* strains lysogenized with either *glo*$^+$ or *glo*$^-$ K139 phage showed that the *glo*$^+$ strains were at least 10-fold more virulent. Thus, kappa phage ge-nomes present in some El Tor O1 and O139 strains and all O1 classical strains, probably also enhance the virulence of *V. cholerae* through expression of Glo. The mechanism of Glo-enhanced virulence, however, remains to be determined.

Resistance of the O139 strains to multiple antibiotics was found to be mediated by the SXT element, a 62-kb chromosomal region containing genes providing resistance to streptomycin, trimethoprim, and sulfamethoxazole (100). The SXT element is self-transmissible by conjugation, and it then integrates in a site-specific manner into a single chromosomal site (100). This element may contain additional genes that contribute positively to the environmental fitness or virulence of *V. cholerae*, although it does not enhance colonization as assessed in the infant mouse model.

Genes encoding the O139 serogroup antigen also appear to be carried on a gene cluster that was acquired by horizontal transfer. O-Antigen biosynthesis in O1 strains is controlled by the *rfb* genes (26, 82, 101). In O139 strains, 22 kb of this *rfb* region has been replaced by a 36-kb insertion of O139-specific DNA that presumably mediates production of the O139 capsular antigen (6, 7, 18, 19, 81, 103). As with the SXT element and the *tcp* pathogenicity island, it is not known how this O139-specific region was acquired by El Tor O1 strains.

UNRESOLVED QUESTIONS CONCERNING THE EMERGENCE OF VIRULENT *V. CHOLERAE*

Given the above information, it is possible to propose a model for the emergence of virulent *V. cholerae* strains (Fig. 1). While this is a good working model, it also raises many unresolved questions. Most strains of *V. cholerae* contain the *toxR* regulatory gene, so in theory, any strain of *V. cholerae* could be the ancestral strain. However, we do not know whether El Tor and classical strains evolved from different ancestral strains. These two biotypes are different enough to suggest that the proposed steps outlined below occurred independently at least twice. The first step in the emergence is probably acquisition of the appropriate serogroup genes (e.g., O1 serogroup genes), perhaps via bacterial conjugation or generalized transduction. We envision this as an important early step in emergence because most phages that infect *V. cholerae* depend on expression of the O1 serogroup. Since the TCP island is not found in many other serogroups of *V. cholerae*, we further speculate that an O1-specific phage is probably involved in moving the TCP island into *V. cholerae* O1 strains. While TCP$^+$, CTX$^-$ strains are rare, such strains do exist in the environment, most notably in the Gulf Coast of the United States. These strains are clonal with toxinogenic strains isolated from patients in the same region and thus probably represent environmental precursor strains of toxinogenic isolates in the region (13).

The next step is the acquisition of CTXϕ by a TCP-dependent transduction event that most likely occurs in vivo within the gastrointestinal tract. This produces the first fully pathogenic *V. cholerae* strains capable of both colonizing the intestine and producing cholera toxin. The origin of CTXϕ is unknown, but its modular structure indicates that it may have been acquired by *V. cholerae* in multiple transfer events (99). Pathogenic strains could subsequently become more virulent by acquiring kappalike phages (72). Although kappa phages plate only on O1 serogroup strains, most nontoxinogenic environmental O1 strains lack kappa (63). This observation suggests that kappa phages provide an evolutionary advantage only for toxinogenic strains.

Finally, an El Tor O1 strain is converted into an O139 strain. Several environmental strains encode antigens related to O139 (7, 95), and one or more of these nonpathogenic strains probably donated the O139 genes to an El Tor O1. This conversion event probably occurred at least twice, because some O139 strains carry kappa phage, while others do not. Since kappa phages do not infect O139 strains, it seems likely that two different O1 strains (differing in kappa lysogeny) were converted to O139 when this strain emerged (72). Additionally, all of the initially isolated O139 strains carried the SXT element, suggesting that there might have been some connection between SXT element transfer and the O139

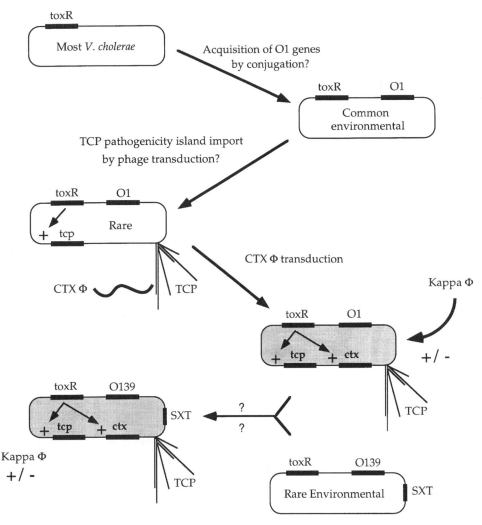

FIGURE 1 Proposed model for the evolution of epidemic strains of *V. cholerae* (indicated by shaded areas).

biosynthetic genes. These two gene clusters are not closely linked physically, but one hypothesis is that the SXT element might have facilitated mobilization of the unlinked O139 genes (100). More recently isolated O139 strains lack the SXT element. Like the O139 strains that lack kappa phage DNA, we do not know whether these are newly emerged O139 strains (i.e., a new lineage) or simply derivatives of earlier O139 strains that have lost the SXT element and/or kappa phage genomes.

Mobile genetic elements clearly contribute to the pathogenesis of *V. cholerae* in several ways. Not only are virulence and colonization factors such as cholera toxin and TCP transmitted via these elements, but it seems that factors that facilitate or prolong infection (e.g., antibiotic resistance and novel surface antigens) can also be horizontally acquired. Transmission of these elements has played a significant role in the emergence of new pathogenic strains. This process, which is at present not well understood, is probably influenced by environmental factors, including the environment within the human host. However, numerous other traits, such as the ability to survive in the extra-host environment, to colonize nonmammalian hosts, to establish asymptomatic carriers, and to survive unfavorable environmental conditions, might all contribute to the epidemic potential of *V. cholerae*. Sequencing of the *V. cholerae* genome is currently well under way. Eventually, genomic comparisons of pathogenic and non-pathogenic environmental strains will provide a complete molecular description of the DNA segments that have been acquired by *V. cholerae* during its emergence as a human pathogen.

ACKNOWLEDGMENTS

This work was supported by NIH grant AI18045 to J. J. M. S. C. is an Illick Fellow of the Ryan Foundation.

REVIEWS AND KEY PAPERS

Kaper, J. B., J. G. Morris, and M. M. Levine. 1995. Cholera. *Clin. Microbiol. Rev.* **8**:48–86.

Mel, S. F., and J. J. Mekalanos. 1996. Modulation of horizontal gene transfer in pathogenic bacteria by *in vivo* signals. *Cell* **87**:795–798.

Rubin, E. J., M. K. Waldor, and J. J. Mekalanos. 1998. Mobile genetic elements and the evolution of new epidemic strains of *Vibrio cholerae*, p. 147–161. *In* R. A. Krause (ed.), *Emerging Infections.* Academic Press, New York.

Wachsmuth, I. K., Ø. Olsvik, G. M. Evins, and T. Popovic. 1994. Molecular epidemiology of cholera, p. 357–370. *In* I. K. Wachsmuth, P. A. Blake, and Ø. Olsvik (ed.), *Vibrio cholerae and Cholera: Molecular to Global Perspectives.* American Society for Microbiology, Washington, D.C.

Waldor, M. K., and J. J. Mekalanos. 1996. Lysogenic conversion by a filamentous phage encoding cholera toxin. *Science* **272**:1910–1914.

REFERENCES

1. Albert, M. J., A. K. Siddique, M. S. Islam, A. S. G. Faruque, M. Ansaruzzaman, S. M. Faruque, and R. B. Sack. 1993. Large outbreak of clinical cholera due to *Vibrio cholerae* non-O1 in Bangladesh. *Lancet* **341**:704.

2. Albright, L. M., E. Huala, and F. M. Ausubel. 1989. Prokaryotic signal transduction mediated by sensor and regulator protein pairs. *Annu. Rev. Genet.* **23**:311–336.

3. Attridge, S. R., E. Voss, and P. A. Manning. 1993. The role of toxin-coregulated pili in the pathogenesis of *Vibrio cholerae* O1 El Tor. *Microbial Pathogen.* **15**:421–431.

4. Bakeeva, L. E., K. M. Chumakov, A. L. Drachev, A. L. Metlina, and V. P. Skulachev. 1986. The sodium cycle. III. *Vibrio alginolyticus* resembles *Vibrio cholerae* and some other vibriones by flagellar motor and ribosomal 5S-RNA structures. *Biochim. et Biophys. Acta* **850**:466–472.

5. Bennish, M. L. 1994. Cholera: pathophysiology, clinical features, and treatment, p. 229–255. *In* I. K. Wachsmuth, P. A. Blake, and Ø. Olsvik (ed.), *Vibrio cholerae and Cholera: Molecular to Global Perspectives.* American Society for Microbiology, Washington, D.C.

6. Bik, E. M., A. E. Bunschoten, R. D. Gouw, and F. Mooi. 1995. Genesis of the novel epidemic *Vibrio cholerae* O139 strain: evidence for horizontal transfer of genes involved in polysaccharide synthesis. *EMBO J.* **14**:209–216.

7. Bik, E. M., A. E. Bunschoten, R. J. L. Willems, A. C. Y. Chang, and F. R. Mooi. 1996. Genetic organization and functional analysis of the *otn* DNA essential for cell-wall polysaccharide synthesis in *Vibrio cholerae* O139. *Mol. Microbiol.* **20**:799–811.

8. Brown, I. I., and L. A. Sirenko. 1997. The role of the sodium cycle of energy coupling in the emergence and persistence of natural foci of modern cholera. *Biochemistry* (Moscow) **62**:225–230.

9. Brown, R. C., and R. K. Taylor. 1995. Organization of *tcp*, *acf*, and *toxT* genes within a ToxT-dependent operon. *Mol. Microbiol.* **16**:425–439.

10. Carroll, P. A., K. T. Tashima, M. B. Rogers, V. J. DiRita, and S. B. Calderwood. 1997. Phase variation in *tcpH* modulates expression of the ToxR regulon in *Vibrio cholerae. Mol. Microbiol.* **25**:1099–1111.

11. Cash, R. A., S. I. Music, J. P. Libonati, M. J. Snyder, R. P. Wenzel, and R. B. Hornick. 1974. Response of man to infection with *Vibrio cholerae*. I. Clinical, serologic, and bacteriologic responses to a known inoculum. *J. Infect. Dis.* **129**:45–52.

12. Champion, G. A., M. N. Neely, M. A. Brennan, and V. J. DiRita. 1997. A branch in the ToxR regulatory cascade of *Vibrio cholerae* revealed by characterization of *toxT* mutant strains. *Mol. Microbiol.* **23**:323–331.

13. **Chen, F., G. M. Evins, W. L. Cook, R. Almeida, N. Hargrett-Bean, and K. Wachsmuth.** 1991. Genetic diversity among toxigenic and nontoxigenic *Vibrio cholerae* O1 isolated from the Western Hemisphere. *Epidemiol. Infect.* **107:** 225–233.

14. **Chiang, S. L., and J. J. Mekalanos.** 1998. Use of signature-tagged transposon mutagenesis to identify *Vibrio cholerae* genes critical for colonization. *Mol. Microbiol.* **27:**797–806.

15. **Clark, C. A., L. Purins, P. Kaewrakon, and P. A. Manning.** 1997. VCR repetitive sequence elements in the *Vibrio cholerae* chromosome constitute a mega-integron. *Mol. Microbiol.* **26:**1137–1138. (Letter.)

16. **Colwell, R. R.** 1996. Global climate and infectious disease: the cholera paradigm. *Science* **274:** 2025–2031.

17. **Colwell, R. R., and A. Huq.** 1994. Vibrios in the environment: viable but nonculturable *Vibrio cholerae*, p. 117–133. *In* I. K. Wachsmuth, P. A. Blake, and Ø. Olsvik (ed.), *Vibrio cholerae and Cholera: Molecular to Global Perspectives.* American Society for Microbiology, Washington, D.C.

18. **Comstock, L. E., J. A. Johnson, J. M. Machalski, J. G. Morris, and J. B. Kaper.** 1996. Cloning and sequence of a region encoding a surface polysaccharide of *Vibrio cholerae* O139 and characterization of the insertion site in the chromosome of *Vibrio cholerae* O1. *Mol. Microbiol.* **19:** 815–826.

19. **Comstock, L. E., D. Maneval, P. Panigrahi, A. Joseph, M. M. Levine, J. B. Kaper, J. G. Morris, and J. Johnson.** 1995. The capsule and O antigen in *Vibrio cholerae* O139 Bengal are associated with a genetic region not present in *Vibrio cholerae* O1. *Infect. Immun.* **63:**317–323.

20. **Coster, T. S., K. P. Killeen, M. K. Waldor, D. Beattie, D. Spriggs, J. R. Kenner, A. Trofa, J. Sadoff, J. J. Mekalanos, and D. N. Taylor.** 1995. Safety, immunogenicity and efficacy of a live attenuated *Vibrio cholerae* O139 vaccine prototype, Bengal-15. *Lancet* **345:**949–952.

21. **DiRita, V. J.** 1995. Three-component regulatory system controlling virulence in *Vibrio cholerae*, p. 351–365. *In* J. A. Hoch and T. J. Silhavy (ed.), *Two-Component Signal Transduction.* American Society for Microbiology, Washington, D.C.

22. **DiRita, V. J., and J. J. Mekalanos.** 1991. Periplasmic interaction between two membrane regulatory proteins, ToxR and ToxS, results in signal transduction and transcriptional activation. *Cell* **64:**29–37.

23. **DiRita, V. J., C. Parsot, G. Jander, and J. J. Mekalanos.** 1991. Regulatory cascade controls virulence in *Vibrio cholerae*. *Proc. Natl. Acad. Sci. USA* **88:**5403–5407.

24. **Everiss, K. D., K. J. Hughes, M. E. Kovach, and K. M. Peterson.** 1994. The *Vibrio cholerae acfB* colonization determinant encodes an inner membrane protein that is related to a family of signal-transducing proteins. *Infect. Immun.* **62:** 3289–3298.

25. **Everiss, K. D., K. J. Hughes, and K. M. Peterson.** 1996. The accessory colonization factor and the toxin-coregulated pilus gene clusters are physically linked in the *Vibrio cholerae* O395 genome. *DNA Seq.* **5:**51–55.

26. **Fallarino, A., C. Mavrangelos, U. H. Stroeher, and P. A. Manning.** 1997. Identification of additional genes required for O-antigen biosynthesis in *Vibrio cholerae* O1. *J. Bacteriol.* **179:** 2147–2153.

27. **Fasano, A., B. Baudry, D. W. Pumplin, S. S. Wasserman, B. D. Tall, J. N. Ketley, and J. B. Kaper.** 1991. *Vibrio cholerae* produces a second enterotoxin which affects intestinal tight junctions. *Proc. Natl. Acad. Sci. USA* **88:**5242–5246.

28. **Finkelstein, R. A.** 1992. Cholera enterotoxin (choleragen): a historical perspective, p. 155–187. *In* D. Barua and W. B. Greenough III (ed.), *Cholera.* Plenum Publishing Corp., New York.

29. **Finkelstein, R. A., M. Boesman-Finkelstein, Y. Chang, and C. C. Häse.** 1992. *Vibrio cholerae* hemagglutinin/protease, colonial variation, virulence, and detachment. *Infect. Immun.* **60:** 472–478.

30. **Finn, T. M., J. Reiser, R. Germanier, and S. J. J. Cryz.** 1987. Cell-associated hemagglutinin-deficient mutant of *Vibrio cholerae*. *Infect. Immun.* **55:**942–946.

31. **Franzon, V. L., A. Barker, and P. A. Manning.** 1993. Nucleotide sequence encoding the mannose-fucose-resistant hemagglutinin of *Vibrio cholerae* O1 and construction of a mutant. *Infect. Immun.* **61:**3032–3037.

32. **Gardel, C., and J. J. Mekalanos.** 1996. Alterations in *Vibrio cholerae* motility phenotypes correlate with changes in virulence factor expression. *J. Bacteriol.* **64:**2246–2255.

33. **Glass, R. I., and R. E. Black.** 1992. The epidemiology of cholera, p. 129–154. *In* D. Barua and W. B. Greenough 3d (ed.), *Current Topics in Infectious Disease: Cholera.* Plenum Publishing Corp., New York.

34. **Goldberg, M. B., V. J. DiRita, and S. B. Calderwood.** 1990. Identification of an iron-regulated virulence determinant in *Vibrio cholerae*, using TnphoA mutagenesis. *Infect. Immun.* **58:**55–60.

35. **Greenough, W. B., 3d.** 1995. *Vibrio cholerae* and cholera, p. 1934–1945. *In* G. L. Mandell, J. E. Bennett, and R. Dolin (ed.), *Principles and Prac-*

tice of Infectious Diseases, 4th ed., vol. 2. Churchill Livingstone, New York.

36. **Harkey, C. W., K. D. Everiss, and K. M. Peterson.** 1994. The *Vibrio cholerae* toxin-coregulated-pilus gene *tcpI* encodes a homolog of methyl-accepting chemotaxis proteins. *Infect. Immun.* **62:**2669–2678.

37. **Hensel, M., J. E. Shea, C. Gleeson, M. D. Jones, E. Dalton, and D. W. Holden.** 1995. Simultaneous identification of bacterial virulence genes by negative selection. *Science* **269:**400–403.

38. **Herrington, D. A., R. H. Hall, G. Losonsky, J. J. Mekalanos, R. K. Taylor, and M. M. Levine.** 1988. Toxin, toxin-coregulated pili, and the *toxR* regulon are essential for *Vibrio cholerae* pathogenesis in humans. *J. Exp. Med.* **168:**1487–1492.

39. **Higgins, D. E., and V. J. DiRita.** 1994. Transcriptional control of *toxT*, a regulatory gene in the ToxR regulon of *Vibrio cholerae*. *Mol. Microbiol.* **14:**17–29.

40. **Higgins, D. E., E. Nazareno, and V. J. DiRita.** 1992. The virulence gene activator ToxT from *Vibrio cholerae* is a member of the AraC family of transcriptional activators. *J. Bacteriol.* **174:**6874–6980.

41. **Häse, C. C., and J. J. Mekalanos.** 1998. TcpP protein is a positive regulator of virulence gene expression in *Vibrio cholerae*. *Proc. Natl. Acad. Sci. USA* **95:**730–734.

42. **Iredell, J. R., and P. A. Manning.** 1994. The toxin-coregulated pilus of *Vibrio cholerae* O1: a model for type 4 pilus biogenesis? *Trends Microbiol.* **2:**187–192.

43. **Iredell, J. R., and P. A. Manning.** 1997. Outer membrane translocation arrest of the TcpA pilin subunit in *rfb* mutants of *Vibrio cholerae* O1 strain 569B. *J. Bacteriol.* **179:**2038–2046.

44. **Johnson, J. A., C. A. Salles, P. Panigrahi, M. J. Albert, A. C. Wright, R. J. Johnson, and J. G. Morris.** 1994. *Vibrio cholerae* O139 synonym Bengal is closely related to *Vibrio cholerae* El Tor but has important differences. *Infect. Immun.* **62:**2108–2110.

45. **Jonson, G., J. Holmgren, and A. M. Svennerholm.** 1991. Identification of a mannose-binding pilus on *Vibrio cholerae* El Tor. *Microb. Pathog.* **11:**433–441.

46. **Jonson, G., M. Lebens, and J. Holmgren.** 1994. Cloning and sequencing of *Vibrio cholerae* mannose-sensitive haemagglutinin pilin gene: localization of *mshA* within a cluster of type 4 pilin genes. *Mol. Microbiol.* **13:**109–118.

47. **Kaper, J. B., A. Fasano, and M. Trucksis.** 1994. Toxins of *Vibrio cholerae*, p. 145–176. *In* I. K. Wachsmuth, P. A. Blake, and Ø. Olsvik (ed.), *Vibrio cholerae and Cholera: Molecular to Global Per-*

spectives. American Society for Microbiology, Washington D.C.

48. **Kaper, J. B., J. G. Morris, and M. M. Levine.** 1995. Cholera. *Clin. Microbiol. Rev.* **8:**48–86.

49. **Karaolis, D. K., R. Lan, and P. R. Reeves.** 1995. The sixth and seventh cholera pandemics are due to independent clones separately derived from environmental, nontoxigenic, non-O1 *Vibrio cholerae*. *J. Bacteriol.* **177:**3191–3198.

50. **Kaufman, M. R., J. M. Seyer, and R. K. Taylor.** 1991. Processing of TCP pilin by TcpJ typifies a common step intrinsic to a newly recognized pathway of extracellular protein secretion by gram-negative bacteria. *Genes Dev.* **5:**1834–1846.

51. **Kaufman, M. R., C. E. Shaw, I. D. Jones, and R. K. Taylor.** 1993. Biogenesis and regulation of the *Vibrio cholerae* toxin-coregulated pilus: analogies to other virulence factor secretory systems. *Gene* **126:**43–49.

52. **Kaufman, M. R., and R. K. Taylor.** 1994. The toxin-coregulated pilus: biogenesis and function, p. 187–202. *In* I. K. Wachsmuth, P. A. Blake, and Ø. Olsvik (ed.), *Vibrio cholerae and Cholera: Molecular to Global Perspectives*. American Society for Microbiology, Washington D.C.

53. **Kenner, J., T. Coster, A. Trofa, D. Taylor, M. Barrera-Oro, T. Hyman, J. Adams, D. Beattie, K. Killeen, J. J. Mekalanos, and J. C. Sadoff.** 1995. Peru-15, a live, attenuated oral vaccine candidate for *Vibrio cholerae* O1 El Tor. *J. Infect. Dis.* **172:**1126–1129.

54. **Klose, K. E., and J. J. Mekalanos.** 1998. Differential regulation of multiple flagellins in *Vibrio cholerae*. *J. Bacteriol.* **180:**303–316.

55. **Kovach, M. E., M. D. Shaffer, and K. M. Peterson.** 1996. A putative integrase gene defines the distal end of large cluster of ToxR-regulated colonization genes in *Vibrio cholerae*. *Microbiology* **142:**2165–2174.

56. **Levine, M. M., R. E. Black, M. L. Clements, C. Lanata, S. Sears, T. Honda, C. R. Young, and R. A. Finkelstein.** 1984. Evaluation in humans of attenuated *Vibrio cholerae* El Tor Ogawa strain Texas Star-SR as a live oral vaccine. *Infect. Immun.* **43:**515–522.

57. **Levine, M. M., J. B. Kaper, D. Herrington, G. Losonsky, J. G. Morris, M. Clements, R. E. Black, B. Tall, and R. Hall.** 1988. Volunteer studies of deletion mutants of *Vibrio cholerae* O1 prepared by recombinant techniques. *Infect. Immun.* **56:**161–167.

58. **Mekalanos, J. J., D. J. Swartz, G. D. Pearson, N. Harford, F. Groyne, and M. deWilde.** 1983. Cholera toxin genes: nucleotide sequence, deletion analysis and vaccine development. *Nature* **306:**551–557.

59. **Mel, S. F., and J. J. Mekalanos.** 1996. Modulation of horizontal gene transfer in pathogenic bacteria by *in vivo* signals. *Cell* **87**:795–798.

60. **Miller, V. L., V. J. DiRita, and J. J. Mekalanos.** 1989. Identification of *toxS*, a regulatory gene whose product enhances *toxR*-mediated activation of the cholera toxin promoter. *J. Bacteriol.* **171**:1288–1293.

61. **Miller, V. L., and J. J. Mekalanos.** 1988. A novel suicide vector and its use in construction of insertion mutations: osmoregulation of outer membrane proteins and virulence determinants in *Vibrio cholerae* requires *toxR*. *J. Bacteriol.* **170**:2575–2583.

62. **Miller, V. L., R. K. Taylor, and J. J. Mekalanos.** 1987. Cholera toxin transcriptional activator ToxR is a transmembrane DNA binding protein. *Cell* **48**:271–279.

63. **Minami, A., S. Hashimoto, H. Abe, M. Arita, T. Taniguchi, T. Honda, T. Miwatani, and M. Nishibuchi.** 1991. Cholera enterotoxin production in *Vibrio cholerae* O1 strains isolated from the environment and from humans in Japan. *Appl. Environ. Microbiol.* **57**:2152–2157.

64. **Nalin, D. R., R. J. Levine, M. M. Levine, D. Hoover, E. Bergquist, J. McLaughlin, J. Libonati, J. Alam, and R. B. Hornick.** 1978. Cholera, non-vibrio cholera, and stomach acid. *Lancet* **2**:856–859.

65. **Ogierman, M. A., S. Zabihi, L. Mourtzios, and P. A. Manning.** 1993. Genetic organization and sequence of the promoter-distal region of the *tcp* gene cluster of *Vibrio cholerae*. *Gene* **126**:51–60.

66. **Osek, J., A. M. Svennerholm, and J. Holmgren.** 1992. Protection against *Vibrio cholerae* El Tor infection by specific antibodies against mannose-binding hemagglutinin pili. *Infect. Immun.* **60**:4961–4964.

67. **Ottemann, K. M., and J. J. Mekalanos.** 1994. Regulation of cholera toxin expression, p. 177–185. *In* I. K. Wachsmuth, P. A. Blake, and Ø. Olsvik (ed.), *Vibrio cholerae and Cholera: Molecular to Global Perspectives*. American Society for Microbiology, Washington, D.C.

68. **Pearson, G. D. N., A. Woods, S. L. Chiang, and J. J. Mekalanos.** 1993. CTX genetic element encodes a site-specific recombination system and an intestinal colonization factor. *Proc. Natl. Acad. Sci. USA* **90**:3750–3754.

69. **Peek, J. A., and R. K. Taylor.** 1992. Characterization of a periplasmic thiol:disulfide interchange protein required for the functional maturation of secreted virulence factors of *Vibrio cholerae*. *Proc. Natl. Acad. Sci. USA* **89**:6210–6214.

70. **Peterson, K. M., and J. J. Mekalanos.** 1988. Characterization of the *Vibrio cholerae* ToxR regulon: identification of novel genes involved in intestinal colonization. *Infect. Immun.* **56**:2822–2829.

71. **Ramamurthy, T., S. Garg, R. Sharma, S. K. Bhattacharya, G. B. Nair, T. Shimada, T. Takeda, T. Karasawa, H. Kurazano, A. Pal, and Y. Takeda.** 1993. Emergence of novel strain of *Vibrio cholerae* with epidemic potential in southern and eastern India. *Lancet* **341**:703–704.

72. **Reidl, J., and J. J. Mekalanos.** 1995. Characterization of *Vibrio cholerae* bacteriophage K139 and use of a novel mini-transposon to identify a phage-encoded virulence factor. *Mol. Microbiol.* **18**:685–701.

73. **Richardson, K.** 1991. Roles of motility and flagellar structure in pathogenicity of *Vibrio cholerae*: analysis of motility mutants in three animal models. *Infect. Immun.* **59**:2727–2736.

74. **Rubin, E. J., W. Lin, J. J. Mekalanos, and M. K. Waldor.** 1998. Replication and integration of a *Vibrio cholerae* cryptic plasmid linked to the CTX prophage. *Mol. Microbiol.* **28**:1247–1254.

75. **Rubin, E. J., M. K. Waldor, and J. J. Mekalanos.** 1998. Mobile genetic elements and the evolution of new epidemic strains of *Vibrio cholerae*, p. 147–161. *In* R. A. Krause (ed.), *Emerging Infections*. Academic Press, New York.

76. **Scholtissek, C.** 1994. Source for influenza pandemics. *Eur. J. Epidemiol.* **10**:455–458.

77. **Shaw, C. E., and R. K. Taylor.** 1990. *Vibrio cholerae* O395 *tcpA* pilin gene sequence and comparison of predicted protein structural features to those of type 4 pilins. *Infect. Immun.* **58**:3042–3049.

78. **Shimodori, S., F. Kojima, K. Amako, M. Ehara, Y. Ichinose, T. Hirayama, Y. Honma, M. Iwanaga, and M. J. Albert.** 1996. Filamentous phages of *Vibrio cholerae* O139 and O1, p. 34–35. Thirty-Second Joint Conference on Cholera and Related Diarrheal Diseases. The U.S.-Japan Cooperative Medical Science Program.

79. **Sigel, S. P., S. Lanier, V. S. Baselski, and C. D. Parker.** 1980. *In vivo* evaluation of pathogenicity of clinical and environmental isolates of *Vibrio cholerae*. *Infect. Immun.* **28**:681–687.

80. **Skorupski, K., and R. K. Taylor.** 1997. Cyclic AMP and its receptor protein negatively regulate the coordinate expression of cholera toxin and the toxin-coregulated pilus in *Vibrio cholerae*. *Proc. Natl. Acad. Sci. USA* **94**:265–270.

81. **Stroeher, U. H., K. E. Jedani, B. K. Dredge, R. Morona, M. H. Brown, L. E. Karageorgos, M. J. Albert, and P. A. Manning.** 1995.

Genetic rearrangements in the *rfb* regions of *Vibrio cholerae* O1 and O139. *Proc. Natl. Acad. Sci. USA* **84:**2833–2837.

82. **Stroeher, U. H., L. E. Karageorgos, R. Morona, and P. A. Manning.** 1992. Serotype conversion in *Vibrio cholerae* O1. *Proc. Natl. Acad. Sci. USA* **89:**2566–2570.

83. **Strom, M. S., and S. Lory.** 1993. Structure-function and biogenesis of the type IV pili. *Annu. Rev. Microbiol.* **47:**565–596.

84. **Svennerholm, A.-M., G. Jonson, and J. Holmgren.** 1994. Immunity to *Vibrio cholerae* infection, p. 257–272. *In* I. K. Wachsmuth, P. A. Blake, and Ø. Olsvik (ed.), *Vibrio cholerae and Cholera: Molecular to Global Perspectives.* American Society for Microbiology, Washington, D.C.

85. **Swerdlow, D. L., and M. Isaäcson.** 1994. The epidemiology of cholera in Africa, p. 297–308. *In* I. K. Wachsmuth, P. A. Blake, and Ø. Olsvik (ed.), *Vibrio cholerae and Cholera: Molecular to Global Perspectives.* American Society for Microbiology, Washington, D.C.

86. **Tacket, C. O., G. Losonsky, J. P. Nataro, S. J. Cryz, R. Edelman, A. Fasano, J. Michalski, J. B. Kaper, and M. M. Levine.** 1993. Safety, immunogenicity, and transmissibility of live oral cholera vaccine candidate CVD112, a ΔctxA Δzot Δace derivative of El Tor Ogawa *Vibrio cholerae. J. Infect. Dis.* **168:**1536–1540.

87. **Tacket, C. O., R. K. Taylor, G. Losonsky, Y. Lim, J. P. Nataro, J. B. Kaper, and M. M. Levine.** 1998. Investigation of the roles of toxin-coregulated pili and mannose-sensitive hemagglutinin pili in the pathogenesis of *Vibrio cholerae* O139 infection. *Infect. Immun.* **66:**692–695.

88. **Tashima, K. T., P. A. Carroll, M. B. Rogers, and S. B. Calderwood.** 1996. Relative importance of three iron-regulated outer membrane proteins for in vivo growth of *Vibrio cholerae. Infect. Immun.* **64:**1756–1761.

89. **Tauxe, R., L. Seminario, R. Tapia, and M. Libel.** 1994. The Latin American epidemic, p. 321–344. *In* I. K. Wachsmuth, P. A. Blake, and Ø. Olsvik (ed.), *Vibrio cholerae and Cholera: Molecular to Global Perspectives.* American Society for Microbiology Washington, D.C.

90. **Taylor, D. N., K. P. Killeen, D. C. Hack, J. R. Kenner, T. S. Coster, D. T. Beattie, J. Ezzell, T. Hyman, A. Trofa, M. H. Sjogren, A. Friedlander, J. J. Mekalanos, and J. C. Sadoff.** 1994. Development of a live, oral, attenuated vaccine against El Tor cholera. *J. Infect. Dis.* **170:**1518–1523.

91. **Taylor, R., C. Shaw, K. Peterson, P. Spears, and J. Mekalanos.** 1988. Safe, live *Vibrio cholerae* vaccines? *Vaccine* **6:**151–154.

92. **Taylor, R. K., V. L. Miller, D. B. Furlong, and J. J. Mekalanos.** 1987. Use of *phoA* gene fusions to identify a pilus colonization factor coordinately regulated with cholera toxin. *Proc. Natl. Acad. Sci. USA* **84:**2833–2837.

93. **Thelin, K. H., and R. K. Taylor.** 1996. Toxin-coregulated pilus, but not mannose-sensitive hemagglutinin, is required for colonization by *Vibrio cholerae* O1 El Tor biotype and O139 strains. *Infect. Immun.* **64:**2853–2856.

94. **Trucksis, M., J. Galen, J. Michalski, A. Fasano, and J. B. Kaper.** 1993. Accessory cholera enterotoxin (Ace), the third toxin of a *Vibrio cholerae* virulence cassette. *Proc. Natl. Acad. Sci. USA* **90:**5267–5271.

95. **Vimont, S., S. Dumontier, V. Escuyer, and P. Berche.** 1997. The *rfaD* locus: a region of rearrangement in *Vibrio cholerae* O139. *Gene* **185:**43–47.

96. **Wachsmuth, I. K., Ø. Olsvik, G. M. Evins, and T. Popovic.** 1994. Molecular epidemiology of cholera, p. 357–370. *In* I. K. Wachsmuth, P. A. Blake, and Ø. Olsvik (ed.), *Vibrio cholerae and Cholera: Molecular to Global Perspectives.* American Society for Microbiology, Washington, D.C.

97. **Waldor, M. K., R. Colwell, and J. J. Mekalanos.** 1994. The *Vibrio cholerae* 0139 serogroup antigen includes O-antigen capsule and lipopolysaccharide virulence determinants. *Proc. Natl. Acad. Sci. USA* **91:**11388–11392.

98. **Waldor, M. K., and J. J. Mekalanos.** 1996. Lysogenic conversion by a filamentous phage encoding cholera toxin. *Science* **272:**1910–1914.

99. **Waldor, M. K., E. J. Rubin, G. D. Pearson, H. Kimsey, and J. J. Mekalanos.** 1997. Regulation, replication, and integration functions of the *Vibrio cholerae* CTX φ are encoded by region RS2. *Mol. Microbiol.* **24:**917–926.

100. **Waldor, M. K., H. Tschäpe, and J. J. Mekalanos.** 1996. A new type of conjugative transposon encodes resistance to sulfamethoxazole, trimethoprim, and streptomycin in *Vibrio cholerae* O139. *J. Bacteriol.* **178:**4157–4165.

101. **Ward, H. M., and P. A. Manning.** 1989. Mapping of chromosomal loci associated with lipopolysaccharide synthesis and serotype specificity in *Vibrio cholerae* O1 by transposon mutagenesis using Tn5 and Tn2680. *Mol. Gen. Genet.* **218:**367–370.

102. **Willumsen, B. M., K. Norris, A. G. Papageorge, N. L. Hubbert, and D. R. Lowy.** 1984. Harvey murine sarcoma virus p21ras protein: biological and biochemical significance of the cysteine nearest the carboxy terminus. *EMBO J.* **3:**2581–2585.

103. **Yamasaki, S., K. Hoshino, T. Shimizu, S. Garg, T. Shimada, S. Ho, R. K. Bhadra, G. B. Nair, and Y. Takeda.** 1996. Comparative analysis of the gene responsible for lipopolysaccharide synthesis of *Vibrio cholerae* O1 and O139 and those of non-O1 non-O139 *Vibrio cholerae*, p. 24–27. Thirty-Second Joint Conference on Cholera and Related Diarrheal Diseases. The U.S.-Japan Cooperative Medical Science Program.

INTRACELLULAR MULTIPLICATION OF *LEGIONELLA PNEUMOPHILA* IN HUMAN AND ENVIRONMENTAL HOSTS

Gil Segal and Howard A. Shuman

14

THE LEGIONNAIRES DISEASE BACTERIUM

Legionella pneumophila, the causative agent of Legionnaires disease and related respiratory ailments, is a facultative intracellular pathogen (35). This organism is ingested by human macrophages and evades the microbicidal defenses of the phagocytes by maintaining the vacuolar pH near neutrality (34) and preventing phagosome-lysosome fusion (32). The organism then grows exponentially within a specialized vacuole (31). Many of these events are similar to those which are observed in a variety of other intracellular parasites such as *Toxoplasma gondii*, *Leishmania donovani*, and *Mycobacterium tuberculosis* (3, 16, 39). In contrast to these organisms, *L. pneumophila* can be cultivated easily in the laboratory using standard microbiological media components (21). As we and others have demonstrated, it is possible to perform a wide variety of genetic manipulations conveniently with *L. pneumophila* (51, 52, 63, 64). This provides a distinct advantage in being able to understand the molecular basis for the ability of *L. pneumophila*

and other intracellular pathogens to interact with host cells. It is our hope that the information obtained concerning the ways in which *L. pneumophila* modifies the endosomal pathway and other aspects of intracellular organelle traffic will provide knowledge of general relevance to the other pathogens that replicate in human mononuclear cells, perhaps even viruses such as human immunodeficiency virus.

Although Legionnaires disease and other forms of legionellosis have probably existed in the past, the clinical entities were not recognized until 1976 when several cases of Legionnaires disease occurred at a national convention of the American Legion in Philadelphia, Pennsylvania. It is now clear that man-made devices such as air-conditioner cooling towers, showers, respirators, and other equipment that generates aerosols of standing water contribute to the spread of the organism from the environment and can cause outbreaks of *Legionella* pneumonia (10, 11).

Occurrence in Natural and Man-Made Environments

It has been possible to isolate *L. pneumophila* and related species from almost any type of freshwater sample (24). Frequently the organism is found in close association with algae

Gil Segal and Howard A. Shuman, Department of Microbiology, College of Physicians & Surgeons, Columbia University, 701 West 168th Street, New York, NY 10032.

Microbial Ecology and Infectious Disease, Edited by Eugene Rosenberg
©1999 American Society for Microbiology, Washington, D.C.

and protozoa. Although it is not definitively known if *Legionellaceae* are able to be free living, several lines of evidence strongly suggest that in natural environments, legionellae grow exclusively within other organisms (22). First, many amoebae are found to have *Legionella*-like organisms growing within them (2). Second, a specific protozoan, *Hartmanella vermiformis*, has been identified in several outbreaks of Legionnaires disease (23). Third, it has been demonstrated that *L. pneumophila* can replicate within both amoebae and ciliated protozoa such as *Tetrahymena pyriformis* (30, 41, 60).

Legionellosis is the direct consequence of the ability of *Legionella* spp. to gain access to human lungs by dispersal in aerosols. This occurs in a variety of ways, all of which involve a man-made device. Perhaps the most common device that has been responsible for introducing the organism into the human environment is the air-conditioning cooling tower (66). In this device, water returning from an air-conditioning system is allowed to evaporate. Due to the increased temperature and exposure to the external environment, water that contains legionellae can be cocolonized by protozoan hosts that under some conditions may facilitate explosive growth of the bacteria. Either bacteria or protozoa infected with bacteria are then aerosolized throughout the air-conditioning system. Experiments in susceptible animals have shown that coinfection of *L. pneumophila* and *H. vermiformis* produces more-acute disease than infection with *L. pneumophila* alone (14).

Standard plumbing devices such as shower heads, pipes, and heat-exchange bumpers have also been shown to harbor the organism (10). In this case, biofilms within these devices allow consortia of organisms to thrive (48). It is likely that here as well, protozoa serve as hosts for *Legionella* spp. In a smaller number of cases, other devices such as whirlpools, respiratory therapy devices, and even grocery store produce misters have been shown to be a source of *Legionella* spp. In all these cases, the potential for legionellosis is realized when water containing legionellae alone or in combination with a protozoan is aerosolized.

Legionellae are frequently present in potable water supplies but pose a health threat only in certain circumstances that favor replication of the organism to large enough numbers. These conditions may include the formation of biofilms that contain a susceptible host, temperature, and the absence of added biocides.

Interaction with Human Monocytic Cells

BINDING AND UPTAKE

The association of *L. pneumophila* with human mononuclear phagocytes has been carefully studied by Marcus Horwitz and coworkers. The interaction of *L. pneumophila* with these cells seems to be a multistep process (summarized in Fig. 1). Attachment of the bacteria to the phagocyte is mediated via complement components C3b and C3bi, which covalently modify and attach to the major outer membrane protein, MOMP, encoded by the *ompS* gene (5, 25, 28, 29). The bacteria are then able to bind to the complement receptors CR1 and CR3. Binding to these receptors is able to promote phagocytosis but does not trigger the respiratory burst that accompanies phagocytosis mediated by the immunoglobulin Fc receptor, FcR. Phagocytosis of *L. pneumophila* is an unusual type of coiling phagocytosis in which a single pseudopod wraps around the bacterium (33). Coiling phagocytosis has been observed during the entry of other pathogens (e.g., *L. donovani*, *Chlamydia psittaci*, *Trypanosoma brucei*, and *Borrelia burgdorferi*). In the case of *L. pneumophila*, heat-killed bacteria are also taken up by the coiling mechanism indicating that coiling per se does not require active participation of the bacterium. Coating *L. pneumophila* with specific antibody promotes uptake by conventional FcR-mediated "zipper phagocytosis." About half of the organisms are killed by the cells, and the remaining viable bacteria are able to replicate intracellularly (36).

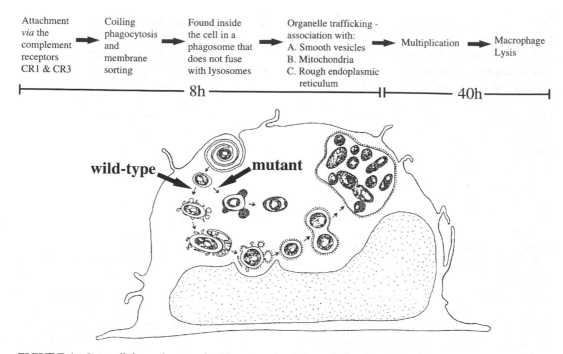

| Attachment *via* the complement receptors CR1 & CR3 | → | Coiling phagocytosis and membrane sorting | → | Found inside the cell in a phagosome that does not fuse with lysosomes | → | Organelle trafficking - association with: A. Smooth vesicles B. Mitochondria C. Rough endoplasmic reticulum | → | Multiplication | → | Macrophage Lysis |

├───────────────── 8h ─────────────────┤├─────── 40h ───────┤

wild-type ... **mutant**

FIGURE 1 Intracellular pathways of wild-type and avirulent mutant *L. pneumophila* in macrophages. Upper part, the series of events that occur in the cell during infection with a wild-type *L. pneumophila*. The scheme represents the differences between wild type and an avirulent mutant. Both wild type and mutant (25D) enter by coiling phagocytosis, but thereafter their pathways diverge. The wild-type phagosome interacts sequentially with smooth vesicles, mitochondria, and rough endoplasmic reticulum; the avirulent mutant does not recruit these organelles. The phagosome of the wild-type *L. pneumophila*, but not of the avirulent mutant, avoids fusion with lysosomes. The wild-type organism multiplies within the ribosome-lined phagosome until the macrophage becomes full of bacteria and disintegrates. The mutant survives but does not multiply in its phagolysosome, and it does not destroy the macrophage.

PHAGOSOME FORMATION AND FATE

Following coiling phagocytosis, the many layers of the coil resolve to form a single-layered membrane-bound compartment. Although the mechanism of resolution is not understood, there is some information about the behavior of individual plasma membrane markers during this process. Clemens and Horwitz examined the distribution of plasma membrane alkaline phosphatase, 5′-nucleotidase, major histocompatibility complex (MHC) class I and class II, and complement receptors CR1 and CR3. They found that some proteins were excluded from the phagosomal membrane (MHC, alkaline phosphatase) while others were enriched (CR1, CR3, 5′-nucleotidase). This implies that the bacteria have exerted some effect on the composition of the incipient phagosomal membrane as it is being formed (17, 18).

Following its formation, the phagosome undergoes a variety of events that distinguish it from typical phagosomes. The most crucial events from the point of view of the bacterium seem to be the failure to acidify and the failure to fuse with secondary lysosomes (32, 34). In addition, the phagosome is surrounded by smooth vesicles and mitochondria (31). Eventually the cytosolic side of the phagosome is surrounded with material that may correspond to, or be derived from, rough endoplasmic reticulum (ER). In support of this idea, Swanson and Isberg have described intense staining for the ER chaperone BiP at this location (56). Because these properties distinguish the phagosome from known compartments within the endosomal pathway, we have chosen to call this compartment the *Legionella*-specific phagosome, or LSP. It is clear from the analysis of mutant forms of *L. pneumophila* with decreased ability to replicate intracellularly that the properties of the LSP are important for the intracellular fate of the bacteria (see below).

INTRACELLULAR MULTIPLICATION

At some point following formation of the LSP, the internalized bacteria begin to replicate. There is typically a lag time of approximately 6 to 8 h postinfection before any increase in bacterial number is detected. During this time, it is possible that the LSP is being formed and the proper conditions for growth are being established. Alternatively, the bacteria are in a "lag phase" of growth and are adapting to the nutritional conditions that prevail within the LSP. It should be possible to distinguish these possibilities by isolating bacteria from host cells at 6 to 8 h postinfection and determining if they undergo the same "lag phase." If they begin to replicate immediately after uptake, it would favor the latter explanation for the observed delay. In contrast, if the delay is still observed, it would argue that it takes a certain time for the LSP to support *L. pneumophila* replication.

Once the bacteria begin to replicate intracellularly, their generation time is approximately 2 h, which is the same as the generation time in bacteriological media. This implies that their nutritional needs are met within the LSP. It is generally considered that *L. pneumophila* require high concentrations of cysteine (400 mg/liter) and iron salts (250 mg/liter) in bacteriological media (20). One might therefore think that these conditions are present within the LSP. Results from our laboratory present a different view. When iron salts and cysteine are mixed in preparation of standard bacteriological media for *L. pneumophila*, they react to form a variety of redox products, including cystine. We found that addition of 40 to 60 mg/liter cysteine to standard media would support *L. pneumophila* growth if no additional iron salts were added. In addition, higher levels of iron were toxic to *L. pneumophila* in the absence of the high cysteine concentrations (A. B. Sadosky and H. A. Shuman, unpublished results). What appears most important is the correct balance of cysteine and iron. *L. pneumophila* are certainly auxotrophic for cysteine and may require slightly higher concentrations than *Escherichia coli* to satisfy their cysteine requirement, but the apparent need for extraordinarily high concentrations of this amino acid and iron salts is an artifact introduced through unnecessary addition of high concentrations of iron. There is no need, therefore, to infer the existence of extraordinary concentrations of either cysteine or iron in the LSP.

Free amino acids are the preferred source of carbon, nitrogen, and energy for *L. pneumophila*. In particular, proline, serine, and threonine seem to be most actively utilized (58, 59). One would therefore expect that these would be available within the LSP. Although *L. pneumophila* secretes an abundant Zn^{2+} protease, MSP, that could in principle generate amino acids from proteins in the LSP, it is not required for intracellular replication. A mutant that lacks MSP and secretes less than 0.1% of the wild-type levels of caseinolytic activity replicates intracellularly with the same generation time as the wild type (45, 57). It should be possible to evaluate which materials are not available in the LSP with the aid of appropriate mutants. For example, thymidine-requiring mutants of *L. pneumophila* are unable to grow in macrophages, indicating that thymidine is unavailable in the LSP (6, 44).

Other conditions are known to be critical for *L. pneumophila* replication in bacteriological media; pH near neutrality, absence of Na^+, and absence of oxidants. These conditions seem to be reflected in the LSP. Indeed, the pH of the LSP was found to be close to pH 6.5 to 6.8 (34). As mentioned above, *L. pneumophila* circumvents the respiratory burst produced by the macrophages. Because Na$^+$ inhibits the growth of wild-type *L. pneumophila* in bacteriological media, it would be expected that the LSP would contain low amounts of this ion (15).

HOST CELL KILLING

Infection of host cells with wild-type *L. pneumophila* results in a dramatic cytopathic effect approximately 18 h postinfection. Initial studies suggested that the secreted MSP protease was a cytotoxin and was responsible for this cytopathic effect. As mentioned above, null mutants in the structural gene for the protease were found to replicate within cells and to produce the same cytopathic effect as wild-type *L. pneumophila* (9). Others had reported that low-molecular-weight compounds secreted from the bacteria had cytotoxic activity. None of these studies rigorously excluded the possibility that lipopolysaccharides derived from the bacteria were responsible for the observed effects (27). The question of whether *L. pneumophila* secretes cytotoxins that are responsible for host cell killing is still unanswered.

An alternative view is that the bacteria induce apoptosis, or programed cell death, in the host. This phenomenon has been described for *Shigella flexneri* and *Bordetella pertussis* (40, 68). Both the teleologic significance and mechanisms for a parasite inducing apoptosis are at present unclear. Muller et al. describe apoptosis in phorbol myristate acetate (PMA)-treated HL-60 cells infected with *L. pneumophila*. The authors conclude that apoptosis is due to the infecting *L. pneumophila* (46). Other groups describe both the induction and attenuation of apoptosis in HL-60 cells by PMA alone (67). Whether *L. pneumophila* truly induces apoptosis in macrophages or other host cells that have not been treated with phorbol esters and other compounds known to induce apoptosis requires clarification.

A third view is that the burden of bacterial replication and the production of NH$_3$ from amino acid metabolism as well as other byproducts of metabolism eventually cause the host cells to die. At the present time, none of the three models can be convincingly ruled out. In theory, study of *L. pneumophila* mutants that are not cytotoxic for the host might indicate something about the mechanisms of cell death.

Other *Legionella* functions that have been suggested to be important in the intracellular development of the organism are (i) phosphatases, (ii) phospholipase C, (iii) protein kinases, and (iv) a low-molecular-weight toxin. The properties of these molecules and their imputed importance has been recently summarized (19). The importance of these molecules for intracellular multiplication, host cell killing, or disease in animals has not been tested. A phenomenon of rapid cytotoxicity was reported by Husmann and Johnson (37). Killing of host cells by large numbers of *L. pneumophila* in close association with the cells was observed after short times. Avirulent mutants were unable to produce the same effect. Very recently, Kirby et al. reported more details about the rapid cytotoxicity and presented evidence for a pore with a specific diameter in the membranes of host cells infected with large numbers of *L. pneumophila* (42). Formation of the pore depended on genes that are known to be required for intracellular multiplication, which correspond to some of the *icm* genes described below. The significance of the rapid cytotoxicity and its relationship to inhibition of phagosome-lysosome fusion and intracellular multiplication is unclear at the present time.

Interaction with Unicellular Amoebae

REPLICATIVE VERSUS
SYMBIOTIC LIFESTYLES

As described above, the ability of *L. pneumophila* to replicate within unicellular protozoa may be a key requirement for their ability to be delivered to the human environment. T. J. Rowbotham has described the ability of *L. pneumophila* to replicate within *Acanthamoeba* and *Naegleria* spp. (49, 50). In addition, other organisms, clearly related to *L. pneumophila* on the basis of rRNA sequence homology, are able to replicate within amoebae and protozoa. A number of other *Legionella*-like amoebal pathogens have been described and classified phylogenetically into 12 groups that may represent five species (2). Independently, Jeon and coworkers had observed bacteria-like forms within *Amoeba discoides* and *Amoeba proteus*. Subsequent isolation of the bacteria and analysis of their genes for 16S rRNA and the GroEL heat shock protein enabled these workers to conclude that the bacteria were related to the taxon *Legionellaceae*. Jeon and coworkers refer to the symbionts as "X-bacteria" and have found them in many isolates of amoebae from nature (38). These results and those cited above indicate that *Legionella* sp. can have either a symbiotic or replicative relationship with the protozoan host. What determines which relationship will take place is unknown at present, but it may depend on factors in both organisms.

COMPARISON OF EVENTS IN PROTOZOAN AND MAMMALIAN HOST CELLS

Several investigators have compared the events in protozoan hosts with those described above for mammalian phagocytes. In general, similar events are observed over a wide range of hosts. The cardinal feature of the *L. pneumophila* lifestyle seems to be avoidance of phagosome-lysosome fusion and replication in a membrane-bound compartment that exhibits unusual features such as association with smooth vesicles, mitochondria, and ER (1, 12, 55).

Important differences between the mammalian and protozoan hosts seem to be the ability of the protozoa to expel "respirable vesicles" (8), membrane-bound compartments that contain large numbers of living *L. pneumophila*, and the ability of the protozoa to encyst and encapsulate the bacteria in a protective particle. The respirable vesicles likely result from the typical functioning of a defecatory system used to eliminate metabolic waste products. Cysts are formed when the protozoa encounter conditions of low moisture and/or poor nutrient availability (4).

The question of receptors for *Legionella* on protozoan hosts is of particular interest since protozoa obviously do not possess components of the complement cascade and their integrin receptors. Abu Kwaik has shown that specific large-molecular-weight receptors for sugars serve as the receptors for *L. pneumophila* on *H. vermiformis*. Indeed, sugars that are known ligands for the receptors block *L. pneumophila* entry (26, 61).

GENETIC ANALYSIS OF FACTORS REQUIRED FOR INTRACELLULAR MULTIPLICATION AND HOST CELL KILLING

Complementation of Avirulent Variants

Several approaches have been taken to understand the genetic basis for intracellular multiplication. The first was based on the properties of avirulent variants that had lost the ability to replicate inside macrophages and were also defective in preventing phagosome-lysosome fusion. We reasoned that introduction of a wild-type region of the *L. pneumophila* genome that restored the ability to replicate within and kill human macrophages would provide information about the genes that were defective in the variants. A library of wild-type *L. pneumophila* DNA was introduced to an avirulent variant, and complemented bacteria that regained the abilities to replicate intracellularly and kill host cells were identified with the aid of a plaque assay (43). The region of the *L. pneumophila* genome present in the complementing plasmid contained several genes that we referred to as *icm* (intracellular multiplication) genes (13). Using an independent approach, Berger and Isberg identified the same region and referred to a large open reading frame (ORF) as *dotA* (defective organelle trafficking) (7).

Transposon-Induced Mutants That Cannot Kill Host Cells

To ask if the *icm/dotA* locus was the only set of genes required for intracellular multiplication and host cell killing, we used random transposon mutagenesis with Tn*903*dII*lacZ* to generate a large collection ($n \sim$ 5,000) of independent random insertion mutations in the *L. pneumophila* genome. Among these mutants, we identified 55 mutants that lost the ability to multiply within and kill HL-60–derived macrophages (51). These mutants grow as well as wild type on bacteriological media, indicating that their defect is specific to the intracellular lifestyle. Initially, the mutants were classified into 16 hybridization groups on the basis of the *Eco*RI fragment that contained the transposon. Subsequently, we have characterized these mutants in several ways to find out about the genes and functions they encode. Mapping and DNA sequence analysis indicate that most of the mutations (38 of 55) define two unlinked regions of the *L. pneumophila* genome, which we refer to as region I and region II.

To characterize the *icm* genes genetically, we have (i) cloned the wild-type DNA that corresponds to the mutant loci; (ii) determined the DNA sequence of these regions; (iii) determined the sequence of the fusion joints between the transposon and *L. pneumophila* DNA, for 53 of 55 mutations; (iv) constructed mutations in ORFs not containing a transposon; (v) analyzed the phenotypes of the mutants; and (vi) conducted complementation tests for mutations in each gene to evaluate its role in intracellular multiplication and host cell killing.

icm/dot GENE COMPLEX: 23 GENES—ONE FUNCTION?

Region I
Region I contains the *icmA/dotA* locus. The previously identified 12-kb *Eco*RI fragment that complemented the avirulent variant "25D" (43), independently identified by Berger and Isberg, corresponds to hybridization group 1. Eleven of the Tn*903*dIII*lacZ* insertions (i.e., group 1) map to this region, including two in the *dotA* gene. The nine other insertions lie in three adjacent genes called *icmV*, *icmW*, and *icmX*. Figure 2 and Table 1 describe the arrangement of these genes and

the properties of the gene products. Results from Ralph Isberg's group indicate the presence of three other genes, *dotBCD*, 8 kb downstream from *dotA* that are required for intracellular multiplication (62). We found that group 5 represents part of a gene that has sequence similarity to components of the "general secretory pathway" in gram-negative bacteria and corresponds to the *dotB* gene.

Region II
Region II (22 kb) comprises 18 genes, 16 of which are required for intracellular multiplication. As a result of sequencing and cosmid mapping, we established that seven of the DNA hybridization groups are contiguous and contain 18 genes. Seven of these genes were not mutated in any of the transposon insertion mutants. For these genes, we constructed mutants by insertion of drug-resistance elements in the *L. pneumophila* genome. Complementation studies indicate that 16 of the 18 genes are required for intracellular multiplication and macrophage killing. Mutations in the other two genes, *lphA* and *tphA* (for lipoprotein homolog and transport protein homolog, respectively) are indistinguishable from wild-type in HL-60–derived macrophages. Work in Isberg's laboratory has also identified some of the genes in this region (62).

THE *icmTSRQPO* CLUSTER
The *icmTSRQPO* gene cluster was identified by cloning the region corresponding to DNA hybridization group 3 (54). The cloned DNA was sequenced (6,432 bp) and found to contain six genes, *icmT–O*. Five of these contained at least one transposon. The *icmS* gene did not contain a transposon and was mutagenized by insertion of a kanamycin resistance cassette. Bacteria with mutations in the *icmS*, *icmR*, and *icmQ* genes retained some detectable ability to kill HL–60 derived macrophages. In contrast, those with mutations in the *icmT*, *icmP*, and *icmO* genes were completely defective in macrophage killing. Complementation tests using plasmids with in-frame deletions of each gene indicated that the *icmTS* genes are

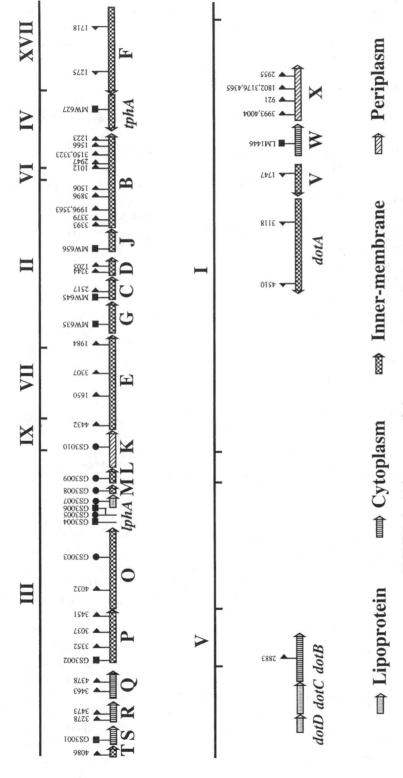

FIGURE 2 Linkage map of the two *icm* regions. Region I containing *icmVWX-dotABCD* genes and region II containing *icmTSRQPO-lphA-icmMLKEGCDJB-tphA-icmF* (*icm* genes are indicated by one-letter code). Coding regions are indicated by bold arrows, the different patterns indicate the predicted location of the protein in the bacterial cell. The DNA hybridization groups are indicated above the strain names. The site of the Tn903dIIlacZ insertions (LELA strains) are indicated by flags (showing the direction of the *lacZ* gene fusion), the site of the kanamycin-resistance cassettes are indicated by circles (for insertions), and squares (for deletion substitutions).

⇧ Lipoprotein   ▥ Cytoplasm   ⇨ Inner-membrane   ⬖ Periplasm

TABLE 1 Protein properties

Protein	Size (aa)	pI	Predicted location[a]	Motifs[b]	Homology
IcmT	87	12.0	IM-1		
IcmS	115	4.4	Cyt		
IcmR	122	4.7	Cyt		
IcmQ	192	9.6	Cyt		
IcmP	376	8.3	IM-2	RGD	TrbA (R64), Sat (pCPP519)
IcmO	783	5.3	IM-2	A/G	TrbC (R64)
LphA	189	9.9	OM-31	Lipoprotein	YiaD
IcmM	94	6.4	IM-1		
IcmL	212	9.4	IM-1	Amphipathic-β	Orf3 (R446), Orf5 (pCPP519)
IcmK	360	5.9	Perp-26		
IcmE	1,048	5.6	IM-1		TrbI (RK2)
IcmG	269	7.8	IM-1	Coiled-coil	
IcmC	194	9.1	IM-4		
IcmD	132	9.8	IM-1		
IcmJ	208	7.5	IM-1		
IcmB	1009	5.4	IM-1	A/G	
TphA	418	9.3	IM-12	Transporter	ProP/CitA
IcmF	973	7.0	IM-2	A/G	
IcmV	151	10.1	IM-2		
IcmW	151	4.9	Cyt		
IcmX	466	6.3	Perp-22		
DotA	1,048	5.8	IM-8		
DotB	378	5.5	Cyt	A/G	PilT
DotC	304	9.2	OM-38	Lipoprotein	
DotD	164	9.2	OM-16	Lipoprotein	

[a] Location was determined by the Psort program; IM, inner membrane—number of transmembrane domains; Cyt, cytoplasm; OM-#, outer membrane; and Perp-#, periplasm—location of the N-terminal signal sequence cleavage site.

[b] Motif search was done with the Prosite program; AG, ATP or GTP binding site; RGD, Arginine-Glycine-Aspartic acid sequence.

likely to be cotranscribed, as are *icmPO*. In addition, the *icmR* and *icmQ* genes are likely to be independently transcribed. Sequence homology was found between the *icmP* (23% over 376 amino acids) and *icmO* (24% over 783 amino acids) genes with the *trbA* and *trbC* genes, respectively, that are involved in gene transfer in the *Salmonella* R64 plasmid.

THE *lphA, icmMLKE* CLUSTER

Region II contains a cluster of four genes (*lphA, icmMLK*) that had not been identified from the transposon insertions (53). The *icmMLKE* genes are required for growth within and killing of macrophages. The *icmE*

gene spans groups 9, 7, and 2. The other genes were mutagenized by allele exchange with a kanamycin-resistance cassette. The *lphA* gene is not required for growth within or killing of macrophages but is partially required when amoebae are used as a host (Table 2). The *lphA* gene product contains a fatty acid acylation site sequence found in lipoproteins as well as an "OmpA" box, an amino acid sequence found in several gram–negative outer-membrane proteins. Complementation tests indicate that the *lphA* gene is transcribed as a single gene and that the *icmMLKE* genes are probably cotranscribed. The *icmE* gene sequence is remarkable because it encodes

TABLE 2 Phenotypes associated with mutations in *icm* genes

Gene	Growth inside and killing of HL-60 cells	Immediate cytotoxicity for HL-60 cells	Growth inside *Acanthamoeba*	Plasmid conjugation
WT	+++	+++	+++	+++
icmT	−	−	−	−
icmS	+	−	−	+++
icmR	+/−	−	−	−
icmQ	+/−	−	−	+++
icmP	−	−	−	+++
icmO	−	−	−	+++
lphA	+++	++	++	+++
icmM	−	−	−	+++
icmL	−	−	−	+++
icmK	−	−	−	+++
icmE	−	−	−	++
icmG	++	+	-	+++
icmC	−	−	−	+
icmD	−	−	−	+++
icmJ	−	−	−	+++
icmB	−	−	−	+++
tphA	+++	+++	+++	ND
icmF	++	+	−	+
icmX	−	−	−	+++
dotA	−	−	−	−

42 repeats of a 10-amino acid sequence. Although the significance of the repeats is unknown at present, it suggests a highly organized repeated structural element. The *icmL* and *icmE* genes also bear significant homology to plasmid genes found to be involved in DNA transfer.

THE *icmGCDJBF, tphA* CLUSTER

The *icmGCDJBF, tphA* cluster of genes in region II was originally identified by complementation of an *icmB* mutation by the pMW100 plasmid, derived from a genomic library in pMMB207 (47). Bacteria with mutations in *icmG* and *icmF* have only slight defects in the abilities to grow within and kill HL-60–derived macrophages but these genes are required for growth in amoebae (Table 2). Mutations in the *tphA* gene result in no detectable defects in either ability. This gene en-

codes a protein that is highly homologous to several amino acid transporters. Strains with mutations in the remaining genes are unable to grow within or kill macrophages. These genes do not exhibit significant sequence homologies to data base entries. The IcmG protein, however, contains a 60-amino acid region that is predicted to form an amphipathic coiled:coil structure. Such structures are known to participate frequently in protein interactions. This type of structural motif is thought to be of primary importance for interactions among the components of the SNARE complex that determines vesicle fusion.

DETACHMENT FROM PLASTIC AND LDH RELEASE AS ASSAYS FOR RAPID CYTOTOXICITY

In the course of setting up synchronized infections of HL-60 cells, we found that when large numbers of wild-type *L. pneumophila* (multiplicity of infection [MOI] > 10) were centrifuged (880 × *g*) onto a monolayer of macrophages, the macrophages lifted off the plastic and formed a compact ball with the infecting bacteria within 4 to 6 min. We found that lifting and formation of the ball did not occur at 4°C and did not require bacterial phagocytosis. All of the *icm* mutants tested had little or no effect on the cell monolayer (Table 2). We considered that the primary event leading to lifting and formation of the ball might be an increase in permeability of the macrophage plasma membrane. Indeed, when we measured release of lactate dehydrogenase (LDH) from the macrophages, we found very similar results with the same time and MOI dependence. We concluded that a tight association between Icm$^+$ *L. pneumophila* and the macrophages damaged the macrophage plasma membrane and led to LDH release as well as lifting and formation of the ball. Recently Ralph Isberg's group provided evidence for the formation of a cytotoxic-pore that depends on similar conditions and the same group of genes (which they call *dot* genes) (42).

CONJUGAL ACTIVITY OF THE Icm/Dot COMPLEX

The striking homology between four of the *icm* genes and plasmid-encoded genes involved in conjugal DNA transfer prompted us to whether *L. pneumophila* could conjugally transfer DNA. We found that indeed, the IncQ plasmid pMMB207 is transferred between *L. pneumophila* strains at a frequency of 10^{-3} per donor (53). Although transfer is absolutely dependent on the *icmR*, *icmT*, and *dotA* genes, mutations in other *icm* genes result in a 50-fold decrease in transfer (Table 2). Interestingly, the *icmP*, *icmO*, and *icmL* genes, which exhibit homology to the plasmid transfer genes, are not at all required for conjugal transfer. We also showed that the *oriT* origin of transfer of pMMB207 and the MobA protein are required for transfer. Because others have shown that the MobA protein (i) pro-

duces a single-stranded nick at *oriT*, (ii) forms a covalent intermediate with the single strand of plasmid DNA, and (iii) is transferred to the recipient as a nucleoprotein complex with single-stranded binding protein (SSB), these results suggest that the Icm transfer apparatus, or a portion of it, can transport the same nucleoprotein complex to the recipient cell. We also have evidence that *L. pneumophila* can transfer chromosomal markers in addition to plasmids. Several strains containing Tn*903*dIII*lacZ* at different locations in the genome were able to transfer the Km^r phenotype to another strain at approximately the same frequency (10^{-6} per donor).

SIMILARITY TO THE *AGROBACTERIUM* SYSTEM

Because several of the *icm* genes bear homology to transfer genes of plasmids and because other systems that are known to be used for macromolecular transfer also contain genes with similarity to plasmid transfer genes, it is worth considering possible parallels between these other systems and the Icm system. The *vir* system of *Agrobacterium tumefaciens*, which transfers T-DNA to plant cells, the pertussis toxin *ptl* exporter, and the *tra* conjugative system of the IncN plasmid pKM101 are closely related to one another (65). Although most of these genes do not share significant sequence similarity with the *L. pneumophila icm* genes, the overall composition and arrangements of the components suggests that the systems may share functional similarities. In the *vir*, *ptl*, and *tra* systems, there are approximately 20 components and a preponderance of proteins with transmembrane domains. However, the IcmE and DotB proteins each contain a region that shows slight similarity to VirB11 and VirB10, respectively. Each system has components with nucleotide binding sites that are thought to be required for energization of the system. Table 3 presents a direct comparison between the Icm/Dot system and the Vir system of *A. tumefaciens*. The finding that the Icm system can conjugate DNA together with its overall resemblance to these well-characterized sys-

TABLE 3 Comparison between the *Legionella icm* and the *Agrobacterium vir* systems

Feature	Legionella	Agrobacterium
Function	Killing of human macrophages	Tumorigenesis in plants
	23 *icm/dot*-genes	19 *vir*-genes
Conjugation of RSF1010 between bacteria	10^{-3} transconjugants/donor	10^{-3} transconjugants/donor
Conjugation substrate	ssDNA-MobA complex	ssDNA-MobA complex
	(nucleoprotein complex)	(nucleoprotein complex)
Genes required for conjugation	*icmT, icmR, dotA*	*virB2-11, virD4*
Genes partially required for conjugation	*icmC, icmE, icmF*	*virB1*
Genes not required for conjugation	14 *icm* genes	*virD1, virD2, virE2*
Inhibition of virulence by RSF1010	+	+
Natural substrate of the virulence system	?	ssT-DNA-VirD2-VirE2
		(nucleoprotein complex)
Transfer of RSF1010 to the host	?	+
Regulators of virulence	?	*virA–virG*

tems prompted us to think that the Icm system may function as a transfer apparatus to deliver effector molecules specifically to the host cell in a manner that is similar to that of the three systems described above. The *L. pneumophila* effectors probably interact with the components of the host cell that mediate phagosome-lysosome fusion (Fig. 3).

FUNCTION OF THE Icm/Dot COMPLEX

Even though the lack of significant homologies between most of the genes defined by the transposons and entries in the data bases did not provide clues to the specific functions of the putative effectors, careful studies of the intracellular phenotypes of the mutant strains have provided a remarkable result that must be included in any model for understanding the mechanisms of intracellular replication and organelle trafficking. Using fluorescein-labeled *L. pneumophila* and host cells in which the lysosomal compartment has been specifically labeled with high-molecular-weight rhodamine-dextran, it has been possible to measure the degree to which phagosomes containing different strains of *L. pneumophila* fuse with lysosomes. This has been accomplished by using the confocal laser-scanning fluorescence microscope and measuring

whether there is colocalization of the green and red fluorescence signals emanating from fluorescein and rhodamine, respectively. The results of these measurements are astonishingly clear. First, 25 to 30% of the phagosomes containing wild-type viable *L. pneumophila* fuse with lysosomes within 30 min after infection. This proportion does not increase over the next 6 h. In the cases of all of the representative transposon-induced mutants examined in the *icmX, dotA, dotB, icmE, icmR,* and *icmB* genes, 70 to 80% of the phagosomes fused with lysosomes by 30 min, (the earliest time that could be examined). This high degree of fusion was the same as that found for paraformaldehyde-killed *L. pneumophila*. Here as well, the proportion did not increase over the next 6 h, indicating that the maximum level of phagosome-lysosome fusion had been observed shortly after infection (62a). A simple interpretation of these results is that the decision whether a particular phagosome is going to fuse or not fuse with lysosomes is made rapidly upon interaction of the bacteria with the host cell. Defects in any of the *icm* or *dotA* genes examined result in high levels of phagosome-lysosome fusion either during or immediately following uptake into the phagosome. If all of the *dotA/icm* genes are required to minimize the levels of phagosome-

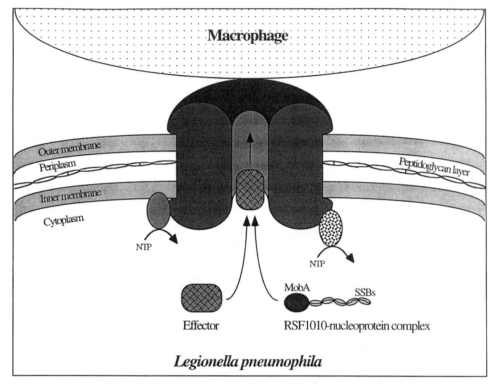

FIGURE 3 A model for the *L. pneumophila* virulence transport system. Some of the *icm* gene products are expected to interact with one another to form a protein complex that will build a channel through the bacterial inner and outer membranes. Other *icm* gene products are expected to be effector molecules. Some of the *icm* gene products may be involved in the assembly of the complex, and the energy required for the assembly or transfer (or both) of the effector molecule may be provided by nucleotide triphosphatase activities of several ATP/GTP binding proteins. The effector molecule is expected to be transferred to the macrophage cytoplasm or to the phagosome space or membrane. Another substrate that moves by the Icm transport system is the RSF1010-nucleoprotein complex that was shown to conjugate between bacteria in an *icm* gene products-dependent manner. (Adapted from Segal, G., and H. A. Shuman, *Trends Microbiol.* **6**:253–255, 1998.)

lysosome fusion at short times following infection, they may play little, if any, role during the later stages of intracellular multiplication. Because the large collection of random insertions was identified on the basis of their inability to kill a host cell, it is unlikely that large numbers of genes specifically required for intracellular multiplication have been ignored. If so, a surprising hypothesis is that the "pathway" of intracellular replication is the necessary consequence of the initial interactions of the Icm/DotA proteins and the host; no other *L. pneumophila* genes may be specif-

ically required for later stages of intracellular multiplication or for ensuring proper organelle trafficking.

UNANSWERED QUESTIONS

Which Icm Proteins Are Effectors and Which Are Components of the Transfer Apparatus?

The current model for how the Icm/Dot complex influences the intracellular fate of *L. pneumophila* is shown in Fig. 3. This model postulates two classes of Icm/Dot gene products. One class of proteins constitutes a "transferosome" or structure similar in composition and arrangement to the type IV secretion system used by *A. tumefaciens*, *B. pertussis*, and pKM101 for delivering DNA to plants, pertussis toxin to host cells, and pilus assembly and conjugation, respectively. The second class are "effector" proteins that are transferred to the host cell and directly interact with the components of the host cell that are involved in phagosome formation and fate. An immediate challenge is to sort out which Icm/Dot components belong to each class. The ability to measure the function of the "transferosome" with the conjugation assay will be key in establishing these assignments. For example, overproduction of effectors may compete with the MobA-nucleoprotein and decrease conjugal efficiency. In addition, direct demonstration of transfer of Icm or Dot products to a host cell would be compelling evidence that the transferred protein has a function in the host.

How Do the Effectors Prevent Phagosome-Lysosome Fusion and Promote Intracellular Multiplication?

Once the effectors and components of the transferosome are identified, the key question of how the effectors determine the fate of the phagosome will need to be addressed. There are several possible mechanisms that could be used to interrupt specifically the fusion of phagosomes with lysosomes. The easiest way to imagine these is in the context of the SNARE hypothesis. This hypothesis is based on the existence and activities of a number of different proteins that are required for fusion in several different systems ranging from synaptic vesicles fusing at nerve junctions to vacuole trafficking in saccharomyces. It seems clear that integral membrane proteins containing a coiled:coil domain are responsible for pairing the compartments that are to be fused and that several classes of cytosolic proteins regulate and/or catalyze the actual events leading to fusion. Among these are ATP-dependent proteins and small, farnesylated

GTP-binding proteins (rabs). The distribution of Ca^{2+} within different compartments may also influence fusion activity. This complexity allows several opportunities for a pathogen to influence whether fusion will take place. In the case of the *L. pneumophila* Icm and Dot products, there are several possible candidates, including those that may form amphipathic pores (IcmL) and influence ion fluxes or coiled:coil domains (IcmG) and compete with the SNARE proteins during pairing of the phagosome with the lysosome.

REVIEWS AND KEY PAPERS

Barker, J., and M. R. Brown. 1994. Trojan horses of the microbial world: protozoa and the survival of bacterial pathogens in the environment. *Microbiology* **140:**1253–1259.

Dowling, J. N., A. K. Saha, and R. H. Glew. 1992. Virulence factors of the family *Legionellaceae*. *Microbiol. Rev.* **56:**32–60.

Fields, B. S. 1996. The molecular ecology of legionellae. *Trends Microbiol.* **4:**286–290.

Horwitz, M. A. 1983. Formation of a novel phagosome by the Legionnaires' disease bacterium (*Legionella pneumophila*) in human monocytes. *J. Exp. Med.* **158:**1319–1331.

Rowbotham, T. J. 1980. Preliminary report on the pathogenicity of *Legionella pneumophila* for freshwater and soil amoebae. *J. Clin. Pathol.* **33:**1179–1183.

Segal, G., M. Purcell, and H. A. Shuman. 1998. Host cell killing and bacterial conjugation require overlapping sets of genes within a 22-kb region of the *Legionella pneumophila* genome. *Proc. Natl. Acad. Sci. USA* **95:**1669–1674.

Shuman, H. A., M. Purcell, G. Segal, L. Hales, and L. A. Wiater. 1998. Intracellular multiplication of *Legionella pneumophila*: human pathogen or accidental tourist? *Curr. Top. Microbiol. Immunol.* **225:**99–112.

Venkataraman, C., B. J. Haack, S. Bondada, and Y. Abu Kwaik. 1997. Identification of a Gal/GalNAc lectin in the protozoan *Hartmannella vermiformis* as a potential receptor for attachment and invasion by the Legionnaires' disease bacterium. *J. Exp. Med.* **186:**537–547.

Vogel, J. P., H. L. Andrews, S. K. Wong, and R. R. Isberg. 1998. Conjugative transfer by the virulence system of *Legionella pneumophila*. *Science* **279:**873–876.

REFERENCES

1. **Abu Kwaik, Y.** 1996. The phagosome containing *Legionella pneumophila* within the protozoan

Hartmannella vermiformis is surrounded by the rough endoplasmic reticulum. *Appl. Environ. Microbiol.* **62**:2022–2028.

2. **Adeleke, A., J. Pruckler, R. Benson, T. Rowbotham, M. Halablab, and B. Fields.** 1996. Legionella-like amebal pathogens—phylogenetic status and possible role in respiratory disease. *Emerg. Infect. Dis.* **2**:225–230.

3. **Armstrong, J. A., and P. D'Arcy Hart.** 1971. Response of cultured macrophages to *Mycobacterium tuberculosis* with observations on fusion of lysosomes with phagosomes. *J. Exp. Med.* **134**:713–740.

4. **Barker, J., and M. R. Brown.** 1994. Trojan horses of the microbial world: protozoa and the survival of bacterial pathogens in the environment. *Microbiology* **140**:1253–1259.

5. **Bellinger, K. C. G., and M. A. Horwitz.** 1990. Complement component C3 fixes selectively to the major outer membrane protein (MOMP) of *Legionella pneumophila* and mediates phagocytosis of liposome-MOMP complexes by human monocytes. *J. Exp. Med.* **172**:1201–1210.

6. **Berger, K. H., and R. R. Isberg.** 1993. Two distinct defects in intracellular growth complemented by a single genetic locus in *Legionella pneumophila*. *Mol. Microbiol.* **7**:7–19.

7. **Berger, K. H., J. J. Merriam, and R. R. Isberg.** 1994. Altered intracellular targeting properties associated with mutations in the *Legionella dotA* gene. *Mol. Microbiol.* **14**:809–822.

8. **Berk, S. G., R. S. Ting, G. W. Turner, and R. J. Ashburn.** 1998. Production of respirable vesicles containing live *Legionella pneumophila* cells by two *Acanthamoeba* spp. *Appl. Environ. Microbiol.* **64**:279–286.

9. **Blander, S. J., L. Szeto, H. A. Shuman, and M. A. Horwitz.** 1990. An immunoprotective molecule, the major secretory protein of *Legionella pneumophila*, is not a virulence factor in a guinea pig model of Legionnaires' disease. *J. Clin. Invest.* **86**:817–824.

10. **Bollin, G. E., J. F. Plouffe, M. F. Para, and B. Hackman.** 1985. Aerosols containing *Legionella pneumophila* generated by shower heads and hot-water faucets. *Appl. Environ. Microbiol.* **50**:1128–1131.

11. **Bornstein, N., D. Marmet, M. Surgot, M. Nowicki, A. Arslan, J. Esteve, and J. Fleurette.** 1989. Exposure to *Legionellaceae* at a hot spring spa: a prospective clinical and serological study. *Epidemiol. Infect.* **102**:31–36.

12. **Bozue, J. A., and W. Johnson.** 1996. Interaction of *Legionella pneumophila* with *Acanthamoeba castellanii*: uptake by coiling phagocytosis and inhibition of phagosome-lysosome fusion. *Infect. Immun.* **64**:668–673.

13. **Brand, B. C., A. B. Sadosky, and H. A. Shuman.** 1994. The *Legionella pneumophila icm* locus: a set of genes required for intracellular multiplication in human macrophages. *Mol. Microbiol.* **14**:797–808.

14. **Brieland, J., M. McClain, L. Heath, C. Chrisp, G. Huffnagle, M. LeGendre, M. Hurley, J. Fantone, and C. Engleberg.** 1996. Coinoculation with *Hartmannella vermiformis* enhances replicative *Legionella pneumophila* lung infection in a murine model of Legionnaires' disease. *Infect. Immun.* **64**:2449–2456.

15. **Catrenich, C. E., and W. Johnson.** 1989. Characterization of the selective inhibition of growth of virulent *Legionella pneumophila* by supplemented Mueller-Hinton medium. *Infect. Immun.* **57**:1862–1864.

16. **Chang, K. P.** 1979. *Leishmania donovani* promastigote-macrophage surface interactions *in vitro*. *Exp. Parasitol.* **48**:175–189.

17. **Clemens, D. L., and M. A. Horwitz.** 1992. Membrane sorting during phagocytosis: exclusion of MHC molecules but not complement receptor CR3 during conventional and coiling phagocytosis. *J. Exp. Med.* **175**:1317–1326.

18. **Clemens, D. L., and M. A. Horwitz.** 1993. Hypoexpression of major histocompatibility complex molecules on *Legionella pneumophila* phagosomes and phagolysosomes. *Infect. Immun.* **61**:2803–2812.

19. **Dowling, J. N., A. K. Saha, and R. H. Glew.** 1992. Virulence factors of the family *Legionellaceae*. *Microbiol. Rev.* **56**:32–60.

20. **Feeley, J. C., R. J. Gibson, G. W. Gorman, N. C. Langford, J. K. Rasheed, D. C. Mackel, and W. B. Baine.** 1979. Charcoal-yeast extract agar: primary isolation medium for *Legionella pneumophila*. *J. Clin. Microbiol.* **10**:437–441.

21. **Feeley, J. C., G. W. Gorman, R. E. Weaver, D. C. Mackel, and H. W. Smith.** 1978. Primary isolation media for Legionnaires' disease bacterium. *J. Clin. Microbiol.* **8**:320–325.

22. **Fields, B. S.** 1996. The molecular ecology of Legionellae. *Trends Microbiol.* **4**:286–290.

23. **Fields, B. S., S. R. Fields, J. N. Loy, E. H. White, W. L. Steffens, and E. B. Shotts.** 1993. Attachment and entry of *Legionella pneumophila* in *Hartmannella vermiformis*. *J. Infect. Dis.* **167**:1146–1150.

24. **Fliermans, C. B., W. B. Cherry, L. H. Orison, S. J. Smith, D. L. Tison, and D. H. Pope.** 1981. Ecological distribution of *Legionella pneumophila*. *Appl. Environ. Microbiol.* **41**:9–16.

25. **Gabay, J. E., M. Blake, W. Niles, and M. A. Horwitz.** 1985. Purification of *Legionella pneumophila* major outer membrane protein and dem-

onstration that it is a porin. *J. Bacteriol.* **162**:85–91.

26. **Harb, O. S., C. Venkataraman, B. J. Haack, L. Gao, and Y. Abu Kwaik.** 1998. Heterogeneity in the attachment and uptake mechanisms of the Legionnaires' disease bacterium, *Legionella pneumophila*, by protozoan hosts. *Appl. Environ. Microbiol.* **64**:126–132.

27. **Hedlund, K. W.** 1981. Legionella toxin. *Pharmacol. Ther.* **15**:123–130.

28. **Hoffman, P. S., M. Ripley, and R. Weeratna.** 1992. Cloning and nucleotide sequence of a gene (*ompS*) encoding the major outer membrane protein of *Legionella pneumophila. J. Bacteriol.* **174**:914–920.

29. **Hoffman, P. S., J. H. Seyer, and C. A. Butler.** 1992. Molecular characterization of the 28- and 31-kilodalton subunits of the *Legionella pneumophila* major outer membrane protein. *J. Bacteriol.* **174**:908–913.

30. **Holden, E. P., H. H. Winkler, D. O. Wood, and E. D. Leinbach.** 1984. Intracellular growth of *Legionella pneumophila* within *Acanthamoeba castellani* Neff. *Infect. Immun.* **45**:18–24.

31. **Horwitz, M. A.** 1983. Formation of a novel phagosome by the Legionnaires' disease bacterium (*Legionella pneumophila*) in human monocytes. *J. Exp. Med.* **158**:1319–1331.

32. **Horwitz, M. A.** 1983. The Legionnaires' disease bacterium (*Legionella pneumophila*) inhibits phagosome-lysosome fusion in human monocytes. *J. Exp. Med.* **158**:2108–2126.

33. **Horwitz, M. A.** 1984. Phagocytosis of the Legionnaires' disease bacterium (*Legionella pneumophila*) occurs by a novel mechanism: engulfment within a pseudopod coil. *Cell* **36**:27–33.

34. **Horwitz, M. A., and F. R. Maxfield.** 1984. *Legionella pneumophila* inhibits acidification of its phagosome in human monocytes. *J. Cell Biol.* **99**:1936–1943.

35. **Horwitz, M. A., and S. C. Silverstein.** 1980. Legionnaires' disease bacterium (*Legionella pneumophila*) multiplies intracellularly in human monocytes. *J. Clin. Invest.* **60**:441–450.

36. **Horwitz, M. A., and S. C. Silverstein.** 1981. Interaction of the Legionnaires' disease bacterium (*Legionella pneumophila*) with human phagocytes. II. Antibody promotes binding of *L. pneumophila* to monocytes but does not inhibit intracellular multiplication. *J. Exp. Med.* **153**:398–406.

37. **Husmann, L. K., and W. Johnson.** 1994. Cytotoxicity of extracellular *Legionella pneumophila. Infect. Immun.* **62**:2111–2114.

38. **Jeon, K. W.** 1995. The large, free-living amoebae: wonderful cells for biological studies. *J. Eukaryot. Microbiol.* **42**:1–7.

39. **Joiner, K. A., S. A. Fuhrman, H. Mietinnen, L. L. Kasper, and I. Mellmena.** 1990. *Toxoplasma gondii*: fusion competence of parasitophorous vacuoles in Fc receptor transfected fibroblasts. *Science* **249**:641–646.

40. **Khelef, N., and N. Guiso.** 1995. Induction of macrophage apoptosis by *Bordetella pertussis* adenylate cyclase-hemolysin. *FEMS Microbiol. Lett.* **134**:27–32.

41. **Kikuhara, H., M. Ogawa, H. Miyamoto, Y. Nikaido, and S. Yoshida.** 1994. Intracellular multiplication of *Legionella pneumophila* in *Tetrahymena thermophila. Sangyo Ika Daigaku Zasshi* **16**:263–275.

42. **Kirby, J. E., J. P. Vogel, H. L. Andrews, and R. R. Isberg.** 1998. Evidence for pore-forming ability by *Legionella pneumophila. Mol. Microbiol.* **27**:323–336.

43. **Marra, A., S. J. Blander, M. A. Horwitz, and H. A. Shuman.** 1992. Identification of a *Legionella pneumophila* locus required for intracellular multiplication in human macrophages. *Proc. Natl. Acad. Sci. USA* **89**:9607–9611.

44. **Mintz, C. S., J. Chen, and H. A. Shuman.** 1988. Isolation and characterization of auxotrophic mutants of *Legionella pneumophila* that fail to multiply in human monocytes. *Infect. Immun.* **56**:1449–1455.

45. **Moffat, J. F., P. H. Edelstein, D. P. J. Regula, J. D. Cirillo, and L. S. Tompkins.** 1994. Effects of an isogenic Zn-metalloprotease-deficient mutant of *Legionella pneumophila* in a guinea-pig pneumonia model. *Mol. Microbiol.* **12**:693–705.

46. **Muller, A., J. Hacker, and B. C. Brand.** 1996. Evidence for apoptosis of human macrophage-like HL-60 cells by *Legionella pneumophila* infection. *Infect. Immun.* **64**:4900–4906.

47. **Purcell, M. W., and H. A. Shuman.** 1998. The *Legionella pneumophila* icmGCDJBF genes are required for killing of human macrophages. *Infect. Immun.* **66**:2245–2255.

48. **Rogers, J., A. B. Dowsett, P. J. Dennis, J. V. Lee, and C. W. Keevil.** 1994. Influence of temperature and plumbing material selection on biofilm formation and growth of *Legionella pneumophila* in a model potable water system containing complex microbial flora. *Appl. Environ. Microbiol.* **60**:1585–1592.

49. **Rowbotham, T. J.** 1980. Preliminary report on the pathogenicity of *Legionella pneumophila* for freshwater and soil amoebae. *J. Clin. Pathol.* **33**:1179–1183.

50. **Rowbotham, T. J.** 1986. Current views on the relationships between amoebae, legionellae and man. *Isr. J. Med. Sci.* **22**:678–689.

51. Sadosky, A. B., L. A. Wiater, and H. A. Shuman. 1993. Identification of *Legionella pneumophila* genes required for growth within and killing of human macrophages. *Infect. Immun.* 61:5361–5373.

52. Sadosky, A. B., J. W. Wilson, H. M. Steinman, and H. A. Shuman. 1994. The iron superoxide dismutase of *Legionella pneumophila* is essential for viability. *J. Bacteriol.* 176:3790–3799.

53. Segal, G., M. Purcell, and H. A. Shuman. 1998. Host cell killing and bacterial conjugation require overlapping sets of genes within a 22-kb region of the *Legionella pneumophila* genome. *Proc. Natl. Acad. Sci. USA* 95:1669–1674.

54. Segal, G., and H. A. Shuman. 1997. Characterization of a new region required for macrophage killing by *Legionella pneumophila*. *Infect. Immun.* 65:5057–5066.

55. Shuman, H. A., M. Purcell, G. Segal, L. Hales, and L. A. Wiater. 1998. Intracellular multiplication of *Legionella pneumophila*: human pathogen or accidental tourist? *Curr. Top. Microbiol. Immunol.* 225:99–112.

56. Swanson, M. S., and R. R. Isberg. 1995. Association of *Legionella pneumophila* with the macrophage endoplasmic reticulum. *Infect. Immun.* 63:3609–3620.

57. Szeto, L., and H. A. Shuman. 1990. The *Legionella pneumophila* major secretory protein, a protease, is not required for intracellular growth or cell killing. *Infect. Immun.* 58:2585–2592.

58. Tesh, M. J., and R. D. Miller. 1982. Growth of *Legionella pneumophila* in defined media: requirement for magnesium and potassium. *Can. J. Microbiol.* 28:1055–1058.

59. Tesh, M. J., S. A. Morse, and R. D. Miller. 1983. Intermediary metabolism in *Legionella pneumophila*: utilization of amino acids and other compounds as energy sources. *J. Bacteriol.* 154:1104–1109.

60. Tyndall, R. L., and E. L. Domingue. 1982. Cocultivation of *Legionella pneumophila* and free-living amoebae. *Appl. Environ. Microbiol.* 44:954–959.

61. Venkataraman, C., B. J. Haack, S. Bondada, and Y. Abu Kwaik. 1997. Identification of a Gal/GalNAc lectin in the protozoan *Hartmannella vermiformis* as a potential receptor for attachment and invasion by the Legionnaires' disease bacterium. *J. Exp. Med.* 186:537–547.

62. Vogel, J. P., H. L. Andrews, S. K. Wong, and R. R. Isberg. 1998. Conjugative transfer by the virulence system of *Legionella pneumophila*. *Science* 279:873–876.

62a. Wiater, L. A., K. Dunn, F. R. Mayfield, and H. A. Shuman. 1998. Early events in phagosome establishment are required for intracellular survival of *Legionella pneumophila*. *Infect. Immun.* 66:4450–4460.

63. Wiater, L. A., A. Marra, and H. A. Shuman. 1994. *Escherichia coli* F plasmid transfers to and replicates within *Legionella pneumophila*: an alternative to using an RP4-based system for gene delivery. *Plasmid* 32:280–294.

64. Wiater, L. A., A. B. Sadosky, and H. A. Shuman. 1994. Mutagenesis of *Legionella pneumophila* using Tn*903*dIIlacZ: identification of a growth-phase-regulated pigmentation gene. *Mol. Microbiol.* 11:641–653.

65. Winans, S. C., D. L. Burns, and P. J. Christie. 1996. Adaptation of the conjugal transfer system for the export of pathogenic macromolecules. *Trends Microbiol.* 4:64–68.

66. Wright, J. B., I. Ruseska, M. A. Athar, S. Corbett, and J. W. Costerton. 1989. *Legionella pneumophila* grows adherent to surfaces *in vitro* and *in situ*. *Infect. Control Hosp. Epidemiol.* 10:408–415.

67. Zhu, W. H., and T. T. Loh. 1996. Differential effects of phorbol ester on apoptosis in HL-60 promyelocytic leukemia cells. *Biochem. Pharmacol.* 51:1229–1236.

68. Zychlinsky, A., M. C. Prevost, and P. J. Sansonetti. 1992. *Shigella flexneri* induces apoptosis in infected macrophages. *Nature* 358:167–169.

MOLECULAR, CELL BIOLOGICAL, AND ECOLOGICAL ASPECTS OF INFECTION BY *LISTERIA MONOCYTOGENES*

Eva M. Busch, Eugen Domann, and Trinad Chakraborty

15

Pathogenic intracellular bacteria cause many severe forms of disease worldwide with devastating morbidity and high mortality rates. Despite the significance of many facultative intracellular pathogens in animal and human diseases, understanding the basis of their different lifestyles within the infected host cell and in their environmental niches is still in its infancy. Thus, conditions that favor growth and persistence of the microorganism in a particular environment are likely to be important in transmission to the infected host. By the same token, understanding the early interactions of parasites with host cell membranes as well as defining (virulence) factors that modulate and promote intracellular survival can lead to novel measures for prevention and treatment. Currently, much of the lack of progress in studying such bacteria is caused by the difficulty of cultivating fastidous microorganisms, deficiency in useful genetic systems to examine and manipulate the bacteria, and a lack of appropriate tissue culture and animal models for assessing virulence. In this respect, the facultative intracellular gram-positive pathogen *Listeria monocytogenes* has emerged as an important model for study of many facets of host-pathogen interactions. Thus *Listeria* remains a model pathogen for assessing immunological aspects of infection (13) and has more recently emerged as a paradigm for the study of the dynamic nature of the actin-based cytoskeleton for cell biologists (17, 23). Foodborne infections by *L. monocytogenes* are favored by the ability of the bacterium to grow and reach high numbers at refrigeration temperatures. The identification of genes that control gene expression in the cold and are required for growth at low temperatures makes *L. monocytogenes* an ideal model for examining the genetic basis of "cold-adapted" growth of microorganisms.

LISTERIA MONOCYTOGENES

Listeria monocytogenes is a ubiquitous gram-positive pathogen. As a foodborne pathogen, it has been implicated in severe systemic infections following consumption of *Listeria*-contaminated food products (8). Although of low incidence, listerial infections have a significant mortality rate (20 to 30%) (1, 9). Listerial infections threaten the unborn, the newborn, and immunocompromised and elderly individuals. Severe clinical listeriosis manifests as meningitis, meningoencephalitis,

Eva M. Busch, Eugen Domann, and Trinad Chakraborty, Institute for Medical Microbiology, University of Giessen, Frankfurterstrasse 107, D-35392 Giessen, Germany.

Microbial Ecology and Infectious Disease, Edited by Eugene Rosenberg
©1999 American Society for Microbiology, Washington, D.C.

or septicemia, and perinatal infections can lead to abortions. Of the survivors of listeriosis, about 11% of the neonates and 30% of the adults suffer from residual symptoms (12). A milder form with symptoms of gastrointestinal illness has been recently described (4, 22); this form is probably dose dependent and does not result in invasive disease.

The presence of *Listeria* spp. in sewage and feces and the fact that these microorganisms multiply readily in decaying vegetable material explain its occurrence in soil. Seasonal variation in the isolation of *Listeria* has been reported; numbers are highest in the summer. Thus, *Listeria* spp. are likely to be associated with most raw food products in low numbers. *L. monocytogenes* can be found particularly on products of animal origin. Its presence in ready-to-eat food usually results from contamination in the production environment (3). Prevalence has been described in meat products (7), fish products (11), dairy products (15), and ready-to-eat food products (20).

Listeria sp. is a robust microorganism that is capable of growth under different conditions, ranging from high salt concentrations (10% NaCl), pH 4.5 to 9, to growth temperatures from 0 to $-45°C$, with generation times varying from 5 to 7 days at $0°C$ on beef (10) to 52 min in tryptic soy broth at $45°C$ (16).

The most important condition favoring contamination in food is the ability of this bacterium to multiply and grow to high numbers in nonsterile food products with a long shelflife. Fermented foods, such as a wide variety of cheeses and milk products that have been considered to be pathogen free because of the combination of inhibitory factors such as low pH, high salt levels, and low storage temperatures, are important sources of *Listeria* contamination. The problem is man made and poses a significant threat to consumers in societies in which there is an increasing demand for "wholesome" and "natural" convenience food, cooked-frozen, cooked-chilled, and minimally processed chilled food. Understanding the factors that allow adaptation and

growth of these bacteria at low temperatures is therefore relevant.

Entry of *L. monocytogenes* into the host normally occurs in the gut after consumption of *Listeria*-contaminated food (10). The precise locus of bacterial invasion is not known, but experimental studies following oral infection of rodents indicate that preferential multiplication following uptake occurs at Peyer's patches (19–21). During an acute infection, many tissues are infected, demonstrating the ability of these bacteria to invade numerous eucaryotic cells in different tissues. Elegant microscopic studies have demonstrated penetration of *L. monocytogenes* into epithelial cells of both the cornea and the intestine in vivo (20, 21). Tissue culture assays of invasion show that *L. monocytogenes* can invade various cell types, including hepatocytes and fibroblasts, albeit with widely different efficiency (14). However, once within the intracellular compartment, the doubling time of these bacteria is about 1 h regardless of cell type. Survival of the internalized bacteria, however, depends on cell type. Following intravenous infection, *L. monocytogenes* appears to be first ingested and rapidly killed by resident macrophages such as the Kupffer cells of the liver (2). A primary aspect of *L. monocytogenes* pathogenesis is the ability of these bacteria to escape from a host vacuole following uptake. Release of bacteria into the cytoplasm requires the concerted action of listeriolysin and phospholipases (18). Once inside the host cytoplasm, bacteria start to grow, a process that can last for more than 8 h. The intracellular environment appears to be a rich milieu for bacterial growth, because even auxotrophic mutants are capable of unrestricted growth.

EXPRESSION OF VIRULENCE FACTORS IS TEMPERATURE AND PrfA DEPENDENT

The establishment of tissue culture infection models (18) and the development of methods for genetic manipulation of *Listeria* spp. were essential for the identification and characterization of various virulence factors, that is, the basis of our current understanding of *Listeria* pathogenesis. To elucidate the function of individual virulence factors and their interplay, biochemical purification schemes, antibodies, and functional assays for these proteins are being developed.

Most of the genes encoding proteins involved in *L. monocytogenes* pathogenesis are clustered in a single 10-kb chromosomal locus containing the *hly* gene flanked by the lecithinase (comprising *mpl*, *actA*, and *plcB* genes) and the *plcA-prfA* operons. The *inlA* and *inlB* genes are located in an independent operon. The involvement of the various gene products in the different stages of the infectious process, summarized in Fig. 1, is detailed below, as is the newly discovered *irpA* gene (5). Successful penetration and survival within host cells as well as spreading throughout tissues and the host itself require coordinate regulation of virulence determinants. The pleiotropic regulator of virulence gene expression, the *prfA* gene, is a transcriptional activator that interacts with a palindromic sequence located within the −44 region of all known virulence factors in *L. monocytogenes* (18). Expression of all virulence genes in complex growth media (such as brain heart infusion) has been shown to be strictly temperature regulated, with an optimum at 37°C (18). Although the *inlA/B* and *irpA*

genes are not part of the virulence gene cluster, their expression was also shown to be regulated by temperature as well as by PrfA (5). The regulation mechanism however differs from those genes in that InlA, InlB, and IrpA are produced not only by isogenic *prfA* mutants but also at lower growth temperatures (20°C) (5, 14). These genes have been shown to harbor additional PrfA-independent promotors. The relative requirement for temperature- and PrfA-dependent regulation may also reflect the compartments in which these genes are required: the *hly*, *plcA*, *mpl*, *actA*, and *plcB* genes are essential for intracellular survival and multiplication, whereas *inlA*, *inlB*, and possibly *irpA* are involved in early interactions with the host cell, such as adhesion (Fig. 2).

EXPRESSION OF GENES AT LOW GROWTH TEMPERATURES

Previous attempts to isolate mutants for genes of *L. monocytogenes* that are essential for growth at low temperatures have not led to a clear identification of any gene(s) required for this phenotype. Thus, isolation of the genes required for growth under these conditions would be of great interest for studying bacterial physiology and metabolism. It has been known for some time that production of flagella, and hence bacterial motility, only occurs

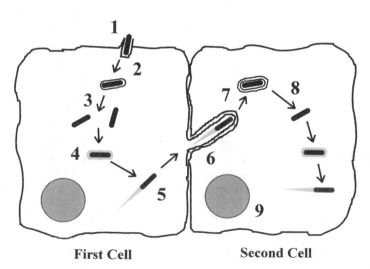

First Cell   **Second Cell**

FIGURE 1 Infection cycle of *L. monocytogenes*. Bacterial genes known to be required in the different steps are summarized; 1, attachment (*inlA*, *inlB*); 2, internalization (*inlA*, *inlB*); 3, escape from endosome (*hly*, *plcA*); 4, actin filament assembly (*actA*); 5, tail generation, motility (*actA*); 6, pseudopod formation (?); 7, pseudopodal uptake (?); 8, escape from double-membrane vacuole (*plcB*, *hly*); 9, apoptosis (*hly*).

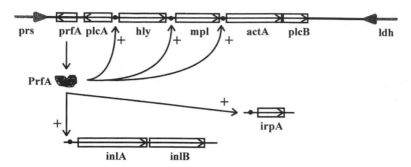

FIGURE 2 Schematic representation of the virulence gene organization and the coordinate regulation by PrfA. Proteins encoded: *prs*, phosphoribosyl-pyrophosphate synthetase; *prfA*, positive regulatory factor A; *plcA*, phosphatidyl inositol-specific phospholipase C; *hly*, listeriolysin; *mpl*, metalloprotease; *actA*, actin-recruiting protein; *plcB*, phosphatidylcholine-specific phospholipase C; *ldh*, lactate dehydrogenease; *irpA*, internalin-related protein A; *inlA*, internalin A; *inlB*, internalin B.

in bacteria grown at temperatures below 30°C. This observation has been confirmed by transcriptional studies on the flagellin *flaA* gene from several *L. monocytogenes* strains (6). The lack of flagellar expression at 37°C makes perfect sense when one considers that during infection of the host cell, intracellular motility and cell-to-cell spread is effected by the ActA protein whose expression is optimal at 37°C and is not expressed at growth temperatures below 30°C.

We initiated a search for novel proteins expressed at low growth temperatures by comparative examination of cell wall extracts from cultures grown at 37 and 20°C. The N-terminal sequence of several proteins that were almost exclusively present in cell wall extracts from cultures grown at 20°C were obtained and used to design oligonucleotides to clone the corresponding gene. N-Terminal sequencing of the two most prominent proteins of 35 kDa and 7 kDa revealed that they corresponded to the flagellin monomer and a protein that is highly homologous to the cold-shock proteins of other bacteria.

The gene encoding the cold-shock protein homolog, designated *cspL1*, encoded a polypeptide of 66 amino acids. Transcriptional analysis showed that the gene was monocistronic and highly transcribed in bacteria grown at 20°C, although basal expression was also observed in cultures grown at 37°C. To examine the role of the *cspL1* gene in *L. monocytogenes*, we created a deletion mutant that removed all but 3 amino acids of the CspL1 polypeptide. Unlike the wild-type bacterial parent strain, the Δ*cspL1* mutant was strongly inhibited for growth at 20°C and did not grow at 4°C at all. Analysis of the cell wall proteins from the mutant grown at 37°C showed that it grew just as well as the wild-type strain and did not reveal any differences in the cell wall extracts. Surprisingly, cell wall extracts derived from the mutant strain grown at 20°C showed that not only was it lacking the CspL1 protein but the expression of flagellin was also completely abrogated. This was confirmed by checking for transcription of the *flaA* gene in the mutant strain. Expression of the *cspL1* and *flaA* genes, as well as growth at low temperatures, was conferred by complementation of a plasmid harboring the *cspL1* gene. Thus, the *cspL1* gene is not only essential for growth at low temperatures but is also clearly a pleiotropic regulator for genes expressed at these growth temperatures.

UNANSWERED QUESTIONS

The diverse environments inhabited by *L. monocytogenes* make it necessary for the bacteria to sense and respond to its immediate surroundings appropriately. We have shown here that disparate sets of genes are required for bacteria in eukaryotic host cells to initiate and maintain infection, as compared to bacteria that are exposed to low growth temperatures as might be expected in *Listeria*'s natural habitat, the soil. Sensing growth temperatures seems a stunningly simple ploy, but currently we have no idea how this is achieved. On the one hand, the master virulence regulator protein PrfA controls expression of all known virulence genes, albeit to varying degrees, and on the other hand, we have identified CspL1 as a pleiotropic regulator for gene expression of cold-adapted genes as well as being essential for growth at these temperatures. Clearly this differential yin-yang gene expression is carefully orchestrated, as evidenced by the different modes of bacterial motility used by the bacteria in different niches: flagellin-based motility in the environment and actin-based motility in the infected host cell. Future research will have to address the control elements that regulate expression of the PrfA and CspL1 proteins and to identify common elements that are integrated into the respective regulatory circuits.

REVIEWS AND KEY PAPERS

Broome, C. V. 1993. Listeriosis: can we prevent it? *ASM News* **59**:444–446.

Chakraborty, T., and J. Wehland. 1997. The host cell infected with *Listeria monocytogenes*, p. 271–290. *In* S. H. E. Kaufmann (ed.), *Host Response to Intracellular Pathogens*. R. G. Landes Co., Austin, Tex.

Farber, J. M., and P. J. Peterkin. 1991. *Listeria monocytogenes*: a foodborne pathogen. *Microbiol. Rev.* **55**:476–511.

Gellin, B. G., and C. V. Broome. 1989. Listeriosis. *JAMA* **261**:1313–1320.

Portnoy, D. A., T. Chakraborty, W. Goebel, and P. Cossart. 1992. Molecular determinants of *Listeria monocytogenes* pathogenesis. *Infect. Immun.* **60**:1263–1267.

REFERENCES

1. Broome, C. V. 1993. Listeriosis: can we prevent it? *ASM News* **59**:444–446.

2. Conlan, J. W., and R. J. North. 1994. Neutrophils are essential for early anti-*Listeria* defense in the liver, but not in the spleen or peritoneal cavity, as revealed by granulocyte-depleting monoclonal antibody. *J. Exp. Med.* **179**:259–268.

3. Cox, L. J., T. Klies, J. L. Cordier, C. Cordellana, P. Konkel, C. Pedrazanni, R. Beumer, and A. Siebenga. 1989. *Listeria* spp. in food processing, non-food, and domestic environments. *Food Microbiol.* **6**:49–61.

4. Dalton, C. B., C. C. Austin, J. Sobel, P. S. Hayes, W. F. Bibb, L. M. Graves, B. Swaminathan, M. E. Proctor, and P. M. Griffin. 1997. An outbreak of gastroenteritis and fever due to *L. monocytogenes* in milk. *N. Engl. J. Med.* **336**:100–105.

5. Domann, E., S. Zechel, A. Lingnau, T. Hain, A. Darji, T. Nichterlein, J. Wehland, and T. Chakraborty. 1997. Identification and characterization of a novel PrfA-regulated gene in *Listeria monocytogenes* whose product, IrpA, is highly homologous to internalin proteins, which contain leucine-rich repeats. *Infect. Immun.* **65**:101–109.

6. Dons, L., F. Rasmussen, and J. E. Olson. 1992. Cloning and characterization of a gene encoding flagellin of *Listeria monocytogenes*. *Mol. Microbiol.* **6**:2919–2929.

7. Farber, J. M., and E. Daley. 1994. Presence and growth of *Listeria monocytogenes* in naturally contaminated meats. *Int. J. Food Microbiol.* **22**:33–42.

8. Farber, J. M., and P. J. Peterkin. 1991. *Listeria monocytogenes*: a foodborne pathogen. *Microbiol. Rev.* **55**:476–511.

9. Gellin, B. G., and C. V. Broome. 1989. Listeriosis. *JAMA* **261**:1313–1320.

10. Grau, F. H., and P. B. Van der Linde. 1990. Growth of *Listeria monocytogenes* on vacuum packaged beef. *J. Food Prot.* **53**:739–741.

11. Jenmi, T. 1993. *Listeria monocytogenes* in smoked fish: an overview. *Arch. Lebensmittelhyg.* **44**:10–13.

12. Jones, E. M., S. Y. McCulloch, D. S. Reeves, and A. P. MacGowan. 1994. A 10 year survey of epidemiology and clinical aspects of listeriosis in a provincial English city. *J. Infect.* **29**:91–103.

13. Kaufmann, S. H. E. 1993. Immunity to intracellular bacteria. *Annu. Rev. Immunol.* **11**:129–163.

14. Lingnau, A., E. Domann, M. Hudel, M. Bock, T. Nichterlein, J. Wehland, and T. Chakraborty. 1995. Expression of the *Listeria monocytogenes* EGD *inlA* and *inlB* genes, whose products mediate bacterial entry into tissue culture cell lines, by PrfA-dependent and

192 ■ BUSCH ET AL.

-independent mechanisms. *Infect. Immun.* **63:** 3896–3903.

15. **Loncarevic, S., M. L. Danielsson-Tham, and W. Tham.** 1995. Occurrence of *Listeria monocytogenes* in soft and semi-soft cheeses in retail outlets in Sweden. *Int. J. Food Microbiol.* **26:**245–250.

16. **Petran, R. L., and E. A. Zottola.** 1989. A study of factors affecting growth and recovery of *Listeria monocytogenes* ScottA. *J. Food Sci.* **54:**45–60.

17. **Pollard, T. D.** 1995. Actin cytoskeleton. Missing link for intracellular bacterial motility. *Curr. Biol.* **5:**837–840.

18. **Portnoy, D. A., T. Chakraborty, W. Goebel, and P. Cossart.** 1992. Molecular determinants of *Listeria monocytogenes* pathogenesis. *Infect. Immun.* **60:**1263–1267.

19. **Pron, B., C. Boumalia, F. Jaubert, S. Sarnacki, J.-P. Monet, P. Berche, and J.-L. Gaillard.** 1998. Comprehensive study of the intestinal stage of listeriosis in a rat ligated ileal loop system. *Infect. Immun.* **66:**747–755.

20. **Racz, P., K. Tenner, and E. Mero.** 1972. Experimental *Listeria* enteritis. I. An electron microscopic study of the epithelial phase in experimental *Listeria* infection. *Lab. Invest. Methods Cell Biol.* **26:**694–700.

21. **Racz, P., K. Tenner, and K. Szivessy.** 1970. Electron microscopic studies in experimental keratoconjunctivitis listeriosa. I. Penetration of *Listeria monocytogenes* into corneal epithelial cells. *Acta. Microbiol. Hung.* **17:**221–236.

22. **Reido, F. X., R. W. Pinner, M. D. Tosca, M. L. Carter, L. M. Graves, M. W. Reeves, R. E. Weaver, B. D. Plikaytis, and C. V. Broome.** 1994. A point-source foodborne listeriosis outbreak: documented incubation period and possible mild illness. *J. Infect. Dis.* **170:**693–696.

23. **Tilney, L. J., and D. A. Portnoy.** 1989. Actin filaments and the growth, movement and spread of the intracellular parasite *Listeria monocytogenes*. *J. Cell Biol.* **109:**1597–1608.

24. **Wilson, I. G.** 1995. Occurrence of Listeria spp. in ready to eat foods. *Epidemiol. Infect.* **115:**519–526.

PATHOGENESIS OF THE INTESTINAL PARASITE *ENTAMOEBA HISTOLYTICA*

David Mirelman and Serge Ankri

16

Amebiasis is defined as an infection with the protozoan parasite *Entamoeba histolytica*. *E. histolytica* is responsible for up to 100,000 deaths per annum, placing it second to malaria in mortality due to a protozoan parasite (69). The amebic trophozoites normally reside in the human large bowel and occasionally invade the intestinal mucosa and disseminate to other organs (52). A number of amebic molecules associated with virulence have been identified, but the factors that trigger invasion are still largely unknown. It has long been known that many people infected with *E. histolytica* never develop symptoms. In recent years, it has become evident that within what was termed *E. histolytica* there are two types of morphologically indistinguishable organisms, the nonpathogenic *Entamoeba dispar* and the pathogenic *E. histolytica*. Amebae isolated from well-established and characterized asymptomatic cyst carriers were termed *E. dispar* and found to differ slightly in various biochemical and molecular characteristics from *E. histolytica* parasites obtained from individuals with clear invasive symptoms (11, 15, 19,

20, 39, 59, 65). However, the spectrum of clinical symptoms seen in amebiasis, especially in less developed countries, is much more complex and difficult to explain than by simple infection of either a pathogenic or a nonpathogenic organism. Recent epidemiological studies that used type-specific polymerase chain reaction (PCR) amplifications directly on stool samples have shown that the extent of infection with *E. histolytica* (between 35 and 78%) is significantly higher than that determined by zymodeme or enzyme-linked immunosorbent assay (ELISA) tests and that a considerable percentage of infected persons (between 20 and 70%, depending on the study) simultaneously harbor both *E. histolytica* and *E. dispar* (1, 21, 44, 57, 68). Furthermore, among the different strains of the pathogenic type *E. histolytica*, there is significant variability in the degree of virulence, and a number of avirulent *E. histolytica* strains have been reported (13). In addition, a number of host factors such as intestinal bacterial flora composition (38), mucus and IgA secretion, as well as changes in the redox potential or pH of the large bowel have been implicated in affecting amebic virulence. The molecular mechanisms by which such host effectors exert their influence on the parasite's behavior in the complex environment of the human colon

David Mirelman and Serge Ankri, Department of Biological Chemistry, The Weizmann Institute of Science, Rehovot 76100, Israel.

Microbial Ecology and Infectious Disease, Edited by Eugene Rosenberg
©1999 American Society for Microbiology, Washington, D.C.

are not yet clear, and available evidence is scanty.

VIRULENCE DETERMINANTS OF E. HISTOLYTICA

E. histolytica should be regarded as a cytotoxic effector cell with an extraordinary capacity for destruction of various types of target cells. Trophozoites also have a very active phagocytic capacity, and they continuously ingest bacteria and cellular debris as a major nutrient source. The histolytica name given to virulent Entamoeba is due to the characteristic lysis it causes to red blood and other target cells. It resembles in some aspects the contact-dependent cytolytic events caused by mammalian cytotoxic lymphocytes. The molecular mechanisms responsible for the pathogenicity of amebae are currently being actively studied in various laboratories, and a number of amebic components involved in the various steps have been identified. Interaction of the parasite with the host can be divided into various steps.

Adherence

The initial step in the encounter between the trophozoite and the mucosal target cells is intimate contact, or the adherence process. The specificity of this process was established 18 years ago, and a number of lectin-like molecules that mediate recognition were identified on E. histolytica trophozoites (25, 37). The binding affinity to distinct carbohydrate-containing receptors on the surface of mucosal cells, blood cells, and bacteria has been characterized (10, 36, 37, 53, 54). The lectin that appears to contribute the most to the initial adherence step is the Gal/GalNAc-specific lectin (36). Various Gal-specific lectins of very similar structure and binding activity have been identified in avirulent E. histolytica strains as well as in the nonpathogenic E. dispar (46). A variety of inhibitors containing Gal or GalNAc molecules inhibit adherence, but none of these, even at high concentrations, inhibit over 70% of the trophozoite adherence. Adherence is a prerequisite for subse-

quent destruction of the mucosal cell, and consequently, the cytopathic effect is also significantly inhibited in the presence of Gal/GalNAc-containing glycoconjugates (53, 54).

Considerable information has become available in recent years on the Gal-specific lectins. Their structure consists of two subunits of 170 and 35 kDa, and a number of gene copies coding for these subunits (which have some structural variations between them) have been identified, both in E. histolytica as well as in E. dispar (50, 66). Very little is known about the relative expression of each of the genes or the binding affinity of each of the various isolectins in different strains to GalNAc-containing glycoconjugates and whether any such differences, if they exist, could affect adherence and amebic virulence. Furthermore, it is still not clear whether the putative complement-binding region identified within the 170-kDa Gal-lectin sequence may have a function in the parasite's resistance to complement (35, 50) or on its ability to inactivate this important host defense mechanism. Recombinant subunits of the 170-kDa Gal-specific subunit of the lectin are currently being studied as potential antigens for an antiamebic vaccine. Preliminary results obtained in the gerbil model indicate that immunizations significantly protected (about 70%) the animals from a direct intrahepatic challenge (7, 36, 47). Moreover, monoclonal antibodies, specific against certain epitopes on the Gal/GalNAc-lectin of E. histolytica, which are not present on E. dispar, have been introduced into diagnostic kits for direct identification of E. histolytica in stools (21, 22). The amounts of Gal-lectin needed for its detection by ELISA (10^3 E. histolytica trophozoites) are, however, over 100-fold higher than the detection levels that can be achieved by PCR amplifications of the structurally different rDNA genes of either E. histolytica or E. dispar (15, 20, 40).

As mentioned above, additional adhesins such as a 220-kDa lectin with a specificity for $(GlcNAc)_n$ (25, 58) and a 112-kDa adhesin have been characterized in E. histolytica (5). It is not yet clear what role each of these adhesins may have in the adherence process, but it is logical to assume that adherence of the trophozoite to a mucosal cell is the result of complementary steps by various adhesins that enable it to bind to alternate receptors on different target cells.

Cytopathic Effect

One of the main goals of amebiasis research has been to identify and characterize the molecular basis of the cytopathic reaction. The working hypothesis was that following the intimate cell-cell contact, which is mediated by the lectins, amebae release into the intercellular space a protein that inserts itself into the membrane of the target cell and forms an ion channel. Over 15 years ago, Lynch et al. (34) and Young et al. (70) independently discovered a very interesting protein component in lysates of *E. histolytica* which they termed the amoebapore. The pore-forming polypeptide spontaneously incorporated into membrane bilayers to form ion channels, and the resulting depolarization caused death of target cells. Subsequently, Leippe and colleagues (28, 29) successfully identified in a virulent strain of *E. histolytica* three isoforms of this amoebapore (A, B, and C), which are expressed in a ratio of approximately 35:10:1. They characterized their primary structure by molecular cloning of the genes and discovered that the mature polypeptides each comprise 77 amino acids with a compact α-helical disulfide-bonded fold. Furthermore, they found that the respective coding regions contain typical signal peptides that allow trafficking to vesicular storage compartments such as cytoplasmic amebic granules (26). The amoebapores are capable of killing metabolically active eukaryotic cells and display antibacterial activity but are not efficient in lysing erythrocytes. Amebae may use amoebapores as effector molecules in a cytolytic reaction that is directed against a broad spectrum of target cells and also to lyse bacteria that are phagocytized by the trophozoites. Amoebapores structurally and functionally resemble the defensins, the recently recognized antibacterial peptides found in granules of mammalian neutrophils. Interestingly, amoebapores also show a marked structural and functional homology to NK-lysins, peptides recently localized to natural killer cells and cytotoxic T cells in pigs (16). Nonpathogenic *E. dispar* possesses structurally similar (95%) amoebapores, which are present at significantly lower levels in the amebic lysates and appear to have a somewhat lower specific activity (60%) than those of *E. histolytica*. It is also not clear whether *E. histolytica* strains that differ in virulence vary in their amoebapore content. At present, the primary function of amoebapores appears to be the killing of phagocytosed bacteria (27), as the destruction of host cells is not an obligatory part of the life cycle of *E. histolytica*. Amoebapores do not appear to be secreted into the medium, and antibodies raised against amoebapores do not protect cells from killing by intact trophozoites. Moreover, vaccination of rodents with amoebapore-derived peptides did not protect the animals from intrahepatic challenge.

Cysteine Proteinases

Cysteine proteinases (CPs) have been implicated as important virulence factors in the pathogenesis of amebiasis and play a key role in tissue invasion and disruption of host tissues, as well as in resistance to the host's immune response (14, 48, 56). In view of their importance in virulence, CPs are currently attracting considerable interest as vaccine candidates and as targets for novel therapeutic agents. Several CPs with molecular masses in the range of 16 to 96 kDa have been observed in lysates of *E. histolytica* (33, 48, 61). Labeling of the amebic CPs with the radiolabeled CP inhibitor ^{125}I-Z-Leu-Tyr-CHN$_2$ and separation on sodium dodecyl sulfate-polyacrylamide gel electrophoresis (SDS-PAGE) confirmed the presence of various CP bands that are also present in the avirulent strain Rahman as well as in *E. dispar* (17). Comparison of the proteinase activities of lysates from the virulent strain HM-1 with those of the less virulent strain HK-9 and avirulent strain Rahman, as determined by digestion of gelatin on SDS-PAGE copolymerized with gelatin, revealed a number of differences in the presence and relative intensity of some of the bands (Fig. 1).

Some correlation has been shown between the level of total CP activities of various strains, as determined by digestion of a chromophoric substrate, and the extent of cytopathic effect of trophozoites on tissue-cultured monolayers of mammalian cells (13, 24). An as yet unexplained exception to this is the *E. histolytica* avirulent strain Rahman, which has levels of CP activity similar to those of virulent strain HM-1 but is incapable of causing damage to mammalian cells or liver lesions in hamsters. CPs are inhibitable at very low concentrations by a variety of inhibitors of thiol proteinases such as leupeptine, cystatin, E-64, Z-Phe-Ala-CHF$_2$ (48), and Z-Leu-Tyr-CHN$_2$ (17). None of these inhibitors is currently being used therapeutically. The role of CPs in virulence has been studied to some extent by following its effects in E-64–treated trophozoites. Li et al. (30) observed that addition of E-64 to strain HM-1 causes only a partial inhibition (50%) of destruction of monolayers suggesting that the activity of cysteine proteinases is not the only cause of the cytopathic effect. On the other hand Stanley et al. (63) showed that trophozoites grown for 24 h with E-64 lost their ability to induce liver lesions in SCID mice. Recently, we have found that allicin, one of the main biologically active molecules present in freshly crushed garlic cloves, strongly inhibits amebic CPs as well as other thiol-containing enzymes such as alcohol dehydrogenases. Preincubation of intact trophozoites of virulent strain HM-1 with allicin (10 μM), strongly inhibits their ability to destroy mammalian cell monolayers (Fig. 2) (3).

The CPs of *E. histolytica* structurally resemble other mammalian CPs. Homologies were found between the sequence of *E. histolytica* CP genes and mammalian cathepsin L as well as papain. Molecular cloning of the amebic CP genes was initially done by PCR amplification using primers based on conserved active-site sequences identified in all members of the eukaryotic CP family (48, 55). Tannich and colleagues have now identified six different CP genes that encode typical papain family proteinases with a high degree of conservation in all active-site residues (12). Homologs for four of the six genes have been identified also in *E. dispar* (12). Significant se-

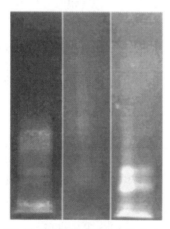

HM1:IMMS HK-9 Rahman

FIGURE 1 Comparison of gelatinase activities of *E. histolytica* HM1:IMMS, HK-9, and Rahman strains.

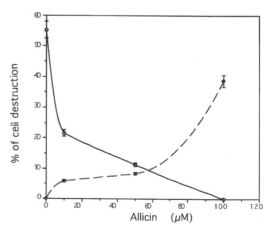

FIGURE 2 Effect of allicin on BHK monolayer cell destruction by *E. histolytica* strain HM-1:IMSS. Empty symbols, assays performed with trophozoites; filled symbols, assays performed without trophozoites.

quence differences (>40%) were identified between EhCP3 and the other CP genes. One of the genes reported to be totally missing in *E. dispar* is EhCP5 (12, 39). Some of the gene sequences suggest that the proteins are translated as preproenzymes. Significant differences have also been found in the levels of transcription of the different CPs in various strains. No correlation could be seen between the levels of CP transcripts and virulence of the particular strain (12). For example, the levels of the EhCP3 transcript of virulent strain HM-1 appear to be three times lower than those of the less virulent strain HK-9 (Ankri et al., unpublished results), whereas the levels of EhCP5 appear to be similar in all strains tested (12) (Ankri et al., unpublished results). At the moment, it is not clear what the physiological roles of each of the CPs are and if they are present in different locations in the cell. Recent reports have localized amebic CPs to lysosome-like vacuoles or proteasomes, suggesting that they also play a role in the basic metabolism of amebae, most likely in intracellular protein degradation (51, 60). Recently, EhCP5 has been identified as a membrane-associated protease. This CP could have a potential role in host tissue destruction of *E. histolytica*, as it is totally missing in the nonpathogenic *E. dispar* (23). Its presence, however, in the avirulent *E. histolytica* strain Rahman clearly indicates that we do not yet fully understand its role in the parasite's virulence.

The recent development of stable transfection methods and vectors (2, 64, 67) has opened the possibility of studying the role of CPs in virulence. Preliminary studies in our laboratory of stable transfectants of strain HK-9 transfected with a hybrid vector (pSA2) containing the EhCP3 gene under the selection of neomycin resistance have shown that it is impossible to obtain a high copy number of EhCP3, as it is toxic to the cells (Ankri et al., unpublished results). A measurable increase in the level of total CP activity was observed in low-copy-number EhCP3 transfectants of strain HK-9 as well as an increased intensity

of bands in SDS-PAGE gelatin in comparison with those of nontransfected HK-9. Interestingly, no significant difference was observed between the transfected and nontransfected trophozoites of strain HK-9 in the rate of destruction of tissue-cultured mammalian cells (Fig. 3).

Transfections of virulent strain HM-1 with a construct encoding antisense EhCP-5 mRNA (Fig. 4) show that the transcription and activity of most of the cysteine proteinases was significantly (~90%) inhibited (Fig. 5), indicating that the antisense mRNA, because of its significant homology, prevented the expression of most of the CP genes (4).

Interestingly, the transfected trophozoites were not deficient in their cytopathic activity, as determined by their ability to destroy mammalian cell monolayers (Fig. 6). The antisense transfected trophozoites were, however, significantly affected in their phagocytic capabilities (Fig. 7). The reason for the deficient phagocytosis in the EhCP5 antisense tropho-

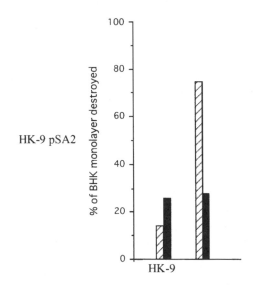

FIGURE 3 Cysteine proteinase activity and BHK monolayer destruction by HK-9 and HK-9 pSA2-transfected trophozoites. Filled boxes, mammalian cell (BHK) monolayer destruction by intact trophozoites; hatched boxes, cysteine proteinase activity of trophozoite lysates on chromophoric substrate (Z-Arg-Arg-pNA).

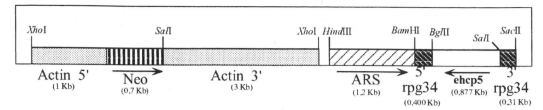

FIGURE 4 Schematic depiction of plasmid pSA8. pSA8 is derived from plasmid pEhAct-Neo (Samuelson J., personal communication, and [2]). The size of plasmid pSA8 is 10.3 kbp. Arrows indicate orientation of transcription. Numbers in brackets represent the size of each segment.

zoites is not clear, especially since addition of CP inhibitors such as E-64 and Leupeptine did not affect phagocytosis of controls. On the other hand, the ability of the transfected trophozoites to lyse red blood cells remained unaffected. This indicates that the hemolysin is a different activity, and its transcript is apparently not inhibited by the antisense EhCP5 mRNA.

These observations confirm that CPs are not essential for the cytopathic activity of *E. histolytica*. The ability of trophozoites to damage host tissues and cells appears to be mutifactorial. The hemolysin together with the remaining cysteine proteinase activity as well as the amoebapores (see above) and the phospholipase activity could all participate in the pathogenic process. Answers to important questions regarding the specific contribution to virulence of each of the CPs, amoebapores, hemolysins, and phospholipases can now be addressed by use of the antisense technology recently developed in our laboratory (2, 4).

Lipophosphoglycans

Another type of molecule on trophozoite surfaces that seems to be involved in amebic virulence is the lipophosphoglycan (LPG) (9, 41, 42, 62). We have recently shown in our laboratory that there appears to be a correlation between the abundance of LPG and the virulence of a particular strain. Virulent trophozoites of strain HM-1:IMSS have high amounts of two types of closely related LPGs, whereas strain Rahman as well as strains of *E. dispar* are deficient in the composition and

content of their cell surface lipophosphoglycan and have less than 10% of the LPG content present in virulent strains (41–43). Interestingly, a less virulent trophozoite subculture of strain HM-1:IMSS, grown in cholesterol-poor serum, also showed a deficiency in LPG components (41–43). The molecular mechanisms by which LPG contributes to the parasite virulence and how its synthesis and appearance on trophozoite surfaces is regulated are not yet known. Growth of the amebae in the presence of certain bacteria appears to modulate the structure of the carbohydrate-containing surface antigen (8). An interesting possibility is that there may be a connection between the composition and structure of the LPG in the outer trophozoite surface and the presence of the putative toxic molecules such as hemolysins, amoebapore, and CPs that appear to participate in the cytopathic effect. In trophozoites that are deficient in LPG, the assembly or exposure of such toxic molecules may be impaired and they may fail to interact efficiently with target cells. A similar observation was recently reported for bacteria that lack lipopolysacharides (49). Obviously much more work is needed for better characterization of the LPGs and their biosynthetic pathways.

UNRESOLVED QUESTIONS AND FUTURE RESEARCH

Variations in Pathogenicity

The mechanisms that regulate the expression of virulence of the parasite are not yet well

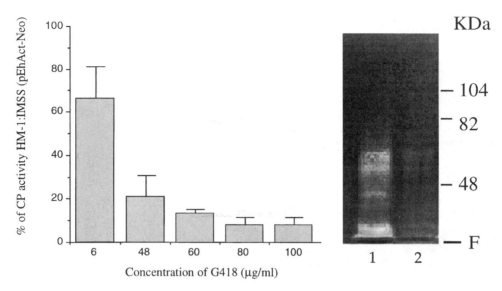

FIGURE 5 Correlation between resistance to G418 concentration and cysteine proteinase activity of *E. histolytica* strain HM-1:IMSS transfected with pSA8. Left panel, Proteinase activity was determined in trophozoite lysates by following the digestion of the chromophoric substrate Z–Arg–Arg–pNA. Right panel, Proteinase activity was determined by following the gelatinase activities on SDS-polyacrylamide gel-gelatin of the control pEhActNeo and the antisense transfectant pSA8.

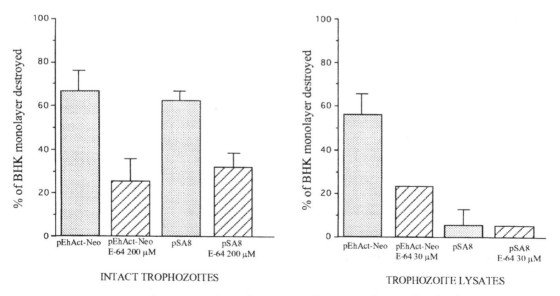

FIGURE 6 Destruction of BHK monolayers by intact trophozoites or lysates of *E. histolytica* strain HM-1:IMMS (pEhAct-Neo used as control) or HM-1:IMSS (pSA8) transfected trophozoites. No effect of E-64 (200 μM) on BHK monolayer viability was observed (data not shown). When indicated (hatched boxes), the assay was performed in the presence of E-64 (200 μM) (for intact trophozoites) or E-64 (30 μM) (for trophozoite lysates).

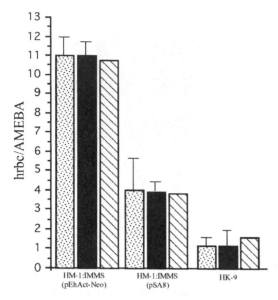

FIGURE 7 Comparison of erythrophagocytosis rates of *E. histolytica* HM-1:IMMS (pEhAct-Neo used as control), pSA8-transfected cells, and nontransfected strain HK-9. The assay was performed without cysteine proteinase inhibitors (dotted boxes) or in the presence of E-64 (200 μM) (filled boxes) and leupeptin (200 μM) (hatched boxes).

understood. Numerous external factors such as growth conditions, nutrients, redox potential, and bacterial flora are known to affect virulence of cloned strains. Thorough examination and investigation of the regulators of certain genes involved in virulence will be needed to help us clarify the complexity of the activation and deactivation mechanisms and responses.

Symptomatic and Asymptomatic Infections

One of the most intriguing questions in amebiasis is the clinical picture seen especially in endemic areas in less-developed countries. Epidemiological studies have shown that only 10% of infected individuals are symptomatic, whereas 90% are considered asymptomatic carriers. Whether this is due to amebic strains of different pathogenicity or due to different host factors has not yet been fully resolved. Differences in pathogenicity of infecting strains have been identified. On the other

hand, quite a number of asymptomatic carriers were found to be infected with potentially virulent strains. Moreover, quite a significant proportion (between 20 and 70%, depending on the study) have been found to harbor pathogenic and nonpathogenic strains simultaneously. Nothing is known about the variations in the proportion of these different amebae growing in the intestine of infected persons, and this could perhaps be one of the reasons for the reported variations in symptoms.

The Amebic Genome

At the molecular level, a lot of open questions require in-depth investigation. The genome organization of amebae is still a complete mystery. We do not know how and why the DNA content and organization of an ameba changes dramatically under different growth conditions (32). As was shown for other protozoa, the genome of *E. histolytica* appears to have considerable plasticity. Genomic polymorphisms and phenotypic variabilities have been reported (18, 45). We still do not know the ploidy of the ameba and whether the large DNA molecules, which were shown to separate in pulsed-field gels, indeed represent linear chromosomes or big circular DNA molecules (6, 31). Neither telomers nor centromers have been identified as yet, so the organization of the nuclear material needs to be clarified. As described above, stable expression of foreign genes has been recently demonstrated in amebae. What we still lack is the ability to integrate foreign genes into the amebic chromosomal DNA by homologous recombination. Recombination will enable establishment of knockout transgenic strains that will be most helpful for further studies of the biology and pathogenicity of the parasite.

ACKNOWLEDGMENTS

The investigations from the authors' laboratory were supported in part by two internal grants of the Weizmann Institute of Science, the Forchheimer Center for Molecular Genetics and the Center for Molecular Biology of Tropical Diseases, as well as by a grant from the Center for the Study of Emerging Diseases. S. A. was supported in his first year by a postdoctoral grant "Bourse Lavoisier" from the Ministère Français des Affaires Etrangères.

REVIEWS AND KEY PAPERS

1. **Martinez-Palomo, A., and M. Espinosa-Cantellano.** 1998. Amoebiasis: New understanding and new goals. *Parasitol. Today* **14:**1–3.
2. **Stanley, S. L., Jr.** 1997. Progress towards development of a vaccine for amebiasis. *Clin. Microbiol. Rev.* **10:**637–649.

REFERENCES

1. **Acuna-Soto, R., J. Samuelson, P. Girolami, L. de Zarate, F. Millan-Velasco, G. Schoolnick, and D. Wirth.** 1993. Application of the polymerase chain reaction to the epidemiology of pathogenic and nonpathogenic *Entamoeba histolytica. Am. J. Trop. Med. Hyg.* **48:**58–70.
2. **Alon, R., R. Bracha, and D. Mirelman.** 1997. Inhibition of expression of the lysine-rich 30 kDa surface antigen of *Entamoeba dispar* by the transcription of its antisense RNA. *Mol. Biochem. Parasitol.* **90:**193–201.
3. **Ankri, S., T. Miron, A. Rabinkov, M. Wilchek, and D. Mirelman.** 1997. Allicin from garlic strongly inhibits cysteine proteinases and cytopathic effects of *Entamoeba histolytica. Antimicrob. Agents Chemother.* **41:**2286–2288.
4. **Ankri, S., T. Stolarsky, and D. Mirelman.** 1998. Antisense inhibition of expression of cysteine proteinases in *Entamoeba histolytica* does not affect cytopathic or hemolytic activity but inhibits phagocytosis. *Mol. Microbiol.* **28:**777–785.
5. **Arroyo, R., and E. Orozco.** 1987. Localization and identification of an *Entamoeba histolytica* adhesin. *Mol. Biochem. Parasitol.* **23:**151–158.
6. **Baez-Camargo, M., A. M. Riveron, D. M. Delgadillo, E. Flores, T. Sanchez, G. Garcia-Rivera, and E. Orozco.** 1996. *Entamoeba hystolitica*: gene linkage groups and relevant features of its karyotype. *Mol. Gen. Genet.* **13:**289–296.
7. **Beving, D. E., C.-J. G. Soong, and J. I. Rav-din.** 1996. Oral immunization with a recombinant cysteine-rich section of the *Entamoeba histolytica* galactose-inhibitable lectin elicits an intestinal secretory immunoglobulin A response that has in vitro adherence inhibition activity. *Infect. Immun.* **64:**1473–1476.
8. **Bhattacharya, A., R. Ghildyal, J. Prasad, S. Bhattacharya, and L. S. Diamond.** 1992. Modulation of a surface antigen of *Entamoeba histolytica* in response to bacteria. *Infect. Immun.* **60:**1711–1713.
9. **Bhattacharya, A., R. Prasad, and D. L. Sacks.** 1992. Identification and partial characterization of a lipophosphoglycan from a pathogenic strain of *Entamoeba histolytica. Mol. Biochem. Parasitol.* **56:**161–168.
10. **Bracha, R., and D. Mirelman.** 1983. Adherence and ingestion of *Escherichia coli* serotype O55 by trophozoites of *Entamoeba histolytica. Infect. Immun.* **40:**882–887.
11. **Bracha, R., Y. Nuchamowitz, and D. Mirelman.** 1995. Molecular cloning of a 30-kilodalton lysine-rich surface antigen from a nonpathogenic *Entamoeba histolytica* strain and its expression in a pathogenic strain. *Infect. Immun.* **63:**917–925.
12. **Bruchhaus, I., T. Jacobs, M. Leippe, and E. Tannich.** 1996. *Entamoeba histolytica* and *Entamoeba dispar*: differences in numbers and expression of cysteine proteinases genes. *Mol. Microbiol.* **22:**255–263.
13. **Burchard, G. D., and D. Mirelman.** 1988. *Entamoeba histolytica*: Virulence potential and sensitivity to metronidazole and emetine of four isolates possessing nonpathogenic zymodemes. *Exp. Parasitol.* **66:**231–242.
14. **Campell, D., and K. Chadee.** 1997. Survival strategies of *Entamoeba histolytica*: Modulation of cell-mediated immune response. *Parasitol. Today* **13:**184–190.
15. **Clark, C. G., and L. S. Diamond.** 1991. Ribosomal RNA genes of "pathogenic" and "nonpathogenic" *Entamoeba histolytica* are distinct. *Mol. Biochem. Parasitol.* **49:**297–302.
16. **Dandekar, T., and M. Leippe.** 1996. Molecular modeling of amoebapore and NK-lysin: A four-α-helix bundle motif of cytolytic peptides from distantly related organisms. *Folding Des.* **2:**47–52.
17. **De Meester, F., E. Shaw, H. Scholze, T. Stolarsky, and D. Mirelman.** 1990. Specific labelling of cysteine proteinases in pathogenic and non pathogenic *Entamoeba histolytica. Infect. Immun.* **58:**1396–1401.
18. **De Menezes Feitosa, L., L. M. Salgado, M. A. Rodriguez, M. A. Vargas, and E. Orozco.** 1997. Phenotype variability and genetic polymorphism in *Entamoeba histolytica* clonal populations. *Arch. Med. Res.* (Mexico) **28:**27–29.
19. **Edman, U., M. A. Meraz, S. Rausser, N. Agabian, and I. Meza.** 1990. Characterization of an immuno-dominant variable surface antigen of pathogenic and non pathogenic *Entamoeba histolytica. J. Exp. Med.* **172:**879–888.
20. **Garfinkel, L. I., M. Giladi, M. Huber, C. Gitler, D. Mirelman, M. Revel, and S. Rozenblatt.** 1989. DNA probes specific for *Entamoeba histolytica* having pathogenic and non

pathogenic zymodemes. *Infect. Immun.* **57:**926–931.

21. **Haque, R., I. K. M. Ali, S. Akther, and W. A. J. Petri.** 1998. Comparison of PCR, iso-enzyme analysis, and antigen detection for diagnosis of *Entamoeba histolytica* infection. *J. Clin. Microbiol.* **36:**449–452.

22. **Haque, R., K. Kress, S. Wood, T. F. H. G. Jackson, D. Lyerly, T. Wilkins, and W. A. Petri, Jr.** 1993. Diagnosis of pathogenic *Entamoeba histolytica* infection using a stool ELISA based on monoclonal antibodies to the galactose-specific adhesin. *J. Infect. Dis.* **167:**247–249.

23. **Jacobs, T., I. Bruchhaus, T. Dandekar, E. Tannich, and M. Leippe.** 1998. Isolation and molecular characterization of a surface-bound proteinase of *Entamoeba histolytica. Mol. Microbiol.* **27:**269–276.

24. **Keene, W. E., M. E. Hidalgo, E. Orozco, and J. H. McKerrow.** 1990. *Entamoeba histolytica*: correlation of the cytopathic effect of virulent trophozoites with secretion of a cysteine proteinase. *Exp. Parasitol.* **71:**199–206.

25. **Kobiler, D., and D. Mirelman.** 1980. Lectin activity in *Entamoeba histolytica* trophozoites. *Infect. Immun.* **29:**221–225.

26. **Leippe, M.** 1997. Amoebapores. *Parasitol. Today* **13:**178–183.

27. **Leippe, M., J. Andrä, and H. J. Müller-Eberhard.** 1994. Cytolytic and antibacterial activity of synthetic peptides derived from amebapore, the pore-forming peptide of *Entamoeba histolytica. Proc. Natl. Acad. Sci. USA* **91:**2602–2606.

28. **Leippe, M., J. Andrä, R. Nickel, E. Tannich, and H. J. Müller-Eberhard.** 1994. Amoebapores, a family of membranolytic peptides from cytoplasmic granules of Entamoeba histolytica: Isolation, primary structure, and pore formation in bacterial cytoplasmic membranes. *Mol. Microbiol.* **14:**895–904.

29. **Leippe, M., S. Ebel, O. L. Schoenberger, R. D. Horstmann, and H. J. Müller-Eberhard.** 1991. Pore-forming peptide of pathogenic *Entamoeba histolytica. Proc. Natl. Acad. Sci. USA* **88:**7659–7663.

30. **Li, E., W. F. Stenson, C. Kunz-Jenkins, P. E. Swanson, R. Duncan, and S. L. Stanley, Jr.** 1994. *Entamoeba histolytica* interactions with polarized human intestinal Caco-2 epithelial cells. *Infect. Immun.* **62:**5112–5119.

31. **Lioutas, C., C. Schmetz, and E. Tannich.** 1995. Identification of various circular DNA molecules in *Entamoeba histolytica. Exp. Parasitol.* **80:**349–352.

32. **Lopez-Revilla, R., and R. Gómez.** 1978. *Entamoeba histolytica, E. invadens,* and *E. moskovskii*: Fluctuations of the DNA content of axenic tro-phozoites. *Exp. Parasitol.* **44:**243–248.

33. **Luaces, A. L., and A. J. Barrett.** 1988. Cysteine proteinase of *Entamoeba histolytica.* I. Partial purification and action on different enzymes. *Mol. Biochem. Parasitol.* **18:**103–112.

34. **Lynch, E. C., I. M. Rosenberg, and C. Gitler.** 1982. An ion-channel forming protein produced by *Entamoeba histolytica. EMBO J.* **1:**801–804.

35. **Mann, B. J., C. Y. Chung, J. M. Dodson, L. S. Ashley, L. L. Braga, and T. L. Snodgrass.** 1993. Neutralizing monoclonal antibody epitopes of the *Entamoeba histolytica* galactose adhesin map to the cysteine-rich extracellular domain of the 170-kilodalton subunit. *Infect. Immun.* **61:**1772–1778.

36. **McCoy, J. J., B. J. Mann, and W. A. Petri, Jr.** 1994. Adherence and cytoxocity of *Entamoeba histolytica*, or, how lectins let parasites stick around. *Infect. Immun.* **62:**3045–3050.

37. **Mirelman, D., and J. I. Ravdin.** 1986. Lectins in *Entamoeba histolytica*, p. 319–334. *In* D. Mirelman (ed.), *Microbial Lectins and Agglutinins: Properties and Biological Activity.* John Wiley & Sons, New York.

38. **Mirelman, D.** 1987. Ameba-bacterium relationship in amebiasis. *Microbiol. Rev.* **51:**272–284.

39. **Mirelman, D., Y. Nuchamowitz, B. Bohm-Gloning, and B. Walderich.** 1996. A homologue of the cysteine proteinase gene (ACP_1 or $Eh\text{-}CPp_3$) of pathogenic *Entamoeba histolytica* is present in non-pathogenic *E. dispar* strains. *Mol. Biochem. Parasit.* **78:**47–54.

40. **Mirelman, D., Y. Nuchamowitz, and T. Stolarsky.** 1997. Comparison between ELISA based kits and PCR of rRNA genes for the simultaneous detection of *Entamoeba histolytica* and *Entamoeba dispar. J. Clin. Microbiol.* **35:**2405–2407.

41. **Moody, S., S. Becker, Y. Nuchamowitz, M. J. McConville, and D. Mirelman.** 1997. The lipophosphoglycan-like molecules of virulent and avirulent *E. histolytica* as well as of *E. dispar* differ in both composition and abundance. *Arch. Med. Res.* (Mexico) **28:**98–102.

42. **Moody, S., S. Becker, Y. Nuchamowitz, and D. Mirelman.** 1997. Virulent and avirulent *Entamoeba histolytica* and *E. dispar* differ in their cell surface phosphorylated glycolipids. *Parasitology* **114:**95–104.

43. **Moody, S., S. Becker, Y. Nuchamowitz, and D. Mirelman.** 1998. Identification of significant variation in the composition of lipo-phosphoglycan-like molecules of *E. histolytica* and *E. dispar. J. Eukaryot. Microbiol.* **45:**179–182.

44. Newton-Sanchez, O. A., K. Sturm-Ramirex, J. L. Romero-Zamora, J. I. Santos-Preciado, and J. Samuelson. 1997. High rate of occult infection with *Entamoeba histolytica* among non-dysenteric Mexican children. *Arch. Med. Res.* **28:**311–313.

45. Orozco, E. 1997. A novel cytoplasmic structure containing DNA networks in *Entamoeba histolytica* trophozoites. *Mol. Gen. Genet.* **254:**250–257.

46. Petri, W. A., T. F. H. G. Jackson, V. Gathiram, K. Kress, L. D. Saffer, T. L. Snodgrass, M. D. Chapman, Z. Keren, and D. Mirelman. 1990. Pathogenic and nonpathogenic strains of *Entamoeba histolytica* can be differentiated by monoclonal antibodies to the galactose-specific adherence lectin. *Infect. Immun.* **58:**1802–1806.

47. Petri, W. A., Jr., and J. I. Ravdin. 1991. Protection of gerbils from amebic liver abscess by immunization with the galactose-specific adherence lectin. *Infect. Immun.* **59:**97–101.

48. Que, X., and S. L. Reed. 1997. The role of extracellular cysteine proteinases in pathogenesis of *Entamoeba histolytica* invasion. *Parasitol. Today* **13:**190–194.

49. Rahman, M. M., J. Guard-Petter, and R. W. Carlson. 1997. A virulent isolate of *Salmonella enteritidis* produces a *Salmonella typhi*-like lipopolysaccharide. *J. Bacteriol.* **179:**2126–2131.

50. Ramakrishnan, G., B. D. Ragland, J. E. Purdy, and B. J. Mann. 1996. Physical mapping and expression of gene families encoding the *N*-acetyl D-galactosamine adherence lectin of *Entamoeba histolytica*. *Mol. Microbiol.* **19:**91–100.

51. Ramos, M. A., R. P. Stock, R. Sanchez-Lopez, F. Olvera, P. M. Lizardi, and A. Alagon. 1997. The *Entamoeba histolytica* proteasome α-subunit gene. *Mol. Biochem. Parasitol.* **84:**131–135.

52. Ravdin, J. I. 1988. Human infection by *Entamoeba histolytica*, p. 166–176. *In* J. I. Ravdin (ed.), *Amebiasis: Human Infection.* John Wiley & Sons, New York.

53. Ravdin, J. I., and R. L. Guerrant. 1981. Role of adherence in cytopathogenic mechanisms of *Entamoeba histolytica* . Study with mammalian tissue culture cells and human erythrocytes. *J. Clin. Invest.* **68:**1305–1313.

54. Ravdin, J. I., C. F. Murphy, R. A. Salata, R. L. Guerrant, and E. L. Hewlett. 1985. N-Acetyl-D-galactosamine-inhibitable adherence lectin of *Entamoeba histolytica*. I. Partial purification and relation to amoebic virulence *in vitro. J. Infect. Dis.* **151:**804–815.

55. Reed, S., J. Bouvier, A. S. Pollack, J. C. Engel, M. Brown, K. Hirata, X. Que, A. Eakin, P. Hagblom, F. Gillin, et al. 1993. Cloning of a virulence factor of *Entamoeba histolytica. J. Clin. Invest.* **91:**1532–1540.

56. Reed, S. L., J. A. Ember, D. S. Herdman, R. G. DiScipio, T. E. Hugli, and I. Gigli. 1995. The extracellular neutral cysteine proteinase of *Entamoeba histolytica* degrades anaphylatoxins C3a and C5a. *J. Immunol.* **155:**266–274.

57. Romero, J. L., S. Descoteaux, S. Reed, E. Orozco, J. Santos, and J. Samuelson. 1992. Use of polymerase chain reaction and nonradioactive DNA probes to diagnose *Entamoeba histolytica* in clinical samples. *Arch. Med. Res.* (Mexico) **23:**277–279.

58. Rosales-Encinas, J. L., I. Meza, P. Lopez de Leon, P. Talamas-Rohana, and M. Rojkind. 1987. Isolation of a 220 kDa protein with lectin properties from a virulent strain of *Entamoeba histolytica. J. Infect. Dis.* **156:**790–797.

59. Sargeaunt, P. G., J. E. Williams, and J. D. Grene. 1978. The differentiation of invasive and non invasive *E. histolytica* by isoenzyme electrophoresis. *Trans. R. Soc. Trop. Med. Hyg.* **72:**519–521.

60. Scholze, H., S. Frey, Z. Cejka, and T. Bakker-Grunwald. 1996. Evidence for the existence of both proteasomes and a novel high molecular weight peptidase in *Entamoeba histolytica. J. Biol. Chem.* **271:**6212–6216.

61. Scholze, H., and E. Werries. 1986. Cysteine proteinase of *Entamoeba histolytica*. I. Partial purification and action on different enzymes. *Mol. Biochem. Parasitol.* **18:**103–112.

62. Stanley, S. L., Jr., H. Huizenga, and E. Li. 1992. Isolation and partial characterization of a surface glycoconjugate of *Entamoeba histolytica. Mol. Biochem. Parasitol.* **50:**127–138.

63. Stanley, S. L. J. 1995. Role of the *Entamoeba histolytica* cysteine proteinase in amebic liver abscess formation in severe combined immunodeficient mice. *Infect. Immun.* **63:**1587–1590.

64. Tannich, E. 1996. Recent advances in DNA-mediated gene transfer in *Entamoeba histolytica. Parasitol. Today* **12:**198–200.

65. Tannich, E., I. Bruchhaus, R. D. Walter, and R. D. Horstman. 1991. Pathogenic and nonpathogenic *Entamoeba histolytica*: identification and molecular cloning of an iron-containing superoxide dismutase. *Mol. Biochem. Parasitol.* **49:**61–71.

66. Tannich, E., F. Ebert, and R. D. Horstmann. 1992. Molecular cloning of cDNA and genomic sequences coding for the 35-kilodalton subunit of the galactose-inhibitable lectin of pathogenic *Entamoeba histolytica. Mol. Biochem. Parasitol.* **55:**225–228.

67. Vines, R. R., J. E. Purdy, B. D. Ragland, J. Samuelson, B. J. Mann, and W. A. Petri.

1995. Stable episomal transfection of *Entamoeba histolytica. Mol. Biochem. Parasitol.* **71:**265–267.

68. **Walderich, B., L. Muller, G. D. Burchard, and D. Mirelman.** 1995. Patients infected with *Entamoeba histolytica* and *Entamoeba dispar* as detected by isoenzymes and two different PCR systems, abstr. L119. European Conference on Tropical Medicine, Hamburg. Blackwell Science, Düsseldorf.

69. **Walsh, J. A.** 1988. Prevalence of *Entamoeba histolytica* infection. p. 93–105. *In* J. I. Ravdin (ed.), *Amebiasis: Human Infection by Entamoeba histolytica.* Wiley Medical, New York.

70. **Young, J., T. M. Young, P. L. Lu, J. C. Unkeless, and Z. A. Cohn.** 1982. Characterization of a membrane pore-forming protein from *Entamoeba histolytica. J. Exp. Med.* **156:**1677–1690.

IS TUBERCULOSIS REALLY AN EMERGING OR A REEMERGING DISEASE?

Hervé Bercovier

17

THE CLASSICAL HISTORY AND SOME QUESTIONS

Mycobacterium tuberculosis evolved from *Mycobacterium bovis* among milk-drinking Indo-Europeans, who then spread the disease during their invasion or migration into Western Europe and Eurasia. This statement, based on a hypothetical phylogeny of *M. bovis* and *M. tuberculosis*, on anthropology, and on a correlation between lactose malabsorbers and incidence of tuberculosis morbidity and macrophage permissivity to *M. tuberculosis*; has never been proved with hard data (6) and in fact holds very little scientific validity. On the contrary, the finding of *M. tuberculosis* in pre-Columbian mummies in the Americas and data on tuberculosis in the Jewish population and in Japan (low incidence of tuberculosis in both populations with a high lactose intolerance rate) negate this theory at least in part. New data are needed to understand the global historical epidemiology of tuberculosis. This paper does not address the evolutionary bounds between *M. bovis* and *M. tuberculosis*; it concerns the epidemiology of tuberculosis

in Europe from the Middle Age until today and asks whether a similar evolution can be predicted in countries that currently structurally mimic the changes that occurred in Europe from the Renaissance to modern times.

RECENT HISTORY OF TUBERCULOSIS

It is generally accepted that tuberculosis culminated in the 18th to 19th centuries in Europe, with a continuous decrease in the 20th century even before vaccination and antibiotic treatment were available (Table 1). Cycles of 50 to 75 years of tuberculosis epidemics have been described and were used to establish that the tuberculosis epidemic in Europe must have peaked in the early 19th century, because tuberculosis was already decreasing at the end of the 19th century. These cycles were found in recent epidemics in North American Indians in situations difficult to compare with that of the industrial revolution in Europe. Nevertheless, in the 19th century and at the beginning of the 20th century, one can find data showing a high prevalence of tuberculosis and the beginning of its decrease (Fig. 1 and Table 1). For example, Bayle found 250 cases of tuberculosis in a series of 696 autopsies at the beginning of the 19th century. It is reported that 50% of the population in England in the

Herve Bercovier, Department of Clinical Microbiology, The Hebrew University-Hadassah Medical School, Ein Karem, Jerusalem 91120, Israel.

Microbial Ecology and Infectious Disease, Edited by Eugene Rosenberg
©1999 American Society for Microbiology, Washington, D.C.

TABLE 1 Evolution of tuberculosis since 1865 (mortality/100,000)

Country	1865	1910	1936	1952	1971	1994
France	500	228	74	43	7	2
Netherlands				12	1.5	1.5
England	153	100	60	20	2	2
Ireland	470	300	100			
Poland				106	8	
Burma			300		150	100

19th century had scrofula, and at the same time, 53% of the orphans in a Berlin orphanage had scrofula. In New York, the death rate from tuberculosis was 750 per 100,000 in 1805 and decreased to 400 per 100,000 in 1870 (9). This dramatic decrease is not fully explained by improved life conditions or by public health measures.

I hypothesize that the epidemic of tuberculosis in the Western world did not start at the end of the 18th century to reach the observed dramatic decrease at the end of the 19th century, but rather this epidemic began at least three centuries earlier and, over four centuries, exerted selection in the European population that was at high risk. A correlate of this hypothesis is that the social changes that happened in the late Middle Ages were a major factor in the epidemization of tuberculosis. Society in Europe changed from an agricultural, scattered, fixed society to a mobile bourgeois (from "bourg," a small city, a burg, or a borough), artisan, corporate structure. Nonexposed European populations that remained rural, such as that in Ireland, remained susceptible to tuberculosis even in the 20th century.

Revisiting the data yields no general report on the morbidity of tuberculosis in the 15th to 17th centuries, which explains why one refers to the beginning of the epidemics during the 18th century or at the beginning of the 19th century, when tuberculosis is well documented. Plague, devastating Europe in the Middle Ages and the Renaissance, probably masked the importance of tuberculosis and therefore prevented its description and the ob-

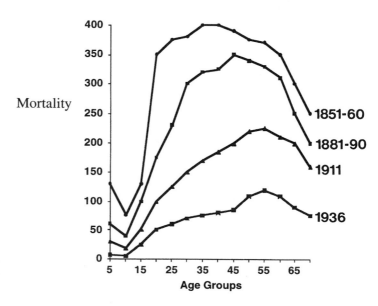

FIGURE 1 Decrease of tuberculosis in England and Wales (mortality shown per 100,000).

servation of the beginning of the epidemic of tuberculosis. However, traces of the importance of tuberculosis can be found prior to the 18th century.

In the 17th century, some precise data on tuberculosis exists. For instance, the registries in England and Wales in 1650 show that "pulmonary phthisis" accounted for 20% of all deaths, mainly in cities (9). If all these cases were really cases of tuberculosis, tuberculosis mortality rates in the 17th century were at least 20 times higher than the accepted peak mortality in the 18th century. The Republic of Luccia in Italy legislated the first decree of prophylaxis against tuberculosis in 1699. A society takes some years before recognizing a specific problem and legislating it, which suggests that tuberculosis was already a serious health problem during the 17th century.

Documentation of tuberculosis in the 16th century can be found in descriptions of sociological events. Scrofula was believed to be cured by the touch of the king's hand. Entering Paris in 1594, the French king Henri IV touched 600 scrofulous persons, a record beaten by Louis XIV, who touched 1,600 scrofulous persons in one session 150 years later. Furthermore, the prevalence of human tuberculosis on the basis of pathological findings and ancient DNA analysis (10) in a late medieval population of Lithuania indicates that between 25 and 50% of the population was infected with *M. tuberculosis*, making a 10 to 20% death rate credible.

In addition to ancient DNA data, the history of *Mycobacterium leprae* in Europe may also provide a way to date the beginning of the European epidemics of tuberculosis at the 15th century. In Europe, leprosy was epidemic in the early Middle Ages but stopped its progress and declined significantly during the Renaissance. A simplistic theory to explain the decreased leprosy was improved hygiene and general cooling of the weather. Sporadic cases of leprosy occurred in Europe until the 20th century, but the last European indigenous case of leprosy occurred in clean and cold Norway in 1953, rendering these theories doubtful. Exclusion of leprosy by tuberculosis, a hypothesis proposed by Chaussinaud 50 years ago (3), seems a better explanation. Dubos and Dubos (9) evoked this hypothesis, stating that no experimental data supported it. Recently, however, experimental data in mice (19) proved that live BCG or BCG extracts were protective against *M. leprae* infection, preventing the multiplication of *M. leprae* inoculated in the footpad. Additional studies in humans in Africa (14), Asia (2), and South America (15) have shown that BCG-vaccinated populations are protected not against adult tuberculosis but against leprosy. If this theory is correct, tuberculosis would have had to be epidemic in the early 15th century to produce a herd immunity extensive enough to eradicate leprosy.

What social changes may have helped tuberculosis become epidemic in the 15th century? In Europe, the main structural changes in the 15th century include the end of feudalism, with the development of a strong state structure with a strong king and with a new bourgeois society reflecting the development of larger communities or small cities ("bourgs"). Farmers, the vast majority of the population were no longer restricted in their movement, by the feudal power and could freely move from the countryside to cities. Industrialization is beginning with the development of some large factories. Commerce also was developing (the first stock exchange was founded in 1460 in Antwerp), allowing more exchanges between cities. The change from a completely scattered population depending on the local feudal power to a more structured society with a centralized power, favoring small cities, probably implanted tuberculosis. The development of commerce, at the same time, favored the large diffusion of the disease.

As a result, tuberculosis was very prevalent in the early 17th century, as shown by kings very busy treating scrofula by hand touch. If the tuberculosis epidemic was already active in the 16th century, it must have started in the 15th century. These partial data indicate the historical pattern of tuberculosis in Western

Europe. More data, based on ancient DNA studies, should be added to confirm this hypothesis.

IS TUBERCULOSIS EMERGING OR REEMERGING AND WHERE?

On the basis of case notifications and estimation, the World Health Organization (WHO) estimates that 88 million new cases of tuberculosis occurred or will occur during the decade 1990–1999. Among those 88 million new cases of tuberculosis, 30 million died or will die (5). The vast majority of tuberculosis case presently occur among inhabitants of Asia and Africa, whereas less than 2% of all new cases concern residents from industrialized countries (Table 2).

Epidemiological data show that the decrease of the already low incidence of tuberculosis has stopped in industrialized countries (Table 2). In certain Western countries, the incidence of tuberculosis has even increased in the last 10 years, but the incidence is so low that the risk of a new epidemic seems low at the moment. Human immunodeficiency virus (HIV) and multiply drug-resistant strains of *M. tuberculosis* are the main factors in the actual relative increase of tuberculosis in industrialized countries. A large segment of the population in industrialized countries maintains a herd immunity due to exposure to *M. tuberculosis* in the 40s. However, within 20 years, most of the exposed population will disappear, and as a result, we could see new foci of epidemics in the Western world if the public health institutions are not prepared to detect and treat the disease rapidly. Such a situation has been recently seen with an epidemic of diphtheria in Eastern Europe. Other factors related to political unstability, resulting in a lack of working institutions, can explain the rise of tuberculosis in countries of the former Communist block (Table 3). Published data show clearly that tuberculosis is reemerging in Eastern Europe (4, 27).

On the other hand, epidemiological data show a high incidence of tuberculosis in Africa and in Asia, similar to that found in the Western world in the 1930s (Tables 1, 2, and 3, 4) (8, 21, 23). Exact evaluation of the prevalence of tuberculosis in Asia and Africa is not possible using the WHO data. Tables 2 and 5 illustrate this lack of consistency in data based on notification to WHO. The decrease of tuberculosis in the 1930s and 1950s in the Western world resulted from public health measures, new antibiotic treatments, and, as suggested above, genetic selection and herd immunity. Is the epidemic in Africa and Asia at a declining phase as it was in the 1930s in Europe or are we witnessing a real emerging disease with a rising epidemic? Will public health measures and new antibiotic treatments reduce and stop tuberculosis in Africa and in Asia or will the incidence of tuberculosis increase?

TABLE 2 Evolution of tuberculosis incidence since 1970

Continent	1970s		1980s: no. of cases	1990		1995: no. of cases	2000[a]	
	No. of cases[b]	Reference		No. of cases	Reference		No. of cases	Reference
Africa	56	23	67	80		242	293	
	283	16		191	8			
Asia	73		87	85	23	241	247	5
	131		115	146	21			
				237	8			
Western Europe/ North America	45		35	23		23	24	

[a] Projected.
[b] Number of new cases of tuberculosis per 100,000 population per year.

TABLE 3 Change of regime changes tuberculosis incidence and mortality

Country	1990		1994/5	
	Incidence[a]	Mortality (%)	Incidence	Mortality (%)
Romania	60	7	94.2	11
Latvia	28.7	6.4	50.5	14.1

[a] Number of cases of tuberculosis per 100,000 population per year.

The data presented in Table 4, where Burma-Myanmar is taken as an example, seems to indicate that the epidemic of tuberculosis is in its declining phase, and we can hope that as in Europe in the 20th century, the incidence of tuberculosis will be reduced with no one really understanding how. Unfortunately, the trustworthiness of the data available from WHO (Tables 3 and 5) does not allow the conclusion that the high incidence of tuberculosis in these continents is at the peak, plateau, or descending phase of an epidemic curve. Another example of this lack of reliability can be seen by comparing the data presented by an independent investigator who studied more than 1 million Chinese (13) and the WHO data on China based on notification (Table 5). On the one hand, incidence of tuberculosis seems to plateau; on the other hand, the incidence of tuberculosis seems to have increased by 50% in less than 10 years.

Therefore, to analyze the current situation and to predict the future, we must try to figure out if the major changes that could be related to the development of the epidemic of tuberculosis in Europe, as analyzed above, are occurring now in Africa and Asia. From this analysis, we could predict whether the epidemics of tuberculosis in Africa and Asia have already reached their apogee or if they are still developing. Are Asia and Africa following a small urbanization from agriculture to small cities, as occurred in Europe in the late Middle Ages? The data presented in Table 6 indicate some similarities in population structure between Asia at the end of the 20th century and Europe in the middle of the 19th century. If large city populations exist along with a large majority of the population living in agricultural settlements, it would be of interest to evaluate whether smaller urban entities centered on small factories are expanding. These small urbanization centers usually lack the medical structure and medical care found in large cities. If such is the case, then the Asian tuberculosis epidemic could mimic that of Europe and could result in an increasing incidence of tuberculosis in the future. Will selection occur in Africa and Asia as it may have occurred in Europe, and will it take four centuries to produce a more resistant population? Will HIV and multiply drug-resistant *M. tuberculosis* strains complicate the epidemiological evolution of tuberculosis? This presenta-

TABLE 4 Comparative tuberculosis data in Asia and Europe

Country	Year	Mortality (%)	PPD/Prevalence (%)	Incidence[a]
Burma	1933	2		
	1937	3	65	3,000
	1970	1	51	450
Europe	1926	0.7–2		300
(Great Britain,	1935	0.6–1		180
France, Denmark)	1952	0.1–0.4	50	40
	1990	0.02		23

[a] Number of cases per 100,000 population per year.

TABLE 5 Incidence of tuberculosis in Asia[a]

	1974–9	1980–86
WHO (incidence)	73	87[b]/115[c]
China[d] (prevalence of active TB)	578	550
(estimated incidence)	200	200
Real incidence if 12% reported to WHO	583	725

[a] Number of cases of tuberculosis per 100,000 population per year.
[b] Reference 23.
[c] Reference 21.
[d] According to Hsu-Yu (13), only 12% of patients with active tuberculosis were recorded by authorities.

tion shows the necessity to generate new data not provided by WHO (Table 2), to monitor the situation. In any case, the best option is to be ready to control tuberculosis better than we do it today. An effective vaccine that would also prevent carrier stage could resolve many problems due to tuberculosis.

DNA VACCINES

The only vaccine available against *M. tuberculosis* is BCG, a live attenuated vaccine. BCG (bacille Calmette-Guérin), an attenuated strain of *M. bovis*, has been used worldwide as a human vaccine against tuberculosis (22). Although the use of BCG has been successful in England and the United States, it has been less effective in other countries. The protective efficacy of the BCG vaccine varied in different trials from 0 to 80% (22). Moreover, this live attenuated strain cannot be used in immunocompromised patients. Cellular immunity and delayed-type hypersensitivity are key processes in the course of mycobacterial infection and are involved in both primary and secondary infection as well as in the induction of protective immunity in the host (11, 20). Only acellular vaccines can provide both safety and immunogenicity to protect immunocompromised and normal patients. Data on acellular vaccines against tuberculosis are meager and based on excreted proteins (1, 12). Acellular vaccines against intracellular multiplying bacteria are yet to be established. Naked DNA has been used for vaccination against viral diseases (influenza, hepatitis B, HIV, rabies, hepatitis C, and herpes simplex), parasitic diseases (malaria, leishmaniasis, schistosomiasis), and bacterial diseases (7, 24–26). The results are encouraging, demonstrating distinct advantages of DNA vaccines over conventional vaccines: processing through the major histocompatibility complex I and II pathways; induction of humoral and cytotoxic lymphocyte responses increased by the presence of CpG sequences; requirement for small amounts of DNA (microgram range) compared with the milligram level needed for proteins and peptides; a long protective immunity

TABLE 6 Demographic data

	Europe-U.S.A.			Romania	Burma	China	
	1850	1950	1995	1995	1995	1975	1995
Population (%)							
Agriculture	65	20–40	2.3–5	30	70	80	65
Urban	35	50	70–87	56	26	17	30
Physicians per 1000 inhabitants			2–4	1.8	0.08	0.7	0.9

after a single inoculation; and easy preparation and preservation of plasmid DNA, which may eliminate the need for the "cold chain" required for conventional vaccines. The DNA is not immunogenic by itself, and it remains episomal. However, in spite of the great potential of DNA vaccination, it still faces safety uncertainties. So far, only the intramuscular injection of naked DNA into the tibialis anterior muscle has proven effective and reproducible in mice.

Recently, promising results were reported: by vaccinating mice with a plasmid DNA encoding the *M. tuberculosis* 85 antigen complex (18) resulted in a Th1 helper cell T-cell response. The level of protection obtained by these DNA vaccines can be measured by a decrease in the bacterial load in certain organs (spleen, lung) of 1 log, or a maximum of 2 log, of the bacterium used for challenge. These results are equal or inferior to the level of protection obtained when using BCG. Similar results were obtained by Lowrie et al. (17) and by us (Bercovier, unpublished data) using plasmid DNA encoding additional *M. tuberculosis* proteins (Hsp65, Hsp70, 36 kDa, 6 kDa, L7/L12). Moreover, these vaccines induce good cellular immunity (increase in both antigen-specific $CD4^+$ $CD8^-$ and $CD4^-$ $CD8^+$ T cells and presence of cytotoxic T lymphocytes) concomitant with the production of gamma interferon, interleukin-2, interleukin-12, and tumor necrosis factor α. Although the DNA vaccines have not yet been proven to be superior in their protective activity to the BCG vaccine, we suggest that in accordance with their immunogenic properties, they should be used as therapeutic vaccines. To control the spread of tuberculosis efficiently, the scientific community must face the challenge of developing a therapeutic vaccine against tuberculosis that can stop the transmission of the disease.

REFERENCES

1. **Andersen, P., and I. Heron.** 1993. Specificity of protective memory immune response against *Mycobacterium tuberculosis*. *Infect. Immun.* **61:** 844–851.
2. **Bertolli, J., C. Pangi, R. Frerichs, and M. E. Halloran.** 1997. A case-control study of the effectiveness of BCG vaccine for preventing leprosy in Yangon, Myanmar. *Int. J. Epidemiol.* **26:** 888–896.
3. **Chaussinaud, R.** 1948. Tuberculose et lepre. Maladies antagonistes. Eviction de la lepre par la tuberculose. *Int. J. Leprosy* **16:**430.
4. **Corlan, E.** 1995. The incidence of tuberculosis in Romania in 1994. *Pneumoftiziologia* **44:**9–16.
5. **Cosivi, O., J. M. Grange, C. J. Daborn, M. C. Raviglione, T. Fujikura, D. Cousins, R. A. Robinson, H. F. A. K. Huchzermeyer, I. de Kantor, and F. X. Meslin.** 1998. Zoonotic tuberculosis due to Mycobacterium bovis in developing countries. *Emerg. Infect. Dis.* **4:**http://www.cdc.gov/ncidod/EID/vol4no1/cosivi.htm.
6. **Daniel, T. M., J. H. Bates, and K. A. Downes.** 1994. History of tuberculosis, p. 13–24. *In* B. R. Bloom (ed.), *Tuberculosis: Pathogenesis, Protection and Control.* American Society for Microbiology, Washington, D.C.
7. **Davis, H. L., M.-L. Michel, and R. G. Whalen.** 1993. DNA-based immunization induces continuous secretion of hepatitis B surface antigen and high levels of circulating antibody. *Hum. Mol. Genet.* **2:**1847–1851.
8. **Dolin, P. J., M. C. Raviglione, and A. Kochi.** 1994. Global tuberculosis incidence and mortality during 1990–2000. *Bull. W.H.O.* **72:** 213–220.
9. **Dubos, R., and J. Dubos.** 1952. *Tuberculosis, Man, and Society: The White Plague.* Little, Brown & Co., Boston.
10. **Faerman, M., R. Jankauskas, A. Gorski, H. Bercovier, and C. L. Greenblatt.** 1997. Prevalence of human tuberculosis in a medieval population of Lithuania studied by ancient DNA analysis. *Ancient Biomolecules* **1:**205–214.
11. **Fishman, Y., and H. Bercovier.** 1995. Involvement of L7/L12 in DTH reaction in mycobacterial infections *J. Cell Biochem. Suppl.* **19B:** 77, abstr. B3–229.
12. **Horwitz, M. A., E. L. Byong-Wha, B. J. Dillon, and G. Harth.** 1994. Protective immunity against tuberculosis induced by vaccination with major extracellular vaccine of *M. tuberculosis. Proc. Natl. Acad. Sci. USA* **92:**1530–1534.
13. **Hsu-yu, H.** 1993. The epidemiologic status of lung tuberculosis in China 1979 and 1984/85. The result of the 2nd nationwide randomized prevalence study. *Pneumologie* **4:**450–455.

14. **Karonga Prevention Trial Group.** 1996. Randomised controlled trial of single BCG, repeated BCG or combined BCG and killed Mycobacterium leprae vaccine for prevention of leprosy and tuberculosis in Malawi. *Lancet* **348:** 17–24.

15. **Lombardi, C., E. S. Pedrazzani, J. C. Pedrazzani, P. F. Filho, and F. Zicker.** 1996. Protective efficacy of BCG against leprosy in Sao Paulo. *Bull. Pan. Am. Health Org.* **30:**24–30.

16. **Lowlell, A. M.** 1984. Tuberculosis: its social and economic impact and some thoughts on epidemiology. *Microbiol. Ser.* **15:**1021–1055.

17. **Lowrie, D. B., C. L. Silva, M. J.Colston, S. Ragno, and R. E. Tascon.** 1997. Protection against tuberculosis by a plasmid DNA vaccine. *Vaccine* **15:**834–838.

18. **Lozes, E., K. Huygen, J. Content, O. Denis, D. L. Montgomery, A. M. Yawman, P. Vandenbussche, J. P. Van Vooren, A. Drowart, J. F. Ulmer, and M. A. Liu.** 1997. Immunogenicity and efficacy of tuberculosis DNA vaccine encoding the components of the secreted antigen 85 complex. *Vaccine* **15:**830–833.

19. **Matsuoka, M., H. Nomaguchi, H. Yukitake, N. Ohara, S. Matsumoto, S. Mike, and T. Yamada.** 1997. Inhibition of multiplication of Mycobacterium leprae in mouse foot pads by immunization with ribosomal fraction and culture filtrate from Mycobacterium bovis BCG. *Vaccine* **15:**1214–1217.

20. **Orme, I. M., E. S. Miller, A. D. Roberts, S. K. Furney, J. P. Griffin, K. M. Dobos, D. Chi, B. Rivoire, and P. J. Brennan.** 1992. T lymphocytes mediating protection and cellular cytolysis during the course of *Mycobacterium tuberculosis* infection. Evidence for different kinetics and recognition of a wide spectrum of protein antigens. *J. Immunol.* **148:**189–196.

21. **Raviglione, M. C., Snider, D. E, Jr., and A. Kochi.** 1995. Global epidemiology of tuberculosis. Morbidity and mortality of worldwide epidemic. *JAMA* **273:**220–226.

22. **Smith, D. W.** 1984. BCG. *Microbiol. Ser.* **15:** 1057–1070.

23. **Sudre, P., G. ten-Dam, and A. Kochi.** 1992. Tuberculosis: A global overview of the situation today. *Bull. W.H.O.* **70:**149–159.

24. **Tang, D. C., M. DeVit, and S. A. Johnston.** 1992. Genetic immunization is a simple method for eliciting an immune response. *Nature* **356:** 152–154.

25. **Ulmer, J. B., J. J. Donnely, S. E. Parker, G. H. Rhodes, P. L. Felgner, V. J. Dwarki, S. H. Gromkowski, R. R. Deck, C. M. Leander, D. Martinez, H. C. Perry, J. W. Shiver, D. L. Mongomery, and M. A. Liu.** 1993. Heterologous protection against influenza by injection of DNA encoding a viral protein. *Science* **259:**1745–1749.

26. **Wang, B., K. E. Ugen, V. Srikantan, M. G. Agadjanyan, K. Dang, Y. Refaeli, A. I. Sato, J. Boyer, W. V. Williams, and D. B. Weiner.** 1993. Gene inoculation generates immune responses against human immunodeficiency virus type 1. *Proc. Natl. Acad. Sci. USA* **90:**4156–4160.

27. **Zalesky, R., J. Leimans, and I. Pavloska.** 1997. The epidemiology of tuberculosis in Latvia. *Monaldi Arch. Chest Dis.* **52:**142–146.

MICROBE-HOST
ASSOCIATIONS

INTRODUCTION

Ronald Weiner

Some important paradigms of the infectious disease process come from the ecological study of microbe-host interactions. Symbiotic associations range from the obligately mutualistic to the lethally parasitic in a dynamic relationship in which the partners "dance" in continuously evolving interplay. The papers in this session mention examples falling within the broad spectrum of symbioses. They include those that are mutualistic (rhizobia), commensalistic (agrobacteria) and parasitic (*Vibrio shiloi*).

Ann Matthysse's paper, "Interactions of Agrobacteria with Plants," reports that three genes, involved in (i) host-bacterium signaling, (ii) bacterial attachment via an exopolysaccharide, and (iii) cellulose synthesis, leading to tight adhesion, each play "an important role in the colonization of tomato roots by *A. tumefaciens*." Furthermore, the agrobacteria are shown to have a broader host range than legume-limited rhizobia, possibly having two root colonization systems, one for legumes and another for some nonlegumes. Eugene Rosenberg reports on the effect of tempera-

ture on bacterial bleaching of corals. In benchmark coral ecology, it is shown that a specific species of bacteria, *Vibrio shiloi*, is the etiological agent of the bleaching disease, much as specific human diseases are caused by specific pathogens. Moreover, it is shown that both the disease epidemiology and the ability of *V. shiloi* to adhere to the coral are temperature dependent.

It is interesting that each of the papers emphasizes the specificity of microbe-host interactions and shows that specificity results from highly evolved molecular interactions. For example, for both agrobacteria (crown galls) and *V. shiloi* (coral bleaching), the infection process is highly dependent on host cell-specific bacterial adhesins. This also applies to many mammalian diseases such as gastroenteritis caused by enteropathogenic *Escherichia coli*, discussed elsewhere in this volume.

Edward Ruby discusses another noteworthy symbiosis and shows the precision in the interactions between cooperative *Vibrio fischeri* and sepiolid squids. The luminous organ of the squid is a potent bacterial growth chamber supporting high *V. fischeri* cell and autoinducer densities, and it optimizes the bacterial bioluminescence. The squid gains important survival advantages when harboring *V. fischeri* and expels it during times when there is no

Ronald Weiner, Department of Cell Biology and Molecular Genetics, University of Maryland, College Park, MD 20742.

apparent advantage to maintaining the symbionts. It may be that mechanisms of some
human diseases are rooted in ancient symbiosis
between microorganisms and less highly
evolved biota such as marine invertebrates.

ECOLOGY OF A BENIGN "INFECTION": COLONIZATION OF THE SQUID LUMINOUS ORGAN BY *VIBRIO FISCHERI*

Edward G. Ruby

18

Very few pathogenic associations have been examined as ecological phenomena, and few aspects of microbial ecology are understood mechanistically to the extent that many bacterial infections of mammals are. Nevertheless, it has become increasingly clear that each of these two fields could gain significantly from an understanding and application of the strengths and approaches of the other. There are not many examples of bacterial interactions with host tissues that have been examined at levels that would be familiar to Serge Winogradsky on one hand and Robert Koch on the other, but in some cooperative associations, the bacterial symbiont has a well-described ecological cycle alternating between its host and other niches in the environment and, when it is associated with the host, exhibits specific signaling processes that change the pattern of gene expression in both partners. One such association (62), that between the sepiolid squid *Euprymna scolopes* (2, 69) and the luminous marine bacterium *Vibrio fischeri* (56), is the subject of this review.

THE *EUPRYMNA SCOLOPES-VIBRIO FISCHERI* SYMBIOSIS

All animals have, and perhaps require, intimate associations with a specific complement of bacteria (21, 28, 55). In most cases, the initial interplay with these cooperative microbial partners begins during the early postembryonic period, when the juvenile animal is first exposed to the ambient environment. During this crucial period, a coordinated program of interactions between the proper bacterial species and the developing host must occur (43). This program results in the establishment of a healthy, stable set of associations without compromising the animal's nonself recognition systems. Such coordination between host and symbionts must involve a complex, reciprocal signaling between these distinct genomes that may be as intricate as that occurring among the cells of an animal during embryogenesis or between a pathogen and its host. Studies of gnotobiotic animals have revealed that not only do hosts fail to thrive without the essential nutrients normally supplied by their indigenous microbiota, but also these microorganisms participate in the normal maturation of both the immune system and the tissues with which they closely associate (8, 21, 68, 72). However, we understand relatively little about the mechanisms

Edward G. Ruby, Pacific Biomedical Research Center, University of Hawaii, Manoa, Honolulu, HI 96813.

Microbial Ecology and Infectious Disease, Edited by Eugene Rosenberg underlying this reciprocal host–bacterial signaling because of the complexity of the interactions existing between and among the typically multispecies microbial consortia of animals. For this reason, development of experimentally approachable model systems can be of great utility.

Adult *E. scolopes* have a complex light-emitting organ in the center of their mantle cavity (45, 46). The organ harbors a monospecific culture of *V. fischeri* (3), whose bioluminescence is used by the host in its antipredatory behavior (41, 59). The light organ consists of two lobes, each with three distinct epithelia-lined crypts that house the extracellular symbionts (45). The three crypts present within each lobe of the adult organ join in a common duct that leads to a single pore on the lateral face of the lobe. Emission of bacterial luminescence is controlled in two ways: (i) by a host-modulated, diel restriction on the luminescent output per bacterial cell (6) and (ii) by a series of accessory tissues (51). These accessory tissues are functionally analogous to the tissues that modulate light quality in the eye. A thick reflector directs luminescence ventrally by surrounding the dorsal and lateral faces of the crypts. The ink sac covers the dorsal surface of the organ to absorb stray light, and diverticula of the ink sac dynamically rotate over the crypts to modulate the intensity of emitted light. Finally, the entire ventral surface of the light organ is covered with a thick, muscle-derived lens that refracts the point-source bacterial light into the environment (51, 85).

Bacterial cell number in the crypts is, at least in part, controlled by a daily venting of about 90% of the bacterial culture through these lateral pores, into the mantle cavity, and out into the surrounding seawater (6). This behavior produces a sufficiently high population density of symbiosis-competent *V. fischeri* in the environment to ensure colonization of the next generation of juvenile squid (34). During embryogenesis, the squid develops an incipient light organ morphology that appears to poise the organ to interact, upon hatching, with *V. fischeri* cells in seawater (52). This

morphology includes formation of the three independent crypts on each side of the nascent organ, and complex ciliated, microvillous epithelial surfaces (CMS) on the exterior of the organ. These structures appear to move ambient seawater past the crypt pores, thereby potentiating inoculation of the organ (42).

Within hours after hatching, the juvenile squid (about 2 mm in length) has been colonized by *V. fischeri* cells, a process that triggers subsequent morphogenesis of the light organ (11, 46). In response to interactions with the bacteria, the cells lining the crypts, which appear to have undergone terminal differentiation, begin to increase in volume, and the crypt space continues to grow by divisions of only a few cells at the blind end of each crypt. In addition, the CMS on the surface of the organ regress over a 4-day period as a result of the bacteria-induced cell death of these superficial epithelial cells (55). Studies in which the light organ infection was cured with antibiotic treatment revealed that the host must be exposed to the bacteria for only 12 h to irreversibly induce the entire 4-day morphogenetic program (11). Curing the organ before that time results in no subsequent morphogenesis. Interestingly, 12 h after initiation of colonization, the symbiotic bacteria themselves undergo differentiation, resulting in the loss of flagellation, reduction of cell size, diminution of growth rate, and enhancement of cell-specific luminescence (3, 12, 63).

In addition to the cell-death-mediated regression of the CMS, during the first week of the symbiosis the light organ begins to form and modify tissues that will be essential in the mature, functional association; i.e., the ink sac begins to control the intensity of light emission, the reflector thickens, and the lens starts to form over the ventral surface of the organ (45). The extent to which bacteria are involved in the induction of these late-development events remains to be determined (50).

The embryonic, colonization, and maturation phases through which the light organ association develops constitute a program reminiscent of that described in the leguminous plant-*Rhizobium* symbioses (39). In these bacteria-induced plant associations, dozens of genes have been identified in both partners that are essential for normal signaling of symbiotic development. The coordinated expression of these genes serves to regulate the genetic and biochemical activities that orchestrate the morphogenesis of the N_2-fixing root nodule (75). Efforts are under way to discover a similarly complex set of reciprocal genetic interactions underlying the development of the *Vibrio*-squid association.

A powerful approach to the study of factors controlling the initiation of a bacteria-animal interaction involves identification and characterization of genes and genetic elements that mediate these phenomena. Such an approach is usually more easily accomplished with the bacterial partner, in which metabolically nonessential genes involved in the colonization of the host can be identified using the well-described paradigm of (i) creating a library of mutant clones, (ii) phenotypically screening these clones for mutants expressing symbiotic defects, and (iii) complementing the defect with the isolated gene or gene product (14).

To apply this paradigm to the identification of *V. fischeri* genes that are active and required in the *E. scolopes* symbiosis has required the development of molecular genetic approaches and tools for use in *V. fischeri*. These include transposon insertion (24–26, 78), and gene replacement (79) mutagenesis to produce symbiosis-defective *V. fischeri* strains, as well as conjugation (24) and electroporation (76) methods to manipulate plasmid constructions, and a generalized transduction protocol to transfer transposon and gene replacement mutations into the chromosome of wild-type, symbiosis-competent *V. fischeri* (37, 77). The availability of these techniques has created new and rapidly developing opportunities in the molecular genetics of bacterial host colonization.

THE STANDARD SQUID COLONIZATION ASSAY

Development of the *V. fischeri*-*E. scolopes* association into a model system for the study of

bacterial tissue colonization has been aided by the optimization of conditions for producing and maintaining large numbers of juvenile squids. Newly hatched juveniles of *E. scolopes* can be routinely and continuously produced in large numbers (>20,000 annually) throughout the year in simple brooding and rearing aquarium facilities (46, 47), by use of either flow-through or recirculating seawater systems. In addition, for studies of late development, juvenile squid can be raised to adulthood (29). Taken together, these culturing results have confirmed the utility of this animal as a facile experimental model.

The standard procedure for experimentally initiating a symbiotic association in juvenile *E. scolopes* can be summarized briefly: newly hatched, symbiont-free (aposymbiotic) squids are rinsed in seawater that does not contain symbiosis-competent bacteria (46). The animals are then placed, individually or as a group, in seawater to which has been added between 10^3 and 10^4 symbiosis-competent bacteria per milliliter (63). Within 1 h, an infection is initiated, and the animals can be rinsed again to remove the excess *V. fischeri* cells present in the surrounding seawater. In this way, subsequent development of colonization in groups of juveniles can be synchronized to within a 1-h window of time, thereby allowing more precise and reproducible study of the temporal unfolding of the colonization program and its morphogenetic consequences.

After infection, the juvenile squids are maintained individually in small glass vials or within the wells of microtiter dishes. Periodically, the animals in either of these containers can be manually or automatically placed in front of a photomultiplier tube, and their light emission can be quantified as a measure of the degree of colonization: beginning 8 h after inoculation and for several days thereafter, the amount of light emitted is roughly proportional to the number of bacteria in the symbiotic infection (63). The actual number of bacteria present in the crypts can be easily determined by homogenizing the light organ and spreading a diluted aliquot of the homogenate onto nutrient agar (46). *V. fischeri* CFU arise within 24 h, with essentially 100% plating efficiency (63). Alternatively, bacterial cells in the homogenate can be stained and enumerated by direct microscopic counting.

Even after the symbiotic colonization has been established, the host tissue and symbiotic bacteria are subject to experimental manipulation. Because the crypt spaces remain in contact with the external environment through a pair of lateral pores that persists indefinitely (45), chemicals added to the seawater in which the animals are maintained will diffuse into the crypt spaces. In this way we have reversibly cured infected light organs with several different antibiotics (11), inhibited bacterial attachment in the crypt by use of lectin-binding mannose analogs (44), induced gene expression from *tac* promoters by adding isopropyl-β-D-thiogalactopyranoside (IPTG) to the seawater (82), and infused antibodies for immunolocalization of surface antigens. In the future, this accessibility will also be useful for introducing presumptive signal compounds or antagonists into the crypt environment.

Morphological responses of light organ tissues to a symbiotic colonization are easily revealed by several methods. The onset of cell death, the process by which regression of the external ciliated structures is accomplished, can be visualized in a host animal within 6 h of infection (53). After a brief staining with acridine orange, examination of these structures by epifluorescence microscopy reveals dying cells that appear in a pattern, and to an extent, that is diagnostic of the development of the symbiotic infection process (18). The resulting degree of loss of the ciliated epithelium of the CMS of 4-day-old juvenile *E. scolopes* can be monitored by scanning electron microscopy (11, 46). In addition, the pattern of protein induction later in development (after 4 days) can be easily visualized by gel electrophoresis of tissue homogenates, and specific proteins can be identified by Western blotting (immunoblot) (51). Finally, recent analyses have revealed that the epithelial cells of the crypt swell four-fold in volume and increase their microvillar density by a factor of 4 when they are in contact with *V. fischeri* symbionts (32). Interestingly, this latter effect, unlike the induction of CMS cell death, is reversed when the light organ infection is cured with antibiotics. Using these morphological and biochemical signatures as benchmarks of various stages in the developmental program of the squid, both inducers of, and genetic interruptions in, the reciprocal signaling between the host and its bacterial symbionts can be identified.

MACROECOLOGY OF ANIMAL-BACTERIA ASSOCIATIONS

Much has been written about the dynamics of microorganisms in the environments of soil and water and how abiotic characteristics of their surroundings influence the ecology of microbes. While the constraints placed on microbial growth and distribution by temperature, salinity, pH, water activity, and other factors have been well documented, the role of biotic influences has been less well described; however, these influences are becoming better understood in certain systems, such as the *Vibrio*-sepiolid squid light organ association. In a recent review of the ecology of this animal-bacteria symbiosis (64), a number of conclusions were drawn: (i) host animals are a major source of the *V. fischeri* cells typically present in the bacterioplankton of Hawaiian seawater (33), (ii) symbiont abundance in seawater from different locations correlates directly with host abundance in those locations (34), (iii) more than 90% of the *V. fischeri* in seawater are in a state that is symbiotically infective, but from which they cannot be easily cultured (36), and (iv) light organ symbionts from different geographical locations and host species exhibit distinct population genetic patterns.

The realization that perhaps all forms of animal life carry numerous species of bacteria and that these symbionts constitute a host-specific community is becoming increasingly clear, and this awareness places a broader significance upon the results of these studies of the ecology of the *Vibrio*-squid association. Many animal-associated microbial species are specifically adapted to life with their hosts and are unable to survive outside of the association. Taken together, these points allow one to predict at least two additional ways in which microbial ecology interfaces with, and perhaps even controls, the dynamics of the host's ecological distribution.

First, a major concern of biologists in recent years has been both extinction and invasion of animal species that are prevalent in certain regions of the world, such as the Hawaiian Archipelago (40). What has rarely been addressed in discussions of these concerns is the role that host-specific microorganisms may play in these macroecological phenomena. For instance, required microbial species that must be obtained by the juvenile host from the ambient environment at each generation have to be able to survive in that environment long enough, and in high enough densities, to allow subsequent colonization of the naive host. Any environmental conditions or episodes that negatively affect survival of these microbial species would be expected to reduce the ecological fitness of the host species as well. Considering the fact that with few exceptions, we know almost nothing about the normal, intrinsic microbiotia of most animal species and much less about the role of these microorganisms in the different stages of the host's life history (43), it is impossible to judge how many animal extinctions have been influenced or even precipitated by microbial extinctions (73).

In a similar manner, one might predict that the introduction of a new species of animal into a region of the world in which it has not previously existed, whether that introduction is purposeful or an unwanted invasion, would depend upon the presence of its required symbiotic microbiota. This requirement would be especially critical in those cases in which the symbionts are not directly passed on from the female to her offspring but instead must be obtained from their surroundings (42, 67). The absence of required microbiota in a new environment might account for the paradox that so few species of invertebrates found in ballast water of ships can successfully invade the locations in which that water is routinely discharged (66).

Macroecological forces can also play an important role in bacteria-host interactions in the congruent evolution of the two partners (1, 13, 30, 31). Identification of the symbiotic bacteria isolated from a number of different species of sepiolid squids from regions as distant as Hawaii (3), Japan (63), and France (16) has increased our understanding of the biogeography of these light organ associations. In addition, they have revealed that *Vibrio logei*, a closely related congener of *V. fischeri*, is the predominant symbiont of sepiolid squids in the genus *Sepiola* and that in these light organs, one can find co-existent populations of both *V. fischeri* and *V. logei* (16). The presence of both of these species has been hypothesized to be related to fluctuations in environmental temperatures experienced by these Mediterranean sepiolids.

Recent results of studies of the genetic relatedness of symbiotic *Vibrio* species isolated from seven species of luminous squids have revealed parallel phylogenies between the symbionts and their hosts (57). Because both the squids and their bacterial partners can be easily cultured independently in the laboratory, these studies were coupled with experiments that examined the ability of the different symbiont strains to compete with each other during the colonization of one of the host species. The results of these competition experiments indicated a pronounced dominance of the native symbiont strains over non-native strains and also revealed a hierarchy of symbiont competency that reflected the relative phylogenetic relationships of the partners. These studies are among the first to couple molecular systematics with experimental colonization assays, providing evidence for parallel speciation among a set of animal-bacteria associations. Such investigations are important in linking the evolutionary and biogeographic history of these associations with the molecular mechanisms underlying host specificity, a subject of increasing concern to pathogenic microbiologists and epidemiologists as well.

MICROECOLOGY OF ANIMAL-BACTERIA ASSOCIATIONS

From the viewpoint of the microorganism, perhaps the most immediate and dominant aspect of ecology that it routinely faces is the interface with its host's tissues. This level of interaction has been the primary focus of countless studies of microbial pathogenesis, although their results have rarely been viewed through the prism of ecological theory. In contrast, much less is known about the manner in which cooperative associations between bacteria and animal species are regulated and maintained over the lifetime of the hosts. One reason for this imbalance in understanding is clearly the urgency that has historically been accorded to ending pathogenic infections. However, a greater awareness of the importance of cooperative microbial associations in attaining and maintaining the "wellness" state in animals is now emerging (43), and because such associations are most often consortia of interacting microorganisms such as those in the enteric tract and on the skin, it is likely that this field will develop with a significant awareness of, and emphasis on, microbial community ecology.

Because of the complexity of most animal-bacteria associations, it is not surprising that many investigators have turned to simple model systems in an attempt to define the parameters that characterize establishment of cooperative interactions. Table 1 lists just a few of these systems, most of which are only now becoming experimentally tractable. Among these models is that between *V. fischeri* and *E. scolopes*. This symbiosis, like many of the others listed, has a number of features that render it attractive for experimental studies: (i) the association is specific and involves only one bacterial species (3), (ii) both partners are cul-

turable under laboratory conditions (46), (iii) the initiation of the association is easily placed under experimental control (83), (iv) molecular genetics can be applied to the bacterial partner (24, 79), and (v) the association represents the most common type of interaction between animals and bacteria, i.e., host epithelial tissues colonized by extracellular, gram-negative bacteria.

The microecological interactions between host and bacteria are closely tied to the changing environment of the tissues that are colonized. Within this context, three host developmental stages must be considered in the *V. fischeri*-*E. scolopes* symbiosis: (i) embryogenesis, the period when tissues form that will mediate the infection process and control specificity and recognition; (ii) colonization, the several days after symbiotic infection, characterized by bacteria-triggered transformation of host epithelia; and (iii) maturation, development, and elaboration of those host tissues that support bacterial light emission and modulation, i.e., tissues of the functional symbiosis. Studies of the embryonic developmental biology of the nascent light organ (prehatching) have revealed that organ morphogenesis begins about halfway through embryogenesis (42, 52). Over the last 50% of the embryonic period, six independent epithelia-lined crypts develop that will house the symbionts during the posthatch infection process. Approximately 70% of the way through embryogenesis, the CMS begin to develop that will serve to potentiate infection of the nascent organ of the newly hatched host with *V. fischeri* cells from ambient seawater (42, 52).

During the second, early posthatch, stage of host symbiotic organ morphogenesis (i.e., from hatching through the first 4 days of the juvenile squid's life), colonization by symbiotic bacteria induces terminal differentiation of the host epithelial cells that line the crypt spaces (42, 53, 54). Colonization also induces cell death of the CMS such that within 96 h postinoculation, the CMS have completely regressed (42, 53, 54). Only a transient (10 to 12 h) colonization of the crypts by *V. fischeri*

TABLE 1 Some emerging model systems for the study of benign bacterial colonization of animal tissue

Animal host	Symbiont	Symbiont culturability	Symbiont activity	Reference
Sepiolid squid (*Euprymna scolopes*)	Luminous bacterium (*Vibrio fischeri*)	+	Luminescence	47
Medicinal leech (*Hirudo medicinalis*)	Enteric bacterium (*Aeromonas veronii*)	+	Blood digestion (?)	23
Aphid (*Schizaphis graminum*)	Bacteriome bacterium (*Buchnera aphidicola*)	−	Amino acid synthesis	1
Nematode worm (*Heterorhabditis* spp.)	Luminous bacterium (*Photorhabdus luminescens*)	+	Predation and antibiotic synthesis	17
Shipworm mollusk (*Lyrodus pedicellatus*)	Gill cell bacterium (undescribed)	+	Cellulose digestion and nitrogen fixation	10
Gnotobiotic mouse (*Mus musculus*)	Enteric bacterium (*Bacteroides thetaiotaomicron*)	+	Sugar hydrolysis	8

cells is required to initiate the 4-day morphogenetic program of CMS regression irreversibly (11). After the first 24 h, the host squid begins to control symbiont number and luminescence intensity by a diel expulsion of bacteria from the light organ crypts (6). Infection of the light organ by *V. fischeri* results in a change in the rate of synthesis of mRNA for a gene encoding a peroxidase (71) related to the antimicrobial protein mammalian myeloperoxidase (74, 86).

Maturation of the host organ continues from 4 through 20 days post-hatch. Three-dimensional reconstructions of the light organs of young adults and juveniles have revealed that the crypts enlarge to accommodate the increasing population of *V. fischeri* by forming interconnecting sheets of epithelial cells between which bacteria are housed. Bromodeoxyuridine labeling of the crypt cells indicates that this is accomplished by divisions of cells at the blind ends of the crypts. In addition, accessory structures are modified and elaborated beginning approximately 96 h postcolonization (49, 50). Aldehyde dehydrogenase, the principal light organ lens protein,

is evident by immunocytochemical reactivity within 1 week of the initiation of symbiosis (85).

Symbiosis-competent strains of *V. fischeri* also pass through three stages in the development of the symbiotic infection (Fig. 1): (i) initiation, during which the bacterial cells must express traits that are required to enter the light organ crypts, associate with epithelia, and initiate growth; (ii) colonization, which requires the bacteria to adapt physiologically to the host-supplied nutrients and signals, reaching the typical level of cell density; and (iii) persistence, during which the bacterial cell maintains itself in the host environment over the changing conditions of the host's developing tissues (62).

Examination of these stages has been aided by the recent availability in *V. fischeri* of a number of molecular genetic techniques. Transposon mutagenesis (24, 78) and gene replacement via electroporation and transduction (77) have been developed for genetic manipulation of symbiosis-competent strains of *V. fischeri,* revealing critical events in the developmental program of the symbiosis. Spe-

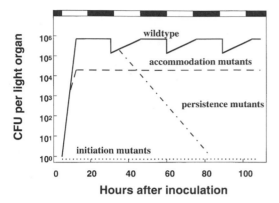

FIGURE 1 Classes of symbiosis-defective mutants of *V. fischeri*. Schematic illustration of the colonization patterns of mutants that either fail to infect ("initiation mutants"), colonize to a diminished extent ("accommodation mutants"), or are unable to maintain a full level of colonization ("persistence mutants"), compared with the wild-type pattern. Representatives of each of these three classes of mutants have been isolated. The daily expulsion each morning of 90% of the wild-type symbionts is depicted, relative to the cycle of day (open bar) and night (black bar) given at the top of the graph.

cifically, examination of the initiation of the symbiosis (i.e., the first 3 h postinoculation) has revealed that the association typically begins with an infection of the crypts by fewer than 10 *V. fischeri* cells from the ambient seawater environment (63). While in natural seawater, most of these cells appear to be in a developmental stage that is nonculturable but remains symbiotically infective (36). Nonmotile strains of *V. fischeri* produced by transposon mutagenesis are completely deficient in the ability to initiate a symbiotic infection (24), suggesting that there is a viscous barrier, perhaps a mucous plug in the pores, through which the *V. fischeri* cells must swim to gain access to the light organ crypts.

Accommodation to the environment of the light organ crypts occurs over the first 12 h after initiation of colonization. During the first 6 to 8 h, at least one homoserine lactone (HSL) quorum-sensing compound (19, 27), or "autoinducer," is released by the growing *V. fischeri* population into the crypts. There, the HSL(s) accumulates to a level (5) that results in induction of the *lux* operon (20, 48) of *V. fischeri*, and the light organ of the juvenile squid becomes bioluminescent (46). After 12 h of rapid growth, competent symbionts have established a colonization of about 10^6 cells (63). *V. fischeri* amino acid auxotrophs can initiate and persist, but in most cases to a level of only 1 to 10% that of the wild-type parent strain (26). These results, as well as analytical studies of the crypt contents, have shown that among the nutrients supplied to the bacterial symbionts by the host are both free amino acids and polypeptides (26).

Beyond the first 12 h postinoculation, the established symbiotic state enters a persistence stage. By 12 h after the symbiosis is established, flagella synthesis by *V. fischeri* cells ceases (63). To persist in the crypts, symbionts must withstand a periodic, host-controlled, expulsion of 90% of the bacterial population that occurs on a 24-h cycle (6) and that results in an abundance of symbiosis-competent *V. fischeri* in the host's habitat (34). A difference in competitive dominance between strains of *V. fischeri* expresses itself only after the first 24 h of a mixed symbiotic colonization (35). Host mechanisms must be maintained to regulate bacterial infection because the crypts of adults remain susceptible to repeated colonization by bacteria from ambient seawater (35). One mechanism for restricting both the types of bacteria and the level of colonization that can occur in the light organ is similar to that limiting pathogenic bacterial infections: reduction of free iron levels in the tissues (84). Although they initiate colonization normally, *V. fischeri* mutants defective in iron sequestration do not persist normally as symbionts for more than 72 h (22, 25).

A number of lines of evidence suggest that the light organ crypts present an oxidatively stressful environment (7, 15, 70) that must be faced by symbiotic *V. fischeri* cells. First, as mentioned above, the tissue of the light organ synthesizes high levels of haloperoxidase, an enzyme that produces the potent oxidant hypochlorous acid (71, 86). Second, *V. fischeri* cells produce a highly active periplasmic catalase, and mutants defective in synthesizing that enzyme have a defect in light organ colonization (79). Finally, while nonluminous strains of *V. fischeri* retain symbiotic competence for at least the first 24 h (77), they lose their ability to persist normally in the light organ after that (76). One hypothesis that could explain this latter phenomenon is that under the oxygen-limiting conditions of the light organ (6), the activity of bacterial luciferase, an enzyme with an unusually high affinity for oxygen (38), maintains the ambient oxygen concentration in the light organ crypts at levels below that necessary to allow host enzymes to generate toxic oxygen radicals (15). Thus, nonluminous bacteria would be more likely to face the detrimental effects of host-generated hypochlorous acid (7).

EVIDENCE FOR STAGE-SPECIFIC GENE EXPRESSION IN SYMBIOTIC *V. FISCHERI*

Similarities between the *E. scolopes* light organ association and better-understood symbioses such as the legume-*Rhizobium* association, (e.g., bacterial species specificity [46]) suggest that certain *V. fischeri* genes will be specifically and obligately induced in a temporal pattern during the development of the symbiosis (65). In fact, evidence for stage-specific *V. fischeri* gene expression has been accumulating and includes (i) the expression of morphological (flagella) and physiological (luminescence) differentiation (36, 63), (ii) the late onset of interstrain competitive dominance (35), and (iii) the identification of mutations (e.g., motility, auxotrophy, and iron acquisition) whose activities are required at different stages in the development of the association (24, 25, 26). Figure 2 is a diagrammatic summary of possible signaling pathways that may function during the development of a symbiotic infection. The interactions depicted include bacterial activities for which mutants have already been identified as well as those hypothesized to have a possible role. While plasmid DNA carriage is a typical characteristic of symbiotic

strains of *V. fischeri*, genes required for symbiotic competence or competitiveness are apparently not carried extrachromosomally (4); thus it should be expected that chromosomally encoded traits will be of greatest interest in the search for colonization factors.

Symbiosis mutants have been produced either by transposon insertion (24, 26, 81) or by gene replacement (77, 79) and were selected to have phenotypes that were predicted to be defective in functions generally required for association with animal tissue (e.g., prototrophy, catalase synthesis, siderophore production). While these initial mutant studies have revealed the importance of such traits to the symbiotic competency of *V. fischeri*, their functions are of a general nature and to date appear to be uninvolved in triggering the several specific events of host morphogenesis that have been assayed (53). Future experiments are needed to identify genes that have a more specific role in the bacterial induction of animal development. These may be best revealed by an approach that allows identification of *V. fischeri* gene promoters that are specifically induced during interaction with host tissue (81).

EFFECT OF THE MUTATIONS ON SYMBIOTIC DEVELOPMENT OF THE HOST

The symbiosis-induced *V. fischeri* strains described above will be useful not only for understanding the response of the bacterium to the symbiotic host environment, but also in determining how the bacterial symbionts may affect host development. There are benchmarks beyond which squid development cannot proceed normally in the absence of the bacteria. For instance, the cell death events that lead to regression of the CMS require the presence of bacteria for at least 12 h (11). Four assays for early developmental benchmarks in the squid light organ can be easily applied; these benchmarks include induction of epithelial cell death (53), changes in oxidative signature of the crypts (70), epithelial cell swelling and microvillar proliferation (32), and induction of the aldehyde dehydrogenase-like

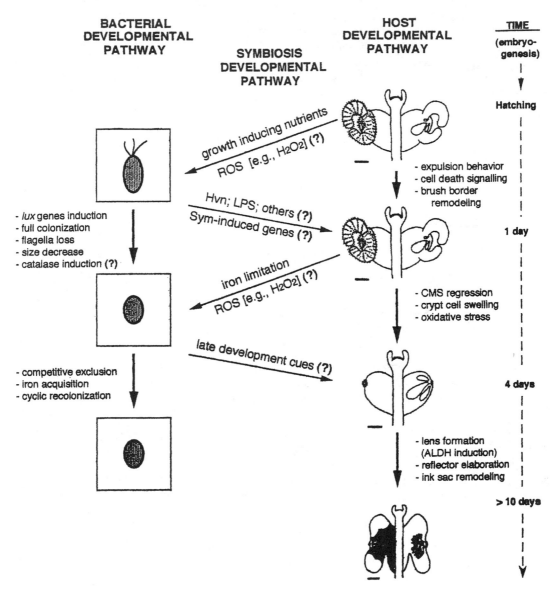

FIGURE 2 Hypothetical reciprocal signaling during development of the *V. fischeri-E. scolopes* symbiosis. Host and bacterial development are characterized by changes in behavior, morphology, and biochemistry in response to interactions with one another. Molecular genetic studies of the bacterial partner and responses of the host to mutant strains of *V fischeri* indicate that a dynamic, programmed dialogue occurs between the two. The result of a successful dialogue is completion of the symbiosis developmental pathway, which leads to the establishment of a stable, mature association. Putative signals produced by the host or by the symbiont may create a biochemical dialogue between the two organisms. This diagram summarizes the possible interactions that future research should clarify. ALDH, aldehyde dehydrogenase, the principal protein of the light organ lens; CMS, ciliated microvillous surface; LPS, lipopolysaccharide surface of the bacterial symbionts; *lux*, genes associated with the bacterial operon encoding luminescence capability; ROS, reactive oxygen species; Sym, symbiosis.

protein (85). If the patterns of development by juvenile squids colonized by mutant strains of *V. fischeri* are distinct from those of wild-type–infected control animals, then the mutated gene is implicated in the signaling process that initiates host morphogenesis. Identification of such genes and their regulators will lead to new discoveries of the dynamics underlying the microecology of tissue colonization (81).

CONCLUSIONS

In this review I have attempted to describe what is currently understood about the *Vibrio*-squid light organ symbioses as an example of the importance of considering bacterial associations with host tissues from both an ecological and a biochemical perspective. The mechanisms underlying the dynamics of these levels of biological interaction are complex and require special approaches and analytical tools. Nevertheless, progress in both areas is becoming increasingly dependent on the other as we converge on the larger emergent properties of bacteria–host associations.

SOME UNRESOLVED QUESTIONS AND FUTURE RESEARCH

1. Increasingly it is becoming clear that there are both homologous (60) and analogous (59, 61) genes that may play a role in the process of host tissue colonization by both pathogenic and cooperative bacteria of the genus *Vibrio*. These similarities bring the term "virulence factors" into a new light and suggest that the evolution of these factors may well have its roots in mechanisms developed for cooperative bacteria–host interactions. To pursue such questions successfully, whole genome-level comparisons between pathogenic *Vibrio* species such as *V. cholerae* and *V. vulnificus* and symbionts such as *V. fischeri* need to be pursued.

2. A striking mechanistic convergence between pathogenic and cooperative bacterial associations has become clear with the discovery of HSL quorum-sensing molecules, first in *V. fischeri*, and then in over 20 other species of animal- and plant-associated bacteria, including numerous pathogens (19, 27). Most recently, the role of these molecules in controlling the development and differentiation of microbial biofilms has been reported (9), opening up an important new field of inquiry that is relevant to many bacteria-tissue associations (80). Such studies emphasize the importance of identifying heretofore undetected genes that are regulated by the levels of HSL signal molecules.

3. An understanding of the complexity of signals and responses that pass between the partners of any bacteria–host association requires a complete description of the environment in which the interaction develops and persists. In the *Vibrio*-squid association, the nature of the crypt contents has begun to be described, with estimates of the levels of molecular oxygen (6), HSL quorum sensors (5), and amino acids (26) already being reported. However, these values constitute only the beginning of our characterization of the crypt environment. Other microchemical conditions of the tissue-bacteria interface that must be determined include the levels of oxygen radicals (70), hydrolytic enzymes (58), and host-derived signal factors and receptors (44).

4. Considering the enormous number of benign bacterial species that normally colonize host tissues, remarkably little is known about the effect of these bacteria, singly and en mass, on host developmental processes (43, 54). Perhaps the best described of these associations is that between the legumes and their N_2-fixing bacterial symbionts (39, 75). Better coordination of collaborative efforts between environmental and pathogenic microbiologists on the one hand and animal biologists on the other must be actively encouraged if we are to bring our understanding of bacteria-animal associations to as advanced a state.

ACKNOWLEDGMENTS

I thank the organizers of the Conference on Microbial Ecology and Infectious Disease for giving me the opportunity to develop the ideas found in this review. I also thank M. McFall-Ngai for insightful discussions, and the members of my laboratory for performing the work I've described.

Portions of this research were funded by National Science Foundation grant IBN96-01155 to M. McFall-Ngai and E.G.R., by the National Institutes of Health through grant RO1-RR12294-02 to E.G.R. and M. McFall-Ngai, and National Research Service Award 1F32GM174724-01A1 to K. Visick.

REVIEWS AND KEY PAPERS

Graf, J, P. V. Dunlap, and E. G. Ruby. 1994. Effect of transposon-induced motility mutations on colonization of the host light organ by *Vibrio fischeri*. *J. Bacteriol.* **176**:6986–6991.

McFall-Ngai, M. J. 1994. Evolutionary morphology of a squid symbiosis. *Am. Zool.* **34**:554–561.

McFall-Ngai, M. J. The development of cooperative associations between animals and bacteria: establishing détente among domains. *Am. Zool.*, in press.

McFall-Ngai, M. J., and E. G. Ruby. 1991. Symbiont recognition and subsequent morphogenesis as early events in an animal-bacterial symbiosis. *Science* **254**:1491–1494.

McFall-Ngai, M. J., and E. G. Ruby. 1998. Bobtail squid and their luminous bacteria: When first they meet. *BioScience* **48**:257–265.

Montgomery, M. K., and M. J. McFall-Ngai. 1994. The effect of bacterial symbionts on early post-embryonic developmental of a squid light organ. *Development* **120**:1719–1729.

Ruby, E. G. 1996. Lessons from a cooperative, bacterial-animal association: the *Vibrio fischeri—Euprymna scolopes* light organ symbiosis. *Annu. Rev. Microbiol.* **50**:591–624.

Ruby, E. G., and K.-H. Lee. 1998. The *Vibrio fischeri-Euprymna scolopes* light organ association: Current ecological paradigms. *Appl. Environ. Microbiol.* **64**:805–812.

Visick, K. L., and E. G. Ruby. 1998. The periplasmic, group III catalase of *Vibrio fischeri* is required for normal symbiotic competence, and is induced both by oxidative stress and by approach to stationary phase. *J. Bacteriol.* **180**:2087–2092.

Visick, K. L., and E. G. Ruby. 1998. Considering the emergent properties of quorum sensing: the consequences to bacteria of autoinducer signaling in their natural environment. *In* G. M. Dunny and S. C. Winans (ed.), *Cell-Cell Signaling in Bacteria.* American Society for Microbiology, Washington, D.C. in press.

REFERENCES

1. **Baumann, P., N. A. Moran, and L. Baumann.** 1997. The evolution and genetics of aphid endosymbionts. *BioScience* **47**:12–20.

2. **Berry, S. S.** 1912. The cephalopoda of the Hawaiian Islands. *Bull. U.S. Bur. Fish.* **32**:255–362.

3. **Boettcher, K. J., and E. G. Ruby.** 1990. Depressed light emission by symbiotic *Vibrio fischeri* of the sepiolid squid, *Euprymna scolopes*. *J. Bacteriol.* **172**:3701–3706.

4. **Boettcher, K. J., and E. G. Ruby.** 1994. Occurrence of plasmid DNA in the sepiolid squid symbiont, *Vibrio fischeri*. *Curr. Microbiol.* **29**:279–286.

5. **Boettcher, K. J., and E. G. Ruby.** 1995. Detection and quantification of *Vibrio fischeri* autoinducer from symbiotic squid light organs. *J. Bacteriol.* **177**:1053–1058.

6. **Boettcher, K. J., E. G. Ruby, and M. J. McFall-Ngai.** 1996. Luminescence in the symbiotic squid *Euprymna scolopes* is controlled by a daily biological rhythm. *J. Comp. Physiol.* **179**: 65–73.

7. **Boettcher, K. J., A. L. Small, and E. G. Ruby.** 1993. Physiological responses of symbiotic *Vibrio fischeri* to oxidative stress. Abstr. 93rd Annu. Meet. Am. Soc. Microbiol. 1993, p. 246.

8. **Bry, L., P. G. Falk, T. Midvedt, and J. I. Gordon.** 1996. A model of host-microbial interactions in an open mammalian ecosystem. *Science* **273**:1380–1383.

9. **Davies, D. G., M. R. Parsek, J. P. Pearson, B. H. Iglewski, J. W. Costerton, and E. P. Greenberg.** 1998. The involvement of cell-to-cell signals in the development of a bacterial biofilm. *Science* **280**:295–298.

10. **Distel, D. L., E. F. DeLong, and J. B. Waterbury.** 1991. Phylogenetic characterization and in situ localization of the bacterial symbiont of shipworms (Teredinidae: Bivalva) by using 16S rRNA sequence analysis and oligodeoxynucleotide probe hybridization. *Appl. Environ. Microbiol.* **57**:2376–2382.

11. **Doino, J. A., and M. J. McFall-Ngai.** 1995. A transient exposure to symbiosis-competent bacteria induces light organ morphogenesis in the host squid. *Biol. Bull.* **189**:347–355.

12. **Dolan, K. M., and E. P. Greenberg.** 1992. Evidence that GroEL, not sigma-32, is involved in transcriptional regulation of the *Vibrio fischeri* luminescence genes in *Escherichia coli*. *J. Bacteriol.* **174**:5132–5135.

13. **Doyle, J. J.** 1994. Phylogeny of the legume family: an approach to understanding the origins of nodulation. *Annu. Rev. Ecol. Syst.* **25**:325–349.

14. **Falkow, S.** 1985. Molecular Koch's postulates applied to microbial pathogenicity. *Rev. Infect. Dis.* **10**(Suppl. 2):S274–S278.

15. **Farr, S. B., and T. Kogoma.** 1991. The oxidative stress responses in *Escherichia coli* and *Salmonella typhimurium*. *Microbiol. Rev.* **55**:561–585.

16. **Fidopiastis, P., S. V. Boletzky, and E. G. Ruby.** 1998. A new niche for *Vibrio logei*, the

predominant light organ symbiont of squids in the genus *Sepiola*. *J. Bacteriol.* **180**:59–64.

17. **Forst, S., and K. Nealson.** 1996. Molecular biology of the symbiotic-pathogenic bacteria *Xenorhabdus* spp. and *Photorhabdus* spp. *Microbiol. Rev.* **60**:21–43.

18. **Foster, J., and M. J. McFall-Ngai.** 1998. Induction of apoptosis by cooperative bacteria in the morphogenesis of host epithelial tissues. *Dev. Genes Evol.*, in press.

19. **Fuqua, W. C., S. C. Winans, and E. P. Greenberg.** 1994. Quorum sensing in bacteria: The LuxR-LuxI family of cell density-dependent transcriptional regulators. *J. Bacteriol.* **176**:269–275.

20. **Gilson, L., A. Kuo, and P. V. Dunlap.** 1995. AinS and a new family of autoinducer synthesis proteins. *J. Bacteriol.* **177**:6946–6951.

21. **Gordon, H. A., and L. Pesti.** 1971. The gnotobiotic animal as a tool in the study of host microbial relationships. *Bacteriol. Rev.* **35**:390–429.

22. **Graf, J.** 1995. Identification of the first symbiotic determinants of *Vibrio fischeri*, the light organ symbiont of *Euprymna scolopes*. Ph.D. thesis. University of Southern California, Los Angeles.

23. **Graf, J.** 1998. The medicinal leech, *Hirudo medicinalis*, a novel animal model for *Aeromonas*. Abstr. Annu. Meet. Am. Soc. Microbiol. 1998, p. 66.

24. **Graf, J., P. V. Dunlap, and E. G. Ruby.** 1994. Effect of transposon-induced motility mutations on colonization of the host light organ by *Vibrio fischeri*. *J. Bacteriol.* **176**:6986–6991.

25. **Graf, J., and E. G. Ruby.** 1994. The effect of iron-sequestration mutations on the colonization of *Euprymna scolopes* by symbiotic *Vibrio fischeri*. Abstr. Annu. Meet. Am. Soc. Microbiol. 1994, p. 76.

26. **Graf, J., and E. G. Ruby.** 1998. Characterization of the nutritional environment of a symbiotic light organ using bacterial mutants and biochemical analyses. *Proc. Natl. Acad. Sci. USA* **95**:1818–1822.

27. **Gray, K. M.** 1997. Intercellular communication and group behavior in bacteria. *Trends Microbiol.* **185**:184–188.

28. **Hackett, K. J., D. E. Lynn, D. L. Williamson, A. S. Ginsberg, and R. F. Whitcomb.** 1986. Cultivation of the *Drosophila* sex-ratio spiroplasma. *Science* **232**:1253–1255.

29. **Hanlon, R. T., M. F. Claes, S. E. Ashcraft, and P. V. Dunlap.** 1997. Laboratory culture of the sepiolid squid *Euprymna scolopes*. *Biol. Bull.* **192**:364–374.

30. **Haygood, M. G. and D. L. Distel.** 1993. Polymerase chain reaction and 16s rRNA gene sequences from the luminous bacterial symbionts of two deep sea anglerfishes. *Nature* **363**:154–156.

31. **Hinkle, G., J. K. Wetterer, T. R. Schultz, M. L. Sogin.** 1994. Phylogeny of the attine ant fungi based on analysis of small subunit rRNA gene sequences. *Science* **266**:1695–1697.

32. **Lamarcq, L. H., and M. J. McFall-Ngai.** 1998. Induction of a gradual, reversible morphogenesis of its host's epithelial brush border by *Vibrio fischeri*. *Infect. Immun.* **66**:777–785.

33. **Lee, K.-H., and E. G. Ruby.** 1992. Detection of the light organ symbiont, *Vibrio fischeri*, in Hawaiian seawater using *lux* gene probes. *Appl. Environ. Microbiol.* **58**:942–947.

34. **Lee, K.-H., and E. G. Ruby.** 1994. Effect of the squid host on the abundance and distribution of symbiotic *Vibrio fischeri* in nature. *Appl. Environ. Microbiol.* **60**:1565–1571.

35. **Lee, K.-H., and E. G. Ruby.** 1994. Competition between *Vibrio fischeri* strains during the initiation and maintenance of a light organ symbiosis. *J. Bacteriol.* **176**:1985–1991.

36. **Lee, K.-H., and E. G. Ruby..** 1995. Symbiotic role of the nonculturable, but viable, state of *Vibrio fischeri* in Hawaiian seawater. *Appl. Environ. Microbiol.* **61**:278–283.

37. **Levisohn, R., J. Moreland, and K. H. Nealson.** 1987. Isolation and characterization of a generalized transducing phage for the marine luminous bacterium *Vibrio fischeri* MJ-1. *J. Gen. Microbiol.* **133**:1577–1582.

38. **Lloyd, D., C. J. James, and J. W. Hastings.** 1985. Oxygen affinities of the bioluminescence systems of various species of luminous bacteria. *J. Gen. Microbiol.* **131**:2137–2140.

39. **Long, S. R.** 1989. *Rhizobium*-legume nodulation: life together in the underground. *Cell* **56**:203–214.

40. **Mack, M. C., and C. M. Dantonio.** 1998. Impacts of biological invasions on disturbance regimes. **13**:195–198.

41. **McFall-Ngai, M. J.** 1990. Crypsis in the pelagic environment. *Am. Zool.* **30**:175–188.

42. **McFall-Ngai, M. J.** 1994. Evolutionary morphology of a squid symbiosis. *Am. Zool.* **34**:554–561.

43. **McFall-Ngai, M. J.** The development of cooperative associations between animals and bacteria: Establishing détente among domains. *Am. Zool.*, in press.

44. **McFall-Ngai, M. J.** 1998. Morphological, biochemical, and molecular responses of *Euprymna scolopes* to interactions with its light organ symbiont, p. 273–276. *In* Y. LeGal and H. O. Halvorson (ed.), *New Developments in Marine Biotechnology*. Plenum Press, New York.

45. **McFall-Ngai, M. J., and M. Montgomery.** 1990. The anatomy and morphology of the adult bacterial light organ of *Euprymna scolopes* Berry (Cephalopoda:Sepiolidae). *Biol. Bull.* **179**:332–339.

46. **McFall-Ngai, M. J., and E. G. Ruby.** 1991. Symbiont recognition and subsequent morphogenesis as early events in an animal-bacterial symbiosis. *Science* **254:**1491–1494.

47. **McFall-Ngai, M. J., and E. G. Ruby.** 1998. Bobtail squid and their luminous bacteria: When first they meet. *BioScience* **48:**257–265.

48. **Meighen, E. A.** 1991. Molecular biology of bacterial bioluminescence. *Microbiol. Rev.* **55:** 123–142.

49. **Montgomery, M. K.** 1993. Development of the symbiotic light organ of *Euprymna scolopes* Berry (*Cephalopoda: Sepiolidae*). Ph.D. thesis. University of Southern California, Los Angeles.

50. **Montgomery, M. K., and M. J. McFall-Ngai.** Unpublished data.

51. **Montgomery, M. K., and M. J. McFall-Ngai.** 1992. The muscle-derived lens of a squid bioluminescent organ is biochemically convergent with the ocular lens. Evidence for recruitment of ALDH as a predominant structural protein. *J. Biol. Chem.* **267:**20999–21003.

52. **Montgomery, M. K., and M. J. McFall-Ngai.** 1993. Embryonic development of the light organ of the sepiolid squid *Euprymna scolopes. Biol. Bull.* **184:**296–308.

53. **Montgomery, M. K., and M. J. McFall-Ngai.** 1994. The effect of bacterial symbionts on early post-embryonic developmental of a squid light organ. *Development* **120:**1719–1729.

54. **Montgomery, M. K., and M. J. McFall-Ngai.** 1995. The inductive role of bacterial symbionts in the morphogenesis of a squid light organ. *Am. Zool.* **35:**372–380.

55. **Nardon, P., and A. M. Grenier.** 1991. Serial endosymbiosis theory and weevil evolution: The role of symbiosis, p. 153–169. *In* L. Margulis and R. Fester (ed.), *Symbiosis As a Source of Evolutionary Innovation.* MIT Press, Cambridge, Mass.

56. **Nealson, K. H., and J. W. Hastings.** 1991. The luminous bacteria, p. 625–639. *In* A. Balows, H. G. Truper, M. Dworkin, W. Harder, and K. H. Schleifer (ed.), *The Prokaryotes, a Handbook on the Biology of Bacteria: Ecophysiology, Isolation, Identification, Applications,* 2nd ed. Springer-Verlag, New York.

57. **Nishiguchi, M. K., E. G. Ruby, and M. J. McFall-Ngai.** Competitive hierarchy among strains of luminous bacteria provides additional evidence for parallel evolution in the sepiolid-*Vibrio* symbioses. *Appl. Environ. Microbiol.* **64:** 3209–3213.

58. **Nyholm, S. V., and M. J. McFall-Ngai.** 1997. The microenvironment surrounding the bacterial symbionts of the *Euprymna scolopes* light organ. *Am. Zool.* **36:**68A.

59. **Reich, K. A., T. Biegal, and G. K. Schoolnik.** 1997. The light organ symbiont *Vibrio fischeri* possesses two distinct secreted ADP-ribosyltransferases. *J. Bacteriol.* **179:**1591–1597.

60. **Reich, K. A., and G. K. Schoolnik.** 1994. The light organ symbiont *Vibrio fischeri* possesses a homolog of the *Vibrio cholerae* transmembrane transcriptional activator ToxR. *J. Bacteriol.* **176:** 3085–3088.

61. **Reich, K. A., and G. K. Schoolnik.** 1996. Halovibrin: A member of a new class of ADP-ribosyltransferases, secreted from the light organ symbiont *Vibrio fischeri. J. Bacteriol.* **178:**209–215.

62. **Ruby, E. G.** 1996. Lessons from a cooperative, bacterial-animal association: the *Vibrio fischeri-Euprymna scolopes* light organ symbiosis. *Annu. Rev. Microbiol.* **50:**591–624.

63. **Ruby, E. G., and L. M. Asato.** 1993. Growth and flagellation of *Vibrio fischeri* during initiation of the sepiolid squid light organ symbiosis. *Arch. Microbiol.* **159:**160–167.

64. **Ruby, E. G., and K.-H. Lee.** 1998. The *Vibrio fischeri-Euprymna scolopes* light organ association: Current ecological paradigms. *Appl. Environ. Microbiol.* **64:**805–812.

65. **Ruby, E. G., and M. J. McFall-Ngai.** 1992. A squid that glows in the night: Development of an animal-bacterial mutualism. *J. Bacteriol.* **174:** 4865–4870.

66. **Ruiz, G. M., J. T. Carlton, E. D. Grosholz, and A. H. Hines.** 1997. Global invasions of marine and estuarine habitats by non-indigenous species—mechanisms, extent and consequences. *Am. Zool.* **37:**621–632.

67. **Saffo, M. B.** 1992. Invertebrates in endosymbiotic associations. *Am. Zool.* **32:**557–565.

68. **Shroff, K. E., K. Meslin, and J. J. Cebra.** 1995. Commensal enteric bacteria engender a self-limiting humoral mucosal immune response while permanently colonizing the gut. *Infect. Immun.* **63:**3904–3913.

69. **Singley, C. T.** 1983. *Euprymna scolopes,* p. 69–74. *In* P. R. Boyle (ed.), *Cephalopod Life Cycles,* vol. 1. *Species Accounts.* Academic Press, Inc., London.

70. **Small, A. L., and M. McFall-Ngai.** 1993. Changes in the oxygen environment of a symbiotic squid light organ in response to infection by its luminous bacterial symbionts. *Am. Zool.* **33:**61A.

71. **Small, A. L., V. Weis, and M. J. McFall-Ngai.** Unpublished data.

72. **Smith, H. W., and W. E. Crabb.** 1961. The faecal bacterial flora of animals and man: Its development in the young. *J. Pathol. Bacteriol.* **82:** 53–66.

73. **Staley, J. T.** 1997. Biodiversity—are microbial species threatened? *Curr. Opin. Biotechnol.* **8:**340–345.

74. **Tomarev, S. I., R. D. Zinovieva, V. M. Weis, A. B. Chepelinsky, J. Piatigorsky, and M. J. McFall-Ngai.** 1993. Abundant mRNAs in the bacterial light organ of a squid encode a protein with high similarity to mammalian antimicrobial peroxidases: Implications for mutualistic symbioses. *Gene* **132:**219–226.

75. **van Rhijn, P., and J. Vanderleyden.** 1995. The *Rhizobium*-plant symbiosis. *Microbiol. Rev.* **59:**124–142.

76. **Visick, K. L., and E. G. Ruby.** Unpublished data.

77. **Visick, K. L., and E. G. Ruby.** 1996. Construction and symbiotic competence of a *luxA*-deletion mutant of *Vibrio fischeri*. *Gene* **175:**89–94.

78. **Visick, K. L., and E. G. Ruby.** 1997. New genetic tools for use in the marine bioluminescent bacterium *Vibrio fischeri*, p. 119–122. *In* J. W. Hastings, L. J. Kricka, and P. E. Stanley (ed.), *Bioluminescence and Chemiluminescence*. John Wiley & Sons, Inc., New York.

79. **Visick, K. L., and E. G. Ruby.** 1998. The periplasmic, group III catalase of *Vibrio fischeri* is required for normal symbiotic competence and is induced both by oxidative stress and by approach to stationary phase. *J. Bacteriol.* **180:**2087–2092.

80. **Visick, K. L., and E. G. Ruby.** 1998. Considering the emergent properties of quorum sensing: the consequences to bacteria of autoinducer signaling in their natural environment *In* G. M. Dunny and S. C. Winans (ed.), *Cell-Cell Signaling in Bacteria*. American Society for Microbiology, Washington, D.C, in press.

81. **Visick, K. L., and E. G. Ruby.** 1998. Tn*luxAB* insertion mutants of *Vibrio fischeri* with symbiosis-regulated phenotypes. Abstr. Annu. Meet. Am. Soc. Microbiol. 1998, p. 277.

82. **Visick, K. L., and E. G. Ruby.** 1998. Temporal control of *lux* gene expression in the symbiosis between *Vibrio fischeri* and its squid host, p. 277–279. *In* Y. LeGal and H. O. Halvorson (ed.), *New Developments in Marine Biotechnology*. Plenum Press, New York.

83. **Wei, S. L., and R. E. Young.** 1989. Development of symbiotic bacterial luminescence in a nearshore cephalopod, *Euprymna scolopes*. *Mar. Biol.* **103:**541–546.

84. **Weinberg, E. D.** 1993. The iron withholding defense. *ASM News* **59:**559–562.

85. **Weis, V. M., M. K. Montgomery, and M. J. McFall-Ngai.** 1993. Enhanced production of ALDH-like protein in the bacterial light organ of the sepiolid squid *Euprymna scolopes*. *Biol. Bull.* **184:**309–321.

86. **Weis, V. M., A. L. Small, and M. J. McFall-Ngai.** 1996. A peroxidase related to the mammalian antimicrobial protein myeloperoxidase in the *Euprymna-Vibrio* mutualism. *Proc. Natl. Acad. Sci. USA* **93:**13683–13688.

INITIAL INTERACTIONS OF
AGROBACTERIUM TUMEFACIENS
WITH PLANTS

Ann G. Matthysse

19

Agrobacteria are gram-negative bacteria found in the soil in association with plants. Some members of this group of bacteria can infect wound sites and cause formation of crown gall tumors (*Agrobacterium tumefaciens*) or hairy roots (*Agrobacterium rhizogenes*). Others *(Agrobacterium vitis)* can cause a prolonged asymptomatic infection of the vascular tissue of grapes. In addition, *A. vitis* can cause formation of tumors at wound sites in infected but otherwise apparently normal grapevines (6). Many of the agrobacteria isolated from the soil are avirulent (*A. radiobacter*) (4, 32). The virulent members of the agrobacteria possess a large plasmid (the Ti or Ri plasmid), which carries a region of DNA bounded by direct repeats and including genes preceded by eukaryotic promoters (the T-DNA). The T-DNA is transferred from the bacteria to the plant host by a mechanism related to the conjugal transfer of certain bacterial plasmids (11, 14, 17, 28). This transferred DNA is integrated into host cell chromosomes where it is stably inherited by daughter cells. It is the expression of the genes carried by T-DNA that

results in formation of tumors or hairy roots (3, 9).

GENES INVOLVED IN INITIAL STEPS IN PATHOGENESIS

Genes Required for Cellulose Synthesis

The mechanism of pathogenesis just described requires intimate contact between the bacteria and the host plant. To study these initial interactions in a situation that is more amenable to biochemical studies and the use of microscopy than infections of wound sites in whole plants, the interaction of *A. tumefaciens* with tissue culture cells was examined. The bacteria were found to be capable of binding to tissue culture cells and of transferring T-DNA to them. The initial binding did not follow the simple second-order kinetics expected for a two-particle interaction and suggested that more than one process was involved. Examination of the bacterial binding to host cells in the scanning electron microscope (SEM) revealed both single bacteria and large aggregates of bacteria attached to the surface of the plant cells (Fig. 1) (21). The large aggregates appeared to be held together by fibrillar material. When the binding of live bacteria to dead plant cells was examined, the fibrillar material

Ann G. Matthysse, Department of Biology, University of North Carolina, Chapel Hill, North Carolina 27599-3280.

Microbial Ecology and Infectious Disease, Edited by Eugene Rosenberg
©1999 American Society for Microbiology, Washington, D.C.

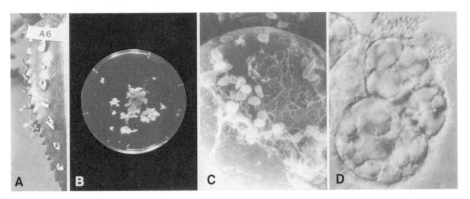

FIGURE 1 Interactions of wild-type *A. tumefaciens* with plants. (A) Tumors formed after 6 weeks on *B. daigremontiana* leaves by inoculating 10^9 bacteria at toothpick wounds. (B) Aggregation of carrot suspension-culture cells by wild-type strain A6 after 24-h incubation. (C and D) Attachment of strain A6 to carrot suspension-culture cells as seen in the SEM (C) and the light microscope using Nomarski optics and living cells (D). Note that both individually attached bacteria and bacterial aggregates are visible. In panel C, cellulose fibrils holding the aggregates together can also be seen. In panels B, C, and D, 10^8 bacteria per ml were inoculated with 10^5 carrot cells per ml in MS medium.

was still present, suggesting that it was made by the bacteria and not by the host. Bacteria incubated in Luria broth with plant extracts produced fibrils visible in the SEM. These fibrils were purified and analyzed chemically. They turn out to be made of cellulose synthesized by the bacteria (21). This would appear to be an effective strategy for a plant pathogen. Cellulose binds very tightly to cellulose, so that the bacteria would be expected to adhere strongly to the host cell surface. In addition, since the host cell is covered with a cellulosic cell wall, the bacteria fibrils can not be removed enzymatically by the host without digestion of its own cell wall.

To examine the role of cellulose in the interaction of the bacteria with the plant, cellulose-minus bacterial mutants were obtained (18). These mutants were isolated by screening transposon mutants for the lack of cellulose synthesis, using the dye cellufluor (a commercial brightener), which stains β-linked polysaccharides to yield a blue-white fluorescence under UV light. Colonies that showed reduced staining with cellufluor were isolated and tested for lack of cellulose production. The genes required for cellulose synthesis

were cloned, using the transposon insertions to select clones of chromosomal DNA containing cellulose synthesis genes. All of the genes identified as required for cellulose synthesis (*cel* genes) mapped to a 10-kb region in one clone from a library of *A. tumefaciens* DNA. This region of DNA was sequenced, and five potential open reading frames (ORFs) were identified. These genes and mutations in them are being used to study the biochemistry of cellulose synthesis in *A. tumefaciens* (22, 24).

When the interaction of cellulose-minus mutants with plants was examined, *cel* mutants were found to retain virulence, although most of them were attenuated to varying extents (18, 27). The cellulose-minus mutants also retained the ability to bind to tissue culture cells. However, no bacterial aggregates were formed, and unlike the wild-type strains, the mutants were unable to cause clumping of the tissue culture cells (Fig. 2). The kinetics of binding of a cellulose-minus mutant to carrot suspension culture cells were simple second order and saturable. The binding of cellulose-minus mutants to tissue culture cells was much weaker than that of the parent strain. The mutant bacteria could be removed from the plant

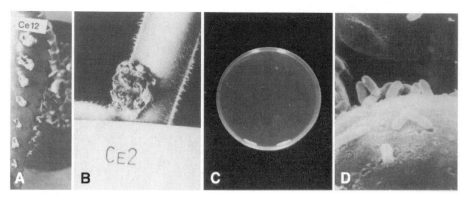

FIGURE 2 Interactions of cellulose-minus mutant bacteria with plants. (A) Tumors formed on *B. daigremontiana* 6 weeks after inoculating a cellulose-minus mutant. (B) Tumor formed on the stem of a tobacco plant at a wound site 6 weeks after inoculation of 10^9 cellulose-minus mutant bacteria. (C) Mutant bacteria incubated with carrot suspension-culture cells. Note the failure of the cellulose-minus bacteria to aggregate carrot suspension-culture cells (compare with Fig. 1B). (D) Attachment of a cellulose-minus mutant to carrot suspension culture cells as seen in the SEM. Note the absence of bacterial aggregates and cellulose fibrils. In panels C and D, 10^8 bacteria per ml were inoculated with 10^5 carrot cells per ml in MS medium, and the mixture was incubated for 24 h.

cells by vortex mixing of the culture; this procedure had no effect on the attachment of the parent cellulose-plus bacteria.

Virulence assays performed in the laboratory are generally carried out under very artificial conditions: the plants are grown in pots in a sheltered environment, the bacteria are introduced into a wound in the leaves or stem, the wound sites are carefully protected, and the plants are watered from the bottom. When infected wound sites on *Bryophyllum daigremontiana* leaves were washed very gently with 10 ml of water 1 h after infection, there was no effect on tumor formation by wild-type bacteria. However, tumor formation by a cellulose-minus mutant was eliminated by this treatment (18). Viable cell counts of bacteria remaining at the wound site suggested that in the absence of cellulose synthesis, the bacteria were washed off the leaf by even this gentle treatment (33). In the real world, rain would easily remove cellulose-minus bacteria from wound sites.

Genes Required for Initial Attachment (*att* Genes)

Although the production of cellulose clearly helps the bacteria adhere to the host, bacterial binding to tissue culture cells still occurs with cellulose-minus mutants. This binding is very loose, but it is important in pathogenesis. Bacterial mutants that could not carry out this initial loose binding were isolated by screening individual transposon mutants for the failure to bind to tissue culture cells (19). All of the nonattaching (*att*) mutants identified were avirulent. The mutants obtained all mapped to one region of the chromosome. When a library clone containing this region of the chromosome was identified, transposon insertions made in it, and those insertions introduced back into the chromosome of the wild-type bacteria, it was found that a region of the chromosome larger than 30-kb contained genes required for the initial binding of the bacteria to plant cells. Mutations anywhere in this region (called the *att* region) rendered the bacteria avirulent as well as nonattaching (Fig. 3). Although we have sequenced more than 30-kb of this chromosomal region, the functions of most of the genes contained in it remain obscure. However, two functions have been associated with some of these *att* genes.

The left end of this region contains a group of six genes all oriented in the same direction.

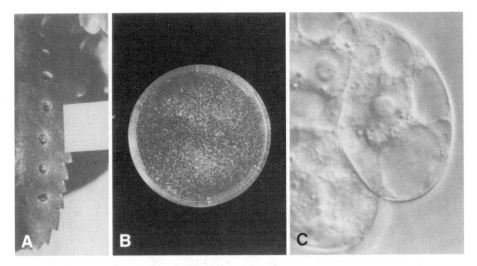

FIGURE 3 Interaction of attachment-minus mutant bacteria with plants. (A) A leaf of *B. daigremontiana* inoculated with an attachment-minus mutant. Note the lack of tumors. (B and C) Carrot suspension culture cells incubated with an attachment-minus mutant. In panel B, note the failure of the bacteria to agglutinate the carrot cells. In panel C, note the failure of the bacteria to attach to carrot cells as seen in the light microscope using Nomarski optics and living cells. In panels B and C, 10^8 bacteria per ml were inoculated with 10^5 carrot cells per ml in MS medium, and the mixture was incubated for 24 h.

These genes probably make up an operon. Four of them have homology to genes of ABC transporters from a variety of other bacteria including *Escherichia coli* (25). ABC transporters are plasma membrane proteins that transport compounds into or out of cells, using ATP hydrolysis for energy. They are widely distributed and have been found in bacteria, fungi, animals, and plants (1, 13). The most famous ABC transporter is probably the cystic fibrosis gene. AttA1 and AttE show homology with the ATP-binding proteins, while AttA2 and AttB are homologous to the membrane-spanning proteins of these transporter systems. AttD is a small protein whose role may be regulatory. AttC has no homologs in the databases at this time. In ABC transporters whose role is the uptake of compounds into gram-negative bacteria, there is often a periplasmic space binding protein that binds the compound to be transported and aids in its uptake. The gene for the binding protein generally is found in the same operon with the rest of the uptake system. AttC may be such

a periplasmic binding protein or it may have some other unexpected role.

Why should an ABC transporter be required for the binding of a bacterium to the surface of a host plant cell? One possibility is that it is involved in signaling between the bacteria and the plant. If signaling occurs between the bacteria and the plant host, one would expect the molecules involved to accumulate in medium in which bacteria and plants were incubated together. To test this hypothesis, conditioned medium was prepared by incubating carrot suspension-culture cells with wild-type bacteria for several hours (20). The bacteria and plant cells were then removed by filter sterilization. Roots of the plant *Arabidopsis thaliana* were placed in the resulting conditioned medium along with a nonattaching mutant (*attD*) of *A. tumefaciens*. Conditioned medium was able to compensate for the defect in the mutant bacteria and allowed them to bind to the roots. Application of conditioned medium to carrot root discs prior to the inoculation of an *attD* mutant also restored the ability of the bacteria to cause tumor formation on the carrot disc. At the present time, the identity of the active substance in conditioned medium is unknown. It is a low-molecular-weight molecule that is relatively hydrophobic.

The other *att* gene whose function has been elucidated is *attR*. This gene encodes a protein that has a high degree of homology to acetyltransferases (30). The defect in AttR mutants is unaffected by the presence of conditioned medium. Indeed AttR mutants are capable of participating in the formation of effective conditioned medium when they are incubated with carrot suspension cells. Thus AttR mutants appear to be blocked at a later step in attachment than signaling. The homology of *attR* to acetyltransferases suggested that the product of this gene might be involved in the synthesis of a surface molecule required for bacterial binding to host cells. When the surface polysaccharides of wild-type bacteria were analyzed and compared with those of an AttR mutant, it was found that the wild-type bacteria had an acetylated capsular polysaccharide (probably a K antigen) that was lacking in the AttR mutant. Purified preparations of this polysaccharide added to carrot suspension culture-cells or *A. thaliana* roots prior to the inoculation of wild-type bacteria blocked bacterial attachment to the plant cell surface. Thus it appears that the *attR* gene product is required for synthesis of surface polysaccharides that participate in bacterial attachment to host cells. Presumably other bacterial genes are also required for the synthesis of this acetylated polysaccharide, but the identity of these genes is presently unknown. The roles of the other *att* genes in the initial interaction of the bacteria with the plant remain to be determined.

Other Genes Affecting Initial Attachment

Two other operons that are found outside the *att* region have been identified which are required for the binding of *A. tumefaciens* to plant cells. These are *chvAB* and *pscA* (also known as *exoC*) (8, 10, 34). The *chvAB* operon encodes the proteins required for the synthesis and export of β-1,2-D-glucans into the periplasmic space. These are cyclic polysaccharides containing about 17 glucose molecules. They appear to function in osmotic regulation by the bacteria and are made when the bacteria are placed in low osmotic strength media (26). Mutations in these genes have pleiotropic effects; the bacteria show reduced motility and overproduction of acidic polysaccharides (succinoglycan) as well as failure to attach to plant cells (29). It may be that all of these defects are due to alterations in the surface of the bacteria caused by problems with osmotic regulation. Several laboratories have examined the effect of exogenously added β-1,2-glucans on the binding of the bacteria to plant cells and have found the polysaccharide to be without effect. The other gene known to be required for bacterial binding to host cells is *pscA*. Mutants in this gene are unable to make glucose 1-phosphate. Mutations in *pscA* affect the synthesis of virtually all of the surface polysaccharides of the bacteria.

Both the signaling between the plant and the bacteria that was lacking in AttA1-H mutants and the binding of the bacteria to the plant cell surface involving an acetylated polysaccharide lacking in AttR mutants were required for bacterial virulence. In addition, bacterial cellulose synthesis appeared to increase bacterial virulence in the laboratory. Indeed our washing experiments suggested that bacterial cellulose synthesis is likely to play a larger role in field situations than in the laboratory. To examine whether *cel* and *att* genes might have a role in the bacterial interaction with the plant even in the absence of pathogenesis, we studied the effect of these genes on root colonization by *A. tumefaciens*.

ROOT COLONIZATION BY AGROBACTERIA

Agrobacteria are found distributed in soil worldwide. They are found in both cultivated and noncultivated soils and, to a lesser extent, in fallow soil (4, 5, 32). In all of these soils, most of the agrobacteria present appear to be nonpathogenic (*A. radiobacter*). In soil cultivated with plants susceptible to particular types of agrobacteria, the number of these bacteria is greater than in other soils. Thus vineyards have greater populations of *A. vitis* and orchard soils contain *A. tumefaciens*. One study found that when a virulent strain of *A. tumefaciens* was inoculated into a susceptible host, the percentage of bacteria that were virulent decreased with increasing time following inoculation (2). Thus, it appears that most agrobacteria may grow in the soil in nonpathogenic associations with plants and that it is rare for the bacteria to be pathogenic.

Role of *cel* and *att* genes in root colonization

To examine the role of *att* and *cel* genes in colonization of roots, we germinated seeds aseptically and inoculated the bacteria onto the plants by dipping roots when they were 1 to 2 cm long into a bacterial suspension. The plants were then sowed in microwaved (pasteurized) soil and harvested after varying lengths of time, and the numbers of viable bacteria found in the soil and on the roots were determined (23).

Tomato roots were readily colonized by wild-type *A. tumefaciens*. The initial population size was about 10^3 bacteria per cm of root length. After 8 days, the number of agrobacteria had increased to about 10^8 bacteria per cm of root length. During this time, the roots had grown from 1–2 cm to 8–10 cm long. When tomato roots incubated in liquid for 8 days were examined in the light microscope, bacteria were observed bound to the root hairs and epidermis throughout the length of the root. In some spots, bacterial colonies were seen on the epidermis and surrounding root hairs. When cellulose-minus mutants were inoculated onto tomato roots in a similar manner, the initial number of bacteria found on the roots was also about 10^3, but the bacteria did not grow well on the roots, and after 10 days, there were only 10^5 bacteria per cm of

root length. Similar results were obtained with *A. thaliana* roots (Fig. 4).

Since water washing of wound sites on *B. daigremontiana* leaves had suggested that bacterial cellulose synthesis was involved in tight binding of the bacteria to the host, we wondered if cellulose played a role in general bacterial binding to roots or was involved only in tight binding. Wild-type and cellulose-minus mutant bacteria were examined for the tightness of their binding to the root surface by comparing the number of bacteria released from the root by shaking the root by hand in buffer and by sonicating the root in buffer in a glassware-cleaning sonicator. The number of bacteria remaining on the root after sonication was determined by placing the root on medium in a petri dish and covering it with soft agar. The number of bacterial colonies formed on the root was determined using a dissecting microscope to count colonies before they grew large enough to coalesce. For both wild-type and cellulose-minus mutants the vast majority of the bacteria could be released from the root by shaking (about 50%) or sonication (about 50%) and less than 0.1% of the bacteria were very tightly bound to the root surface. No difference in tightness of binding was seen between the parent and cellulose-minus mutant strains, suggesting that cellulose synthesis may also play a role in loose binding and/or adherent colony formation. Thus, even in the absence of a wound and a pathogenic interaction, agrobacterial cellulose synthesis was induced by the plant, and this bacterial cellulose aided in root colonization (23).

Root colonization by ChvAB mutants was examined by Hawes and Peuppke (12), who found that these mutations reduced the ability of the bacteria to colonize roots. However, the effects of *chvAB* mutations are so pleiotropic that it is difficult to interpret these results.

Root colonization by AttB and AttD mutants, which lack the ABC transporter system, and by AttR mutants, which lack the acetylated polysaccharide (K antigen), was also examined (23). Both types of *att* mutants were found to be reduced in root colonization. The

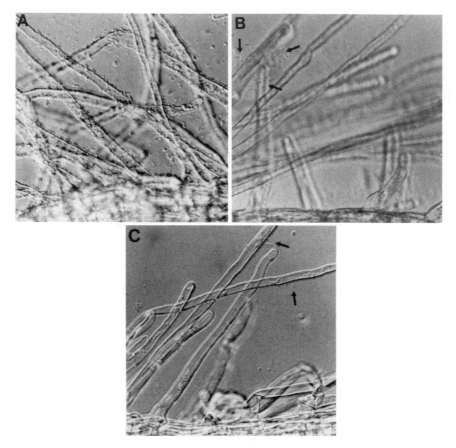

FIGURE 4 Root colonization of *A. thaliana* roots as seen in the light microscope using live roots and Nomarski optics. The roots were incubated with 10^8 bacteria per ml for 24 h in water. (A) Wild-type bacteria. Note the numerous bacteria on the root hairs. (B) A cellulose-minus mutant. Note that very few attached bacteria can be seen (arrows). (C) An attachment-minus mutant. Bacteria around the root hairs are very rare (arrows).

amount of this reduction was similar to that seen with the cellulose-minus mutants. Since AttB and AttD mutants are blocked in signal exchange with the plant, this result suggests that the same type of signaling required for tumor formation by bacteria inoculated directly into a wound site is also required for bacterial colonization of intact roots. The reduction in root colonization by AttR mutants suggests that a similar type of binding mechanism involving an acetylated capsular polysaccharide may be used by the bacteria to bind to intact epidermis, root hairs, and cells exposed in wound sites.

UNANSWERED QUESTIONS CONCERNING THE ECOLOGY OF AGROBACTERIA

Many unsolved questions are raised by our limited knowledge of the ecology of these bacteria. These include the relationship between the avirulent *A. radiobacter* strains that predominate in soils and virulent *A. tumefaciens*, *A. rhizogenes*, and *A. vitis* (15). These three pathogenic species of agrobacteria appear to have different although related chromosomes. Their virulence plasmids (pTi or pRi) also appear to be related but distinct. The chromosomal differences would seem likely to influence the habitats in which each of these organisms could grow well. For example, sensitivity to ionic strength would certainly limit growth of *A. rhizogenes* in some environments. The ability of *A. vitis* to use tartaric acid would appear to aid the growth of this bacterium in grapes that contain this acid (31). In the laboratory, virulent agrobacteria can lose their virulence plasmids to give rise to avirulent strains that would be classified as *A. radiobacter* if they were field isolates. In one study, loss of pTi from a virulent strain of *A. tumefaciens* growing in tumors was observed (2). *A. radiobacter* can also acquire virulence plasmids from virulent strains and become pathogenic. This second process is known to occur in crown gall tumors and was the basis for the original procedure for crossing pTi from one strain to another (16). The frequency of these two processes in the field is unknown, and their contribution to the ecology of agrobacteria remains controversial.

The selective advantage of *A. radiobacter* that causes it to be the predominant agrobacterium in soils is unknown. It is unclear what advantage the virulent agrobacteria gain from the pathogenic process. The opines formed by tumor cells can serve as a sole carbon and nitrogen source for the plasmid-containing bacteria in the laboratory. While it is commonly stated that the production of opines by the plant is the advantage gained by the bacteria from pathogenesis, when various investigators have examined the bacteria found in tumors in nature, the predominant opine utilizers have generally been pseudomonads, not agrobacteria (7). In addition, the advantage to *A. vitis* of tumor formation is very difficult to understand, since these bacteria live in the vascular system of grapes and can utilize the tartrate found there. Nevertheless, when a plant infected with *A. vitis* is wounded, a tumor is generally formed at the wound site.

The fact that *A. tumefaciens* is a very good root colonizer and that some of the same genes and systems required for tumor formation when the bacteria are introduced directly into a wound also play a major role in root colonization suggests that these bacteria may be primarily adapted to grow in association with plants and that the ability to cause disease may have been added onto this fundamental association. Pathogenesis may occur only under particular conditions, while in the absence of these conditions, colonization is the normal state of the interaction between the bacterium and the plant.

REVIEWS AND KEY PAPERS

Binns, A. N., and M. F. Thomashow. 1988. Cell biology of *Agrobacterium* infection and transformation of plants. *Annu. Rev. Microbiol.* **42**:575–606.

Matthysse, A. G. 1995. Observation and measurement of bacterial adhesion to plants. *Methods Enzymol.* **253**:189–206.

Matthysse, A. G. 1996. Adhesion in the rhizosphere, 129–153. *In* M. Fletcher and D. Savage (eds.), *Molecular and Ecological Diversity of Bacterial Adhesion.* John Wiley & Sons, Inc., New York.

Zupan, J. R., and P. Zambryski. 1995. Transfer of T-DNA from *Agrobacterium* to the plant cell. *Plant Physiol.* **107**:1041–1047.

REFERENCES

1. **Ames, G. FL., C. S. Mimura, and V. Shyamala.** 1990. Bacterial periplasmic permeases belong to a family of transport proteins operating from *Escherichia coli* to human: traffic ATPases. FEMS Microbiol. Rev. **75**:429–446.

2. **Belanger, C., M. L. Canfield, L. W. Moore, and P. Dion.** 1995. Genetic analysis of nonpathogenic *Agrobacterium tumefaciens* mutants arising in crown gall tumors. *J. Bacteriol.* **177**:3752–3757.

3. **Binns, A. N., and M. F. Thomashow.** 1988. Cell biology of *Agrobacterium* infection and transformation of plants. *Ann. Rev. Microbiol.* **42**:575–606.

4. **Bouzar, H., and L. W. Moore.** 1987. Isolation of different *Agrobacterium* biovars from a natural oak savanna and tallgrass prairie. *Appl. Environ. Microbiol.* **53**:717–721.

5. **Burr, T. J., B. H. Katz, and A. L. Bishop.** 1987. Populations of Agrobacterium in vineyard and nonvineyard soils and grape roots in vineyards and nurseries. *Plant Dis.* **71:**617–620.

6. **Burr, T. J., C. L. Reid, M. Yoshimura, E. A. Momol, and C. Bazzi.** 1995. Survival and tumorigenicity of *Agrobacterium vitis* in living and decaying grape roots and canes in soil. *Plant Dis.* **79:**677–682.

7. **Canfield, M. L., and L. W. Moore.** 1991. Isolation and characterization of opine-utilizing strains of *Agrobacterium tumefaciens* and fluorescent strains of *Pseudomonas* spp. from rootstocks of *Malus. Phytopathology* **81:**440–443.

8. **Cangelosi, G. A., L. Hung, V. Puvanesarajah, G. Stacey, D. A. Ozaga, J. A. Leigh, and E. W. Nester.** 1987. Common loci for *Agrobacterium tumefaciens* and *Rhizobium meliloti* exopolysaccharide synthesis and their roles in plant interaction. *J. Bacteriol.* **159:**2086–2091.

9. **Chilton, M. D., M. H. Drummond, D. J. Merlo, D. Sciaky, A. L. Montoya, M. P. Gordon, and E. W. Nester.** 1977. Stable incorporation of plasmid DNA into higher plant cells: The molecular basis of crown gall tumorigenesis. *Cell* **11:**263–271.

10. **Douglas, C. J., W. Halperin, and E. W. Nester.** 1982. *Agrobacterium tumefaciens* mutants affected in attachment to plants. *J. Bacteriol.* **152:**1265–1275.

11. **Fullner, K. J., J. C. Lara, and E. W. Nester.** 1996. Pilus assembly by Agrobacterium T-DNA transfer genes. *Science* **273:**1107–1109.

12. **Hawes, M. C., and S. G. Pueppke.** 1989. Reduced rhizosphere colonization ability of *Agrobacterium tumefaciens* chromosomal virulence (*chv*) mutants. *Plant Soil* **113:**129–132.

13. **Higgins, C. F., S. C. Hyde, M. M. Mimmack, U. Gileadi, D. R. Gill, and M. P. Gallagher.** 1990. Binding protein-dependent transport systems. *J. Bioenerg. Biomembr.* **22:**571–592.

14. **Kado, C. I.** 1994. Promiscous DNA transfer system of *Agrobacterium tumefaciens*: Role of the *virB* operon in sex pilus. *Mol. Microbiol.* **12:**17–22.

15. **Kerr, A.** 1987. The genetic basis for virulence, pathogenicity, and host range in *Agrobacterium tumefaciens*, p. 377–387. *In* Anonymous, (ed.), *Current Plant Science and Biotechnology in Agriculture.* Martinus Nijhoff Publishers, Dordrecht, The Netherlands.

16. **Kerr, A., P. Manigault, and J. Tempé.** 1977. Transfer of virulence *in vivo* and *in vitro* in *Agrobacterium. Nature* **265:**569–571.

17. **Lessi, M., and E. Lanka.** 1994. Common mechanisms in bacterial conjugation and Ti-mediated T-DNA transfer to plant cells. *Cell* **77:**321–324.

18. **Matthysse, A. G.** 1983. Role of bacterial cellulose fibrils in *Agrobacterium tumefaciens* infection. *J. Bacteriol.* **154:**906–915.

19. **Matthysse, A. G.** 1987. Characterization of nonattaching mutants of *Agrobacterium tumefaciens. J. Bacteriol.* **169:**313–323.

20. **Matthysse, A. G.** 1994. Conditioned medium promotes the attachment of *Agrobacterium tumefaciens* strain NT1 to carrot cells. *Protoplasma* **183:**131–136.

21. **Matthysse, A. G., K. V. Holmes, and R. H. G. Gurlitz.** 1981. Elaboration of cellulose fibrils by *Agrobacterium tumefaciens* during attachment to carrot cells. *J. Bacteriol.* **145:**583–595.

22. **Matthysse, A. G., R. Lightfoot, and S. White.** 1995. Genes required for cellulose synthesis in *Agrobacterium tumefaciens. J. Bacteriol.* **177:**1069–1075.

23. **Matthysse, A. G., and S. McMahan.** 1998. Root colonization by *Agrobacterium tumefaciens* is reduced in *cel*, *attB*, *attD*, and *attR* mutants. *Appl. Environ. Microbiol.* **64:**2341–2345.

24. **Matthysse, A. G., D. Thomas, and A. R. White.** 1995. Mechanism of cellulose synthesis in *Agrobacterium tumefaciens. J. Bacteriol.* **177:**1076–1081.

25. **Matthysse, A. G., H. A. Yarnall, and N. Young.** 1996. Requirement for genes with homology to ABC transport systems for attachment and virulence of *Agrobacterium tumefaciens. J. Bacteriol.* **178:**5302–5308.

26. **Miller, K. J., E. P. Kennedy, and V. N. Reinhold.** 1986. Osmotic adaptation by gram-negative bacteria: possible role for periplasmic oligosaccharides. *Science* **231:**48–51.

27. **Minnemeyer, S. L., R. Lightfoot, and A. G. Matthysse.** 1991. A semi-quantitative bioassay for relative virulence of *Agrobacterium tumefaciens* strains on *Bryophyllum daigremontiana. J. Bacteriol.* **173:**7723–7724.

28. **Pohlman, R. F., H. D. Genetti, and S. C. Winans.** 1994. Common ancestry between IncN conjugal transfer genes and macromolecular export systems of plant and animal pathogens. *Mol. Microbiol.* **14:**655–668.

29. **Puvanesarajah, V., F. M. Schell, G. Stacey, C. J. Douglas, and E. W. Nester.** 1985. Role for 2-linked-β-D-glucan in the virulence of *Agrobacterium tumefaciens. J. Bacteriol.* **164:**102–106.

30. **Reuhs, B. L., J. S. Kim, and A. G. Matthysse.** 1997. The attachment of *Agrobacterium tumefaciens* to carrot cells and *Arabidopsis* wound sites is correlated with the production of a cell-associated, acidic polysaccharide. *J. Bacteriol.* **179:**5372–5379.

31. **Salomone, J., P. Crouzet, P. De Ruffray, and L. Otten.** 1996. Characterization and distribution of tartrate utilization genes in the grapevine pathogen *Agrobacterium vitis*. *Mol. Plant Microbe Interact.* **9:**401–408.

32. **Schroth, M. N., A. R. Weinhold, A. H. McCain, D. C. Hildebrand, and N. Ross.** 1971. Biology and control of *Agrobacterium tumefaciens*. *Hilgardia* **40:**537–552.

33. **Sykes, L., and A. G. Matthysse.** 1986. Time required for tumor induction by *Agrobacterium tumefaciens*. *Appl. Environ. Microbiol.* **52:**597–598.

34. **Thomashow, M. F., J. E. Karlinsky, J. R. Marks, and R. E. Hurlburt.** 1987. Identification of a new virulence locus in *Agrobacterium tumefaciens* that affects polysaccharide composition and plant cell attachment. *J. Bacteriol.* **169:**3209–3216.

EFFECT OF TEMPERATURE ON BACTERIAL BLEACHING OF CORALS

E. Rosenberg, Y. Ben-Haim, A. Toren, E. Banin,
A. Kushmaro, M. Fine, and Y. Loya

20

Coral reefs are a joy to behold and a highly productive, essential part of marine ecosystems. During the past 15 years, coral bleaching events of unprecedented frequency and global extent have been reported (17–19, 21). Coral bleaching has been defined as the disruption of symbioses between coral animals and their photosynthetic microalgal endosymbionts, the zooxanthellae (23). As a result of the loss of the algae and/or their pigments, the corals turn white. An example of the coral bleaching process is shown in Fig. 1. The sudden loss of zooxanthellae greatly affects the coral host because these photosynthetic symbionts supply up to 63% of the coral's nutrients (16). The energy source derived from the algae facilitates calcification. The causes and consequences of coral bleaching have recently been reviewed (2).

Coral bleaching is generally considered to be a phenomenon caused by environmental stress, such as increased (3, 15, 22, 30, 43) or decreased seawater temperatures (6, 12, 26); increased solar radiation, including UV radiation (11, 13, 37); pollution (31); reduced salinity (9); and combinations of these stresses (4, 30). The evidence supporting stress as the cause of coral bleaching is based on both field studies and laboratory experiments. The field studies involve correlations between environmental parameters and frequency of bleaching. The most common factor believed to be responsible for extensive coral bleaching is elevated sea temperature. This is particularly important because of the possible link between coral bleaching and global warming (1, 15, 16). Hoegh-Guldberg and Salvat (21) reported high frequencies of coral bleaching in sea areas off Phuket, Thailand, and Tahiti, when the surface seawater temperature reached a threshold of 29.2°C. Analysis of satellite-derived sea temperature data has shown that elevated sea temperatures coincide with both onset and duration of major bleaching events in the Carribean Sea and Pacific and Indian Oceans (14).

How does increased seawater temperature cause coral bleaching? In principle, there are three possible targets: the coral animal, the endosymbiotic algae, and potential coral pathogenic microorganisms. There are several reasons to assume that the coral animal is not the prime target. If increased temperature af-

E. Rosenberg, Y. Ben-Haim, A. Toren, and E. Banin, Department of Molecular Microbiology and Biotechnology, Tel Aviv University, Ramat Aviv, 69978, Israel. *A. Kushmaro, M. Fine, and Y. Loya*, Department of Zoology, Tel Aviv University, Ramat Aviv 69978, Israel.

Microbial Ecology and Infectious Disease, Edited by Eugene Rosenberg
©1999 American Society for Microbiology, Washington, D.C.

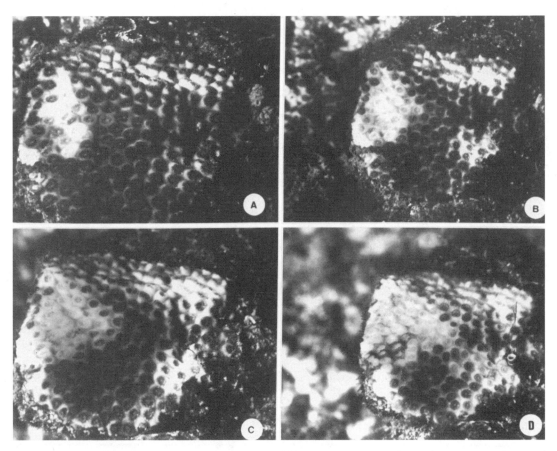

FIGURE 1 The coral O. *patagonica* in the process of bleaching. A–D, Bleaching of 9, 20, 40, and 60% of the surface area after 0, 1, 2, and 4 weeks, respectively.

fected the coral physiology directly, then one would expect that genetically identical coral species exposed to the same temperature stress would all bleach. However, several authors have reported on the patchy spatial distribution and spreading nature of coral bleaching (11, 25, 29, 32). It has been argued that the random mosaic patterns of bleaching observed in coral colonies is difficult to attribute solely to the effect of temperature stress on coral physiology, since neighboring regions of the colony must be exposed to the same extrinsic conditions (20). Furthermore, the correlation between coral bleaching and seawater temperature is not always evident. For example, Oliver (32) and Fisk and Done (11) showed that extensive bleaching in the Great Barrier

Reef during the summer of 1982 was not associated with any major sea surface temperature increase.

The possibility that the endosymbiotic algae are the target of environmental stress, resulting in coral bleaching, was implied in the adaptative bleaching hypothesis of Buddemeir and Fautin (5). They suggested that coral bleaching is a normal regulatory process by which genetic variation among the zooxanthellae is allowed. Accordingly, increased seawater temperature would lead to the loss of algae, allowing more-heat-resistant algae to form stable symbioses with the coral. Moreover, the model of Ware et al. (42) showed how the adaptive bleaching hypothesis could explain some features of bleaching events that are difficult to reconcile with mechanisms based on invariant temperature tolerances of the two symbiotic partners. Recently, it has been shown that corals can host multispecies communities of symbiotic algae (35). The composition of these communities followed a gradient of environmental parameters, and analyses of the symbionts before and after bleaching suggested that some corals were protected from bleaching by hosting an additional symbiont that was more tolerant to the stress condition. The fact that different algae may make corals more resistant to bleaching does not prove that the algae are the primary target of the stress condition. As discussed below, it is possible that pathogenic microorganisms are made more virulent by the stress condition and that different algae show different sensitivities to the pathogen.

The third possible target for an environmental stress condition leading to coral bleaching is potential pathogenic microorganisms. It is known that stress conditions, especially temperature, can cause certain bacteria to become pathogenic by "turning on" virulence genes (7, 33, 42). The surface of living corals is covered by a mucoid material. This surface mucopolysaccharide layer provides a matrix for bacterial colonization, allowing establishment of a "normal bacterial community" that may be characteristic for a particular coral species (8, 31, 34, 38). Thus, the coral animal lives in association with both endosymbiotic algae and a dense heterogenous population of surface bacteria. The role of these bacteria in coral biology is unknown. Based on analogies with other marine animals, the normal bacteria flora may produce antimicrobial compounds that help the coral avoid infection by pathogens (24). It is also possible that some of the bacteria are nitrogen fixers and might stimulate the growth of the corals in their nitrogen-limited marine environment. We suggest that altering the surface bacterial population by even small changes in the environmental conditions can lead to coral bleaching. In the model system that is discussed in this chapter, bleaching of the coral

Oculina patagonica in the Mediterranean Sea, the causative agent of the coral bleaching disease is the bacterium *Vibrio shiloi* (27, 28), and elevated seawater temperatures cause the bacterium to become virulent (40).

BLEACHING OF *OCULINA PATAGONICA* BY *VIBRIO SHILOI*

Bleaching of *Oculina patagonica* in the Mediterranean Sea

The coral *O. patagonica* was first observed in the Mediterranean Sea in 1966 and was assumed to be an immigrant species accidentally introduced from South America (45). Recent surveys show that *O. patagonica* is abundant in wide areas along the Israeli coast of the Mediterranean at a depth range of 1 to 50 m. Most of the bleaching colonies have been found in patchy formations at depths of 1 to 6 m. Bleaching of *O. patagonica* was first observed in 1993 (10) and since then has been continuously monitored. The number of bleached colonies and the extent of bleaching increases rapidly in the summer following rising sea temperatures. The most recent cycles of bleaching and recovery (Dec. 1995–Aug. 1998) are summarized in Fig. 2. In each of the years, Mediterranean seawater temperature off the coast of Israel increased from a minimum of $17 \pm 0.2°C$ in February to a maximum of $29 \pm 0.2°C$ in August. The percentage of colonies that showed bleaching increased from a minimum of less than 10% in February/March to a maximum of 80% in August/September. The frequency of bleaching began to increase in the spring when the water temperature reached 22 to 25°C, and the corals began to recover in the late fall when the temperature again dropped below 25°C. In addition to a higher frequency of colonies that showed bleaching at higher water temperatures, the extent of bleaching within individual colonies was much greater at higher seawater temperatures. For example, in September, more than 50% of the surface was bleached in 40% of the coral colonies, whereas in the winter, very few colonies (>3%) exhibited bleaching over 50%

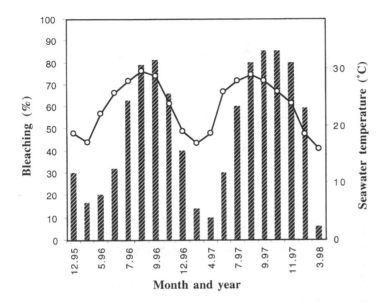

FIGURE 2 Bleaching of the coral *O. patagonica* in the Mediterranean Sea from Dec. 1995 to March 1998 as a function of seawater temperature (○).

of their surface. Thus, there is a high correlation ($r^2 = 0.87$) between seawater temperature and bleaching of *O. patagonica*.

V. shiloi Is the Causative Agent of Bleaching of *O. patagonica*

Koch's postulates were applied to demonstrate that a particular *Vibrio* strain, initially referred to as AK-1, was the causative agent of the coral bleaching disease of *O. patagonica* (27, 28). First, the microorganism was found to be present in all 28 diseased (bleached) corals examined and absent in all 24 healthy corals examined. Second, the bacterium was obtained in pure culture. The bacterium (Fig. 3) was identified as a new species of *Vibrio* by classical biochemical tests (28), fatty acid profile, and 16S rDNA (Fig. 4). The bacterium has been tentatively named *Vibrio shiloi*. Third, pure cultures of *V. shiloi* caused the bleaching disease in controlled aquaria experiments (Table 1). As few as 120 bacteria caused 83% of the corals to bleach in 20 days at 29°C. None of the corals that were not inoculated with bacteria showed any signs of bleaching. Fourth, addition of antibiotics to the aquaria completely blocked the *V. shiloi*-induced bleaching.

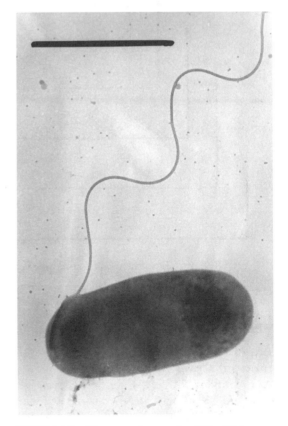

FIGURE 3 Electron micrograph of *V. shiloi*.

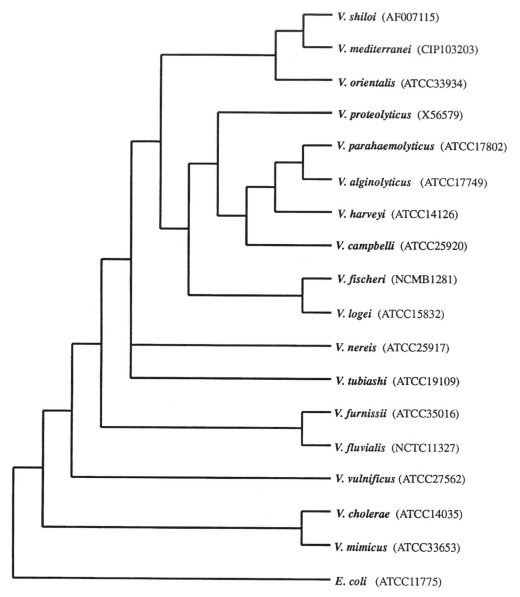

FIGURE 4 Classification of *V. shiloi* by 16S rDNA.

EFFECT OF TEMPERATURE ON BLEACHING AND ADHESION

Effect of Temperature on *V. shiloi*-Induced Coral Bleaching

As mentioned above, bleaching of *O. patagonica* in the Mediterranean Sea is correlated with increased seawater temperatures. To examine whether *V. shiloi* infection of *O. patagonica* is

also temperature regulated, a series of aquarium experiments were performed at different temperatures (Table 2). No bleaching occurred at 16°C. At 20°C, bleaching was slow and reached a maximum of 32% after 45 days. At 25 and 29°C, bleaching was rapid and extensive, reaching 80 and 100%, respectively, after 45 days. Controls with no added bacteria

TABLE 1 Bleaching of the coral *O. patagonica* by *V. shiloi*[a]

V. shiloi AK-1 (cells/coral)	Temp (°C)	Bleaching (%)	
		10 days	20 days
1.2×10^6	23	33	50
1.2×10^4	23	17	50
0	23	0	0
1.2×10^4	29	67	83
1.2×10^2	29	50	83
0	29	0	0

[a] For each temperature, 10 μl of a suspension of washed *V. shiloi* cells in sterile seawater was placed on each of six healthy coral pieces, and the corals were then returned to the aquarium. The 2-liter aerated aquaria containing filtered seawater (0.45 μm) were maintained at constant temperature and illuminated with a fluorescent lamp at 12 h light:12 h dark intervals.

showed no bleaching at all four temperatures tested. Thus, a similar pattern of temperature dependence on bleaching was observed in laboratory infection experiments and field observations.

Adhesion Experiments

In the case of adhesion of *V. shiloi* to *O. patagonica*, the process is both bacteria specific and host specific (40). Approximately 80% of the input *V. shiloi* cells adhered to *O. patagonica* in 6 h, whereas several other marine bacteria failed to adhere to the coral. Several lines of investigation indicated that adhesion of *V. shiloi* to *O. patagonica* involved a β-D-galactoside-containing receptor on the coral surface. First, 50 μM methyl-β-D-galactopyranoside completely inhibited adhesion, whereas several other sugars tested had no effect on the binding of *V. shiloi* to *O. patagonica* (40). Second, addition of methyl-β-D-galactopyranoside solutions to the coral, after the bacteria were allowed to adhere for 6 to 12 h, resulted in desorption of the bacteria from the coral surface. Addition of the inhibitor after 12 h did not release the bacteria, indicating that *V. shiloi* had become irreversibly associated with the coral. Electron micrographs of thin sections of the coral prepared 18 h after the bacteria were allowed to adhere to the coral showed that at least some of the bacteria had penetrated into exodermal cells. Third, *V. shiloi* adhered avidly to Sepharose–β-D-galactopyranoside beads (Table 3).

The observation that *V. shiloi* adhered to Sepharose–β-D-galactopyranoside beads suggested an efficient technique for isolating adhesion-minus mutants. A culture of *V. shiloi* was irradiated with UV for 120 s (99.9% killing) and then grown overnight in Marine

TABLE 2 Bleaching of the coral *O. patagonica* by *V. shiloi* as a function of temperature[a]

Temp (°C)	Bleaching (%) at time:				
	8 days	15 days	22 days	31 days	45 days
16	0	0	0	0	0
20	10	30	30	32	32
25	40	38	42	60	80
29	45	65	90	100	100

[a] The experiment was performed as described in Table 1, except the inoculum was kept constant (10^6 cells/ml.)

TABLE 3 Adhesion of *V. shiloi* to Sepharose beads[a]

Beads	Cells/ml at time:		Adhesion (%)
	Input	1 h	
Sepharose			
100 μl	5.1×10^7	4.7×10^7	7.8
10 μl	5.8×10^7	5.3×10^7	8.6
Sepharose-β-D-galactopyranoside			
5 μl	4.8×10^7	8.7×10^5	98.2
1 μl	5.7×10^7	9.1×10^5	98.4

[a] Sepharose 4B-200 and β-galactopyranoside–sepharose (aminobenzyl-1-thio-β-galacto-pyranoside insolubilized on 4% beaded agarose, spacer 12 atoms) beads were added to 1 ml of *V. shiloi* cells and incubated with gentle shaking for 1 h. The beads were then allowed to settle for 10 min, and the supernatant fluid was diluted and plated on Marine agar.

broth. One milliliter of this culture was then mixed with 100 μl of the β-D-galactopyranoside–Sepharose beads to enrich for mutants unable to bind. After a total of eight adhesion steps with four intervening overnight growth steps (during the last adhesion step, the supernatant remained turbid), the final supernatant was diluted and plated on Marine agar. Three colonies were grown separately and checked for adhesion to the beads (Fig. 5). All three strains, referred to as *V. shiloi* AT1, AT2 and AT3, were adhesion-minus mutants. Mutants AT1 and AT2 were then checked for adhesion to coral. Both mutants

were deficient in adhesion to *O. patagonica*. Mutants *V. shiloi* AT1 and AT2 failed to infect and bleach *O. patagonica* (Table 4), indicating that attachment of *V. shiloi* to a β-galactoside receptor on the coral is a prerequisite for infection.

Temperature-Regulated Adhesion: A Mechanism To Explain How Increased Seawater Temperature Causes Coral Bleaching

In principle, elevated seawater temperature could make corals more sensitive to infection or make the bacterium more virulent. Initially,

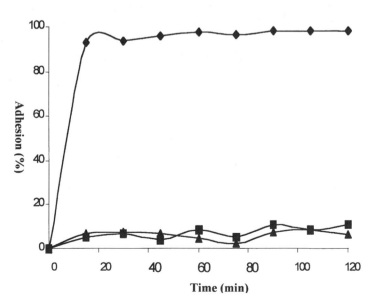

FIGURE 5 Adhesion of wild-type *V. shiloi* (◆) and mutants AT1 (■) and AT2 (▲) to Sepharose beads.

TABLE 4 Bleaching of the coral *O. pagatonica* by *V. shiloi* and nonadhering mutants[a]

Treatment	Bacterial conc (cells/ml)	Bleaching (%) at time:		
		10 days	18 days	24 days
No bacteria	0	0	0	0
V. shiloi	4.8×10^6	23	67	83
V. shiloi AT1	6.5×10^6	0	0	0
V. shiloi AT2	6.5×10^6	0	0	0

[a] For each experiment, 100 μl of an overnight culture of the bacterium was inoculated into four different aquaria and treated as described in Table 1. Percentage bleaching was determined by calculating the fraction of bleached polyps from the total number of coral polyps (ca. 200 per treatment).

it was considered that a possible reason for the failure of *V. shiloi* to infect corals and cause bleaching at temperatures below 20°C is that the bacterium does not grow well at low temperatures. This is not the case, because *V. shiloi* has a doubling time at 16°C in Marine broth of 1.9 h. Even in a more relevant medium prepared from coral mucus, the doubling time of *V. shiloi* was 2.1 h. Therefore, we turned our attention to adhesion as a possible target of the observed temperature effect on infection and bleaching.

As seen in Table 5, when the bacteria were grown at 16°C there was adhesion neither to corals maintained at 16 or 25°C nor to the β-galactoside-containing beads. However, bacteria grown at 25°C adhered to corals

maintained at 16 or 25°C, as well as to the beads. The temperature at which the adhesion experiments were conducted (16 or 25°C) was not a significant factor in the outcome. Thus, adhesion is temperature dependent, and the critical parameter appears to be the temperature of bacterial growth.

The data showing that adhesion is absolutely required for *V. shiloi* to bleach *O. patagonica* and that adhesion does not occur at 16°C provide an explanation for the failure of *V. shiloi* to cause bleaching at 16°C. Furthermore, it emphasizes that the stress condition, elevated seawater temperature, exerts its influence on a virulence factor of the bacterium, rather than on coral or endosymbiotic alga physiology. Regulation of virulence genes by

TABLE 5 Adhesion of *V. shiloi* to *O. patagonica* and Sepharose-β-D-galactopyranoside beads as a function of temperature[a]

Adhesion to:	Temp (°C) of:		Adhesion (%)
	Bacterial growth	Adhesion expt.	
Corals grown at 25°C	16	25	0
	16	16	0
	25	25	79
Corals grown at 16°C	16	16	7
	25	25	47
	25	16	53
β-D-galactopyranoside– Sepharose beads	16	25	7
	25	25	98

[a] The experiment with adhesion to coral was performed as described in Fig. 5 except for the specified temperatures. The experiment with adhesion to beads was performed as described in Table 3.

temperature and adhesion to their host is a well-established principle of medical microbiology. For example, it has recently been reported that cascades of virulence genes are induced following P-pili-mediated binding of *Escherichia coli* to its host cell receptor (44). It will now be interesting to examine whether other virulence factors (e.g., toxins) are expressed after *V. shiloi* adheres to *O. patagonica* (or coated beads) at elevated temperatures.

EFFECT OF EXTRACELLUAR PRODUCTS OF *V. shiloi* ON CORAL ALGAE

To begin to understand the mechanism by which *V. shiloi* infection causes bleaching, i.e., loss of the endosymbiotic algae, a study was carried out on the effect of the bacterium directly on the algae (Table 6). The algae were obtained by disruption of healthy coral and differential centrifugation. After incubation of the algae with the bacterium in sterile seawater for 22 h, 15% of the algae bleached (turned from yellow/brown to colorless), and another 16% lysed. Controls with the algae in seawater under the same conditions but without added bacteria showed no significant bleaching or lysis. Bleaching and lysis of the algae were also observed when the isolated algae were incubated with the extracellular cell-free supernatant fluid of a 24-h culture of *V. shiloi*.

Since the extracellular supernatant fluid of a *V. shiloi* culture contained a product that caused bleaching of the coral algae in 22 h, the effect of this fluid on algal photosynthesis was examined (Table 7). The extracellular cell-free supernatant fluid of *V. shiloi* inhibited the quantum yield of the algae by 72 and 90% in 10 and 60 min, respectively. Most of the product responsible for the inhibition activity had a molecular weight below 10,000 because the ultrafiltrate inhibited the quantum yield by 60 and 88% after 10 and 60 min, respectively. These data suggested that *V. shiloi* produces an extracellular toxin that directly inhibits algal photosynthesis. This toxin is probably the mechanism for the algal bleaching shown in Table 6 and possibly the mechanism of coral bleaching by *V. shiloi*.

Preliminary studies have indicated that inhibition of algal photosynthesis by *V. shiloi* results from a mixture of a nondialyzable material and ammonia. Ammonium is generated during growth on proteins or amino acids. Following a typical growth experiment on Marine broth, the *V. shiloi* cell-free supernatant contained 20 mM NH_4^+ and inhibited the quantum yield of the algae by 80% in 10 min. When 20 mM NH_4Cl was added to fresh Marine broth and incubated under the same conditions as above, inhibition was only 40%, indicating that *V. shiloi* produced an inhibitory product in addition to ammonia. Furthermore, when the *V. shiloi* supernatant fluid was dialyzed, it showed no inhibitory activity by itself, but when added to 20 mM NH_4^+, the initial 80% inhibition was restored. Thus, the bacteria produced an extracellular, nondialyzable material that greatly enhances the

TABLE 6 Bleaching and lysis of zooxanthellae by *V. shiloi*[a]

Addition to the algae	No. of experiments	Bleaching[b] (% ± SD)	Recovery[b] (% ± SD)	Bleaching and lysis (% ± SD)
Seawater	3	3.2 ± 2.1	103 ± 2.9	0.2 ± 1.7
V. shiloi cells[c]	5	14.8 ± 1.9	84.1 ± 6.4	30.6 ± 5.0
Growth medium	5	6.0 ± 2.3	88.0 ± 2.3	18.0 ± 4.1
V. shiloi supernatant[c]	9	19.7 ± 4.9	82.1 ± 6.5	37.6 ± 5.3

[a] Experiments contained 0.1 ml of a crude zooxanthellae preparation (2×10^6 algae ml^{-1}) obtained from healthy *O. patagonica* and 0.1 ml of the fraction to be tested. After mixing, the sample was incubated at 28°C for 22 h in the presence of light.
[b] Bleaching and recovery of algae were the difference in values obtained microscopically after 22 h and at time zero.
[c] Bacteria were harvested after 24 h of incubation in 30°C in MB medium. The supernatant fluid was filtered through a 0.2-μm filter and used in one set of experiments. The cell pellet was washed and resuspended in sterile seawater to 5×10^7 cells/ml^{-1}.

TABLE 7 Inhibition of zooxanthellae photosynthesis by an extracellular toxin of *V. shiloi*[a]

Addition to algae	Photosynthesis (% quantum yield)[b] at time:	
	10 min	60 min
Seawater	94	90
Medium control	92	87
Supernatant fluid[c]	28	10
Ultrafiltrate of supernatant[d]	40	12

[a] Experiments contained 2×10^5 zooxanthellae and 0.1 ml of the fraction to be tested in a final volume of 0.2 ml. After mixing, the samples were incubated at 28°C in the presence of light.

[b] Quantum yield was measured using a mini pulse-amplified-magnitude fluorometer (36, 43). The data are presented as the percent of quantum yield obtained after 10 min and 60 min incubation compared with that at zero time.

[c] *V. shiloi* was grown for 40 h at 29°C in MBT medium. The supernatant fluid was obtained by centrifugation and filtration through a 0.2-μm membrane filter.

[d] The supernatant fluid was filtered through an Amicon filter (cutoff, 10 kDa).

inhibitory activity of ammonia on algal photosynthesis.

UNRESOLVED QUESTIONS AND THE DIRECTION OF FUTURE RESEARCH

The discovery that the causative agent of the bleaching of the coral *O. patagonica* is the bacterium *V. shiloi* and that the infection is temperature regulated, raised four major questions:

1. How general is the phenomenon? Are bacteria the causative agents of coral bleaching in other parts of the world? If so, which bacteria are involved?

2. How do environmental factors such as changes in seawater temperature and radiation trigger the infection?

3. How is the disease transmitted?

4. What are the mechanisms by which bacterial infection causes the loss of the endosymbiotic algae?

Regarding the first question—there have been a few studies that show changes in the bacterial population of corals following bleaching events (34, 41). However, except for the *V.*

shiloi–O. patagonica interaction, there have been no demonstrations that the bacteria associated with the bleached corals are the causative agents of the disease. Part of the problem is that very few laboratories are able to maintain corals in their healthy state for long enough periods to carry out well-controlled infection experiments. Another problem is that there are a large number of different bacterial strains associated with bleached coral, and isolating and testing each of them is a major undertaking. One approach that may be useful is to introduce a recently bleached coral from the sea into an aquarium with healthy corals and explore conditions by which the disease can be transmitted to the healthy corals. If successful, it would provide indirect evidence for an infectious agent. If antibiotics inhibited the transmission of the disease, then it is most likely a bacterial infection. It would then be necessary to isolate the causative agent. Another approach would be to isolate bacteria from within the coral tissue (not the external mucus) during the bleaching process, since at least in the case of *V. shiloi*, the bacteria penetrate into the coral. Finally, the more we learn about the normal bacterial flora of corals, the better will be our chance to isolate the potential pathogen.

How environmental factors influence infectious disease is a general and important problem. The data presented here demonstrate that elevated seawater temperature induces *V. shiloi* to produce an adhesin that allows it to adhere and then bleach *O. patagonica*. However, this is clearly not the whole story. For example, the corals recover in the winter, even though the bacteria must be present in the coral. Certainly, other virulence factors must be temperature regulated. To understand the phenomenon better at the molecular level, it will be necessary to locate and study other virulence genes and their products. Application of the power of molecular genetics to this problem should make it possible to locate potential pathogens in the environment and follow the infection process.

Nothing is known about how *V. shiloi* is transmitted from one coral to another. We have been unable to isolate the organism from seawater surrounding bleached corals, even in the summer. It is possible that the bacterium is transmitted by fish or invertebrates that feed on coral mucus. Understanding the mode of transmission may be of practical significance, because it is one of the ways in which infectious diseases can be controlled.

Finally, the mechanism of bleaching, i.e., the loss of the algae, needs to be investigated further. Loss of zooxanthellae from coral following exposure to extreme temperature shocks in the laboratory was first shown by Steen and Muscatine (39). Subsequently, it was reported that the primary bleaching mechanism in temperature-stressed tropical corals and anemones involved host cell detachment, whereby the coral endodermal cells, containing the zooxanthellae, were discharged (12). Observations on six coral species undergoing bleaching in Thailand in 1991 (4) led to the suggestion that several cellular mechanisms could result in the loss of the algae, the most important of which was in situ degradation of the zooxanthellae. The following working hypothesis is presented to explain how *V. shiloi* bleaches *O. patagonica*: (i) the bacterium attaches to a β-D-galactoside receptor on the coral surface; (ii) the bacterium passes through the mucous layer and enters an exodermal cell; (iii) the bacteria multiply inside the exodermal cell, producing ammonia and an extracellular toxin; (iv) the toxin allows the elevated concentration of ammonia to enter the endodermal cells containing the algae. The toxin and ammonia inhibit algal photosynthesis, leading to degradation of the algae and bleaching. This "ammonia hypothesis" can be tested in a number of ways, including direct measurement of ammonia concentration in exodermal and endodermal cells following infection, and isolation and characterization of the toxin.

ACKNOWLEDGMENTS

This work was supported by BSF grant no. 95-00177, the Porter Super-Center for Ecological and Environmental Studies, the Pasha Gol Chair for Applied Microbiology, and the Center of Emerging Diseases.

REVIEWS AND KEY PAPERS

Brown, B. E. 1997. Coral bleaching: causes and consequences. *Coral Reefs* **16**:S129–S138.

Glynn, P. W. 1993. Coral-reef bleaching—ecological perspectives. *Coral Reefs* **12**:1–17.

Kushmaro, A., E. Rosenberg, M. Fine, and Y. Loya. 1997. Bleaching of the coral *Oculina patagonica* by *Vibrio* AK1. *Mar. Ecol. Prog. Ser.* **147**: 159–165.

Rowan, R., N. Kowlton, A. Baker, and J. Jara. 1997. Landscape ecology of algal symbionts creates variation in episodes of coral bleaching. *Nature* **338**:265–269.

Toren, A., L. Landau, A. Kushmaro, Y. Loya, and E. Rosenberg. 1998. Effect of temperature on the adhesion of *Vibrio* AK-1 to *Oculina patagonica* and coral bleaching. *Appl. Environ. Microbiol.* **64**:1379–1384.

REFERENCES

1. Atwood, D. K., J. C. Hendee, and A. Mendes. 1992. An assessment of global warming stress on Caribbean coral reef ecosystems. *Bull. Mar. Sci.* **51**:118–130.

2. Brown, B. E. 1997. Coral bleaching: Causes and consequences. *Coral Reefs* **16**:S129–S138.

3. Brown, B. E., R. P. Dunne, and H. Chansang. 1996. Coral bleaching relative to elevated seawater temperature in the Andaman Sea (Indian Ocean) over the last 50 years. *Coral Reefs* **15**:151–152.

4. Brown, B. E., M. D. A. Le Tissier, and J. C. Bythell. 1995. Mechanisms of bleaching deduced from histological studies of reef corals sampled during a natural bleaching event. *Mar. Biol.* **122**:655–663.

5. Buddemeier, R. W., and D. G. Fautin. 1993. Coral bleaching as an adaptive mechanism. A testable hypothesis. *BioScience* **43**:320–325.

6. Coles, S. L., and Y. H. Fadlallah. 1991. Reef coral survival and mortality at low temperatures in the Arabian Gulf: new species-specific lower temperature limits. *Coral Reefs* **9**:231–237.

7. Colwell, R. R. 1996. Global climate and infectious disease: the cholera paradigm. *Science* **274**: 2025–2031.

8. Ducklow, H. W., and R. Mitchell. 1979. Bacterial populations and adaptations in the mucus layers on living corals. *Limnol. Oceanogr.* **24**: 715–725.

9. Fang, L. S., C. W. Liao, and M. C. Liu. 1995. Pigment composition in different-colored

scleractinian corals before and during the bleaching process. *Zool. Stud.* **34**:10–17.

10. **Fine, M., and Y. Loya.** 1995. The hermatypic coral *Oculina patagonica*, a new immigrant to the Mediterranean coast of Israel. *Isr. J. Zool.* **41**:84.

11. **Fisk, D. A., and T. J. Done.** 1985. Taxonomic and bathymetric patterns of bleaching in corals, Myrmidon Reef (Queensland). Proceedings of the 5th International Coral Reef Symposium **6**: 149–154.

12. **Gates, R. D., G. Baghdasarian, and L. Mustatine.** 1992. Temperature stress causes host cell detachment in symbiotic cnidarians: implications for coral bleaching. *Biol. Bull.* **182**:324–332.

13. **Gleason, D. F., and G. M. Wellington.** 1993. Ultraviolet radiation and coral bleaching. *Nature* **365**:836–838.

14. **Gleeson, M. W., and A. E. Strong.** 1995. Applying MCSST to coral reef bleaching. *Adv. Space Res.* **16**:151–154.

15. **Glynn, P. W.** 1993. Coral-reef bleaching—ecological perspectives. *Coral Reefs* **12**:1–17.

16. **Glynn, P. W.** 1991. Coral reef bleaching in the 1980s and possible connections with global warming. *Trends Ecol. Evol.* **6**:175–179.

17. **Glynn, P. W.** 1991. Elimination of two reef-building hydrocorals following the 1982–83 El-Nino warming event. *Science* **253**:69–71.

18. **Goreau, T. J.** 1990. Coral bleaching in Jamaica. *Nature* **343**:417.

19. **Goreau, T. J.** 1994. Coral bleaching and ocean "hot spots." *Ambio* **23**:176–180.

20. **Hayes, R. L., and P. G. Bush.** 1990. Microscopic observations of recovery in the reef-building scleractinian coral, *Montastrea annularis*, after bleaching on a Cayman reef. *Coral Reefs* **8**: 203–209.

21. **Hoegh-Guldberg, O., and B. Salvat.** 1995. Periodic mass-bleaching and elevated sea temperatures: bleaching of outer reef slope communities in Moorea, French Polynesia. *Mar. Ecol. Prog. Ser.* **121**:181–190.

22. **Hoegh-Guldberg, O., and G. J. Smith.** 1989. The effect of sudden changes in temperature, light and salinity on the population density and export of zooxanthellae from the reef corals *Stylophora pistillata*. Esper and *Seriatopora hystrix*. Dana. *J. Exp. Mar. Biol. Ecol.* **129**:279–304.

23. **Iglesias-Prieto, R., J. L. Matta, W. A. Robins, and R. K. Trench.** 1992. Photosynthetic response to elevated-temperature in the symbiotic dinoflagellate *Symbiodinium microadriaticum* in culture. *Proc. Natl. Acad. Sci. USA* **89**:302–305.

24. **Jensen, P. R., and W. Fenical.** 1994. Strategies for the discovery of secondary metabolites from marine bacteria: ecological perspectives. *Annu. Rev. Microbiol.* **48**:559–584.

25. **Jokiel, P. L., and S. L. Coles.** 1990. Response of Hawaiian and other Indo-Pacific reef corals to elevated temperature. *Coral Reefs* **8**:155–162.

26. **Kobluk, D. R., and M. A. Lysenko.** 1994. Ring bleaching in Southern Caribbean *Agaricia agaricites* during rapid water cooling. *Bull. Mar. Sci.* **54**:142–150.

27. **Kushmaro, A., Y. Loya, M. Fine, and E. Rosenberg.** 1996. Bacterial infection and coral bleaching. *Nature* **380**:396.

28. **Kushmaro, A., E. Rosenberg, M. Fine, and Y. Loya.** 1997. Bleaching of the coral *Oculina patagonica* by *Vibrio* AK1. *Mar. Ecol. Prog. Ser.* **147**:159–165.

29. **Lang, J. C., H. R. Lasker, E. H. Gladfelter, P. Hallock, W. C. Jaap, F. J. Losada, and R. G. Muller.** 1992. Spatial and temporal variability during periods of "recovery" after mass bleaching on Western Atlantic coral reefs. *Am. Zool.* **32**:696–706.

30. **Lesser, M. P., W. R. Stochaj, D. W. Tapley, and J. M. Shick.** 1990. Bleaching in coral reef anthozoans: effects of irradiance, ultraviolet radiation, and temperature on the activities of protective enzymes against active oxygen. *Coral Reefs* **8**:225–232.

31. **Mitchell, R., and I. Chet.** 1975. Bacterial attack of corals in polluted seawater. *Microb. Ecol.* **2**:227–233.

32. **Oliver, J.** 1985. Recurrent seasonal bleaching and mortality of corals on the Great Barrier Reef. Proceedings of the 5th International Coral Reef Symposium, Tahiti, 1985, **4**:201–206.

33. **Patz, J. A., R. Epstein, A. B. Thomas, and J. M. Balbus.** 1996. Global climate change and emerging infectious diseases. *JAMA* **275**:217–223.

34. **Ritchie, K. B., J. H. Dennis, T. McGrath, and G. W. Smith.** 1994. Bacteria associated with bleached and nonbleached areas of *Montastrea annularis*, p. 75–79. *In* L. Kass (ed.), *Bahamian Field Station*. Proc. 5th Symp. Nat. Hist. Bahamas, San Salvador, Bahamas.

35. **Rowan, R., N. Kowlton, A. Baker, and J. Jara.** 1997. Landscape ecology of algal symbionts creates variation in episodes of coral bleaching. *Nature* **338**:265–269.

36. **Schreiber, U., R. Gademann, P. J. Ralph, A. W. D. Larkum.** 1997. Assessment of photosynthetic performance of prochloron in *Lissoclinum patella* by chlorophyll fluorescence measurements. *Plant Cell Physiol.* **38**:945–951.

37. **Shick, J. M., M. P. Lesser, W. C. Dunlap, W. R. Stochaj, B. E. Chalker, and J. Wu Won.** 1995. Depth-dependent responses to solar ultraviolet radiation and oxidative stress in the

zooxanthellate coral *Acropora microphthalma. Mar. Biol.* **122:**41–51.

38. **Sorokin, Y. I.** 1973. Tropical role of bacteria in the ecosystem of the coral reef. *Nature* **242:**415–417.

39. **Steen, R. G., and L. Muscatine.** 1987. Low temperature evokes rapid exocytosis of symbiotic algae by a sea anemone. *Biol. Bull.* **172:**246–263.

40. **Toren, A., L. Landau, A. Kushmaro, Y. Loya, and E. Rosenberg.** 1998. Effect of temperature on the adhesion of *Vibrio* AK-1 to *Oculina patagonica* and coral bleaching. *Appl. Environ. Microbiol.* **64:**1379–1384.

41. **Upton, S. J., and E. C. Peters.** 1989. A new and unusual species of *Coccidium* (Apicomplexa, Agamococcidiorida) from Caribbean scleractinian corals. *J. Invertebr. Pathol.* **47:**184–193.

42. **Ware, R. J., G. D. Fautin, and W. R. Buddemeier.** 1996. Patterns of coral bleaching: modelling the adaptive bleaching hypothesis. *Ecol. Model.* **84:**199–214.

43. **Warner, M. E., W. J. Fitt, and G. W. Schmidt.** 1996. The effects of elevated temperature on the photosynthetic efficiency of zooxanthellae *in hospite* from four different species of reef coral: a novel approach. *Plant Cell Environ.* **19:**291–299.

44. **Zhang, J. P., and S. Normark.** 1996. Induction of gene expression in *Escherichia coli* after pilus-mediated adherence. *Science* **273:**1234–1236.

45. **Zibrowius, H.** 1974. *Oculina patagonica*, scleractiniaire hermatypique introduit en Mediterranée. *Helgol. Meeresunters.* **26:**163.

DRIVING FORCES IN MICROBIAL ECOLOGY

VI

INTRODUCTION

Elisha Orr

This last, diversified section of the book is devoted to the driving forces in microbial ecology. Microorganisms display remarkable ability to respond to varying environmental conditions, such as nutrients, environmental factors, toxic drugs, etc. These responses are mediated through proteins, which acquired specific domains and/or motifs throughout evolution. Studying such proteins and their corresponding genes should elucidate the mechanisms by which they exert their effects on cell growth, as well as the way they have evolved. They may further assist in solving applied problems, such as antibiotic resistance.

The section includes four chapters, differing in their topics. James Shapiro covers natural genetic engineering systems. These are thought to include all those biochemical systems that bacteria and other cells use to change the information content of DNA molecules. Such systems may be responsible for the incorporation of regulatory elements into different regulons involved in diverse aspects of bacterial physiology and behavior, in the dissemination of multiple antibiotic resistance and complex pathogenicity determinants, and in the evolution of catabolic functions for xenobiotic compounds. Shapiro describes the genetic processes that lead to natural genetic engineering, such as mutations, transpositions, and other genomic rearrangements. He presents examples of these changes and discusses their biological significance.

Eitan Bibi et al. describe the multiple drug resistance (MDR) proteins in *Escherichia coli*. They particularly point to the different systems (at least three) operating in bacteria and to the surprising fact that a component of an MDR system is often capable of handling different drugs, sometimes entirely unrelated in their physical and chemical properties. They raise the important issue of the physiological role(s) of these systems and bring examples of the consequences of disrupting genes encoding components of MDR systems.

David Gutnick and Eshel Ben-Jacob describe an amazing pattern of adaptive microbial behavior that responds to environmental conditions. This behavior is seen in the ability of dynamic microbial colonies of specific strains to develop unique complex patterns on hard surfaces under conditions of energy limitation. These authors discuss the physiological

Elisha Orr, Department of Molecular Microbiology and Biotechnology, Tel Aviv University, Ramat Aviv 69978, Israel.

meanings of these patterns with regard to cell–cell signaling and the dynamics of colony development.

Finally, Albert Taraboulos discusses exciting new discoveries in prion research. Prions may seem to be nonassociated with microorganisms, yet prionlike proteins, e.g., Ure3p and the *SUP35* gene product, have recently been discovered in the yeast *Saccharomyces cerevisiae*. The association of prions with membrane components and its biological importance are presented.

NATURAL GENETIC ENGINEERING, ADAPTIVE MUTATION, AND BACTERIAL EVOLUTION

James A. Shapiro

21

Molecular genetics has taught us many lessons about the "driving forces" in microbial ecology and microbial evolution. Among the most important of these have been lessons about how bacterial genomes are organized as hierarchies of modular components, how bacterial genomes undergo structural change through the action of natural genetic engineering systems, and how natural genetic engineering systems are subject to regulation by cellular control circuits. Moreover, bacterial systems such as antibiotic resistance, xenobiotic degradation, and new pathogenicity combinations provide our most fully documented examples of evolution in action. Thus, prokaryotic molecular genetics provides a dynamic vision of the evolutionary process on the basis of cellular functions rather than localized random genetic change (2, 87, 90).

MODULARITY OF BACTERIAL GENOMES: HIERARCHICALLY ORGANIZED SYSTEMS RATHER THAN UNITS

Beginning in the 1950s with the work of Monod and Benzer, molecular genetics has relentlessly deconstructed individual "genes" into their component parts and revealed the architecture of multilocus genetic determinants underlying the expression of particular phenotypes. At all levels, the genome is composed of nested systems rather than units (Table 1). A few examples will clarify this "systems view" of the genome.

We used to think of proteins as unitary structures with each part of the polypeptide chain integrated with the rest. Thus, the open reading frame (ORF) encoding that protein was conceptually a single unit of function and evolution. Today, however, we realize that proteins comprise separate domains with distinct and separable functions. The alpha and omega segments of *Escherichia coli* β-galactosidase (104) and the DNA-binding and cooperativity regions of lambda cI repressor (72) were recognized early as examples of separable domains. With extensive sequencing, we are able to recognize the signatures of various functional domains, such as ATP- or DNA-binding motifs, and assign proteins to families that share certain domains in common, such as the histidine kinases and response regulators of two-component control systems (96). The fact that domains can be swapped in vitro and retain their functionality shows that they are separable components of

James A. Shapiro, Department of Biochemistry and Molecular Biology, University of Chicago, Cummings Life Sciences Center, 920 East 58th Street, Chicago, Illinois 60637.

Microbial Ecology and Infectious Disease, Edited by Eugene Rosenberg

TABLE 1 Genetic "units" viewed as systems

Units view	Systems view
Protein encoded by single ORF	Composite of linked domains; e.g., –α and ω domains of beta-galactosidase (LacZ) –N-terminal DNA binding and C-terminal cooperativity domains of lambda repressor –Protein kinase and receptor domains of histidine kinase regulatory proteins
Gene	Composite of coding sequence(s), 5′ and 3′ regulatory regions
Promoter (σ^{70})	Composite of −10, −35, spacer and upstream regions with sites for positive transcription factors (e.g., Crp)
Genetic determinant of a cellular activity	Combined action of coordinately regulated products of multiple genetic loci, e.g., –Carbohydrate catabolism –Flagellum biogenesis, motility, and chemotaxis –Iron uptake –Pilus biogenesis –Cell division

the entire protein, whose activity reflects the interactions of its different domains.

The operon theory introduced a new kind of genetic element, the *cis*-acting regulatory site (77). Today we call these elements binding sites for transcription factors or, more generally, for any protein that recognizes a specific oligonucleotide motif (as in replication, recombination or DNA condensation). These binding sites are required both for expression (e.g., promoters) and for proper regulation. For many binding sites, we recognize subcomponents, such as the −10, −35, and spacer regions of canonical σ^{70} promoters (31). Thus, the functional entity of regulated gene expression is not a unit but rather a composite of 5′ and 3′ sites and ORF sequence(s) encoding the multidomain protein(s) of a particular operon (77, 90). Similarly, other kinds of genetic determinants, such as origins of replication or site-specific recombination substrates, display composite organizations composed of multiple recognition sequences (17).

Most transcription factor binding sites are repetitive elements found at multiple locations in the genome. Promoters specific for various

sigma factors and recognition sequences for multilocus control proteins such as Crp (80) and LexA (107) are examples of repeated motifs that integrate different operons into higher-order regulatory networks. In ways that we are now trying to explain, these regulatory connections between different genetic loci define much of the control circuitry that allows bacteria to maintain homeostasis during growth and undergo various cellular differentiations when growth ceases (36, 46, 54, 59). In some cases, regulatory hierarchies are multicellular and not restricted to individual cells. One of the most exciting recent developments in microbial genetics has been the realization that intercellular signaling and quorum-sensing systems have been integrated into the regulatory regimes controlling many distinct bacterial phenotypes (27, 32, 53, 69, 81, 98, 111). In the gram-negative bacteria, the signals are generally acyl homoserine lactones (AHLs) that are synthesized by enzymes encoded by *luxI* homologs and detected by transcription factors encoded by *luxR* homologs. The incorporation of the *luxI* and *luxR* homologs needed for AHL signaling into distinct functional systems is yet another illustration of genomic modularity. Examining the different ways these determinants are organized in each regulon, it appears that the evolutionary process frequently rearranged the orientation and spacing of the *luxI* and *luxR* homologs (Fig. 1) (81).

The modular and hierarchical organization of bacterial genomes has major implications for the fundamental processes of change during evolution. In particular, cellular capacities for rearranging and stitching together different components in a manner analogous to our own genetic engineering are needed to change the functional architecture of a genome (86, 87). How common are such functions in bacteria?

NATURAL GENETIC ENGINEERING SYSTEMS

The basic operations of classical bacterial genetics involve intercellular transfer of genetic information and recombination between DNA molecules, both homology dependent and homology independent. There have long been many indications of the cellular capacities for joining DNA sequences: chromosomal integration of temperate phages and sex factors; cloning of chromosomal markers into episomes by specialized transduction and sex factor excision; formation of deletions, duplications, and genetic fusions; regulation of gene expression by DNA rearrangements; and the movements of transposable elements within and between genomes (4, 83, 84, 89). Although most of these events used to be treated as "illegitimate recombination," we now know that they are regular and adaptively important features of genome flexibility in bacteria. Such flexibility is needed to survive in environments that may change rapidly in predictable or unpredictable ways.

The phrase "natural genetic engineering" is meant to encompass all those biochemical systems that bacteria and other cells use to change the information content of DNA molecules. These systems range from activities that carry out localized mutagenesis to those that generate wholesale rearrangements of major genomic components (Table 2). Natural genetic engineering systems are frequently made up of many components, and there is no correlation between the nature of the genetic change and the biochemical complexity of the responsible proteins. For example, the -1 frameshift that reverses the effect of the *lac33* mutation in response to stress is a single point mutation, but the frameshifting event depends upon the many sequentially acting components of the RecABC pathway (24, 44, 45, 55). The recently sequenced genome of a cyanobacterium contains 99 ORFs with transposase homologies (51), and the genome of *Bacillus subtilis* contains at least ten complete or partial prophages (56).

There are three important points to make about the natural genetic engineering systems listed in Table 2, as follows.

1. They mediate a wide range of DNA changes, from base substitutions and frameshifts through deletions, inversions, duplications, fusions, and transpositions.

2. Many of the systems work independently of genetic homology. Topoisomerases and the unknown activities that mediate in vivo deletions and duplications generally prefer short sequence homologies (1, 109), but they can join completely nonhomologous sequences (10, 13, 49). The action of transposable elements depends on ligating free 3' hydroxyl ends of the donor to 5' phosphate ends of the target (14, 15, 43, 67, 82). This means that target specificity is independent of the ability of donor and target sequences to form a heteroduplex and is determined by the binding affinities of the cognate transposase and accessory proteins.

3. Multiple genetic changes mediated by natural genetic engineering systems often do not occur independently of each other. For example, *Neisseria gonorrhoeae* uses homologous recombination between silent *pilS* cassettes and the expressed *pilE* locus to generate pilus antigenic variation, and multiple base substitutions result from a single recombination event (28, 97). Transposable elements can

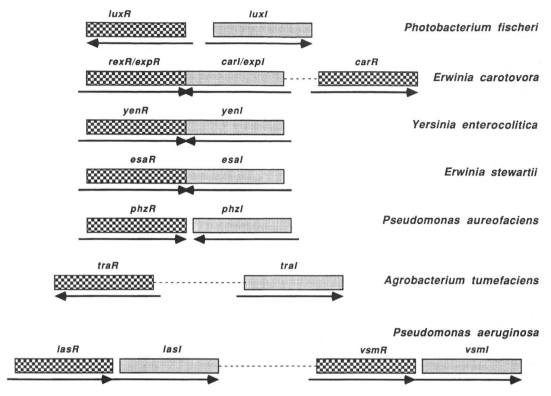

FIGURE 1 Arrangement of *luxR* and *luxI* homologs in different bacterial species controlling distinct functions. The arrows indicate transcripts; merged arrowheads indicate transcriptional overlaps. (Redrawn from reference 81.)

be activated to go through multiple recombination events and accumulate at distinct places in the genome. Most transposable elements duplicate as they mediate DNA rearrangements, either because replication is inherent to the rearrangement process (82) or, in cut and paste events, because the donor site is repaired by recombination with a homolog carrying a copy of the inserted element (14, 40). Thus, related transposition or rearrangement events can occur at multiple genomic locations. It is possible that such coincident events account for the "bursts" of increase in IS element copies observed in dormant cultures of *E. coli* (68).

NATURAL GENETIC ENGINEERING SYSTEMS AT WORK IN REGULATION AND EVOLUTION

The idea of natural genetic engineering systems playing a major role outside the laboratory is no longer new to microbiologists. We are accustomed to thinking about the roles of plasmids, phages, transposons, and integrons in the evolution of antibiotic-resistance determinants that cause real-world problems in medicine and agriculture (e.g., references 42, 74, 108). There are many additional examples of ecologically important phenotypes in which DNA rearrangements play a role in ongoing regulation or participated in the formation of the underlying genetic structures. Looking at pathogenicity and xenobiotic degradation functions provides illustrative examples, as follows.

Antigenic variation of gonococcal pili by gene conversion (97) must occur in nature because of the genetic variability observed in infections, in which mixtures of pilus types are recovered, and in experimental infections, in which recovered pilus types do not corre-

TABLE 2 Some natural genetic engineering systems in bacteria

Genetic engineering system	Functions involved	DNA changes	References
Localized SOS mutagenesis (*E. coli*)	RecA, UmuCD'	Base substitutions, frameshifts	107
Adaptive frameshifting (*E. coli*)	RecABC, RuvAB, PolII, F' Tra	−1 Frameshift	9, 21, 24, 29, 44, 45, 73, 78, 79
Pilus antigenic and phase variation (*N. gonorrhoeae*)	Homologous recombination (Rec)	Gene conversion of coding sequence tracts	97
Surface lipoprotein variation (*B. hermsii*)	Homologous recombination	Reciprocal recombination and gene conversion of coding sequence tracts	3, 76, 114
P.II outer membrane variation (*N. gonorrhoeae*)	Rec independent	Unequal recombination of tandem 5-bp CTTCT repeats; changes coding phase	97
Tn*5*, Tn*9*, Tn*10* precise excision (*E. coli*, *S. typhimurium*)	RecA independent	Reciprocal recombination of flanking 8/9 bp repeats; restores original sequence	4
In vivo deletion, inversion, fusion and duplication formation (*E. coli*)	RecA independent	Generally reciprocal recombination of short sequence repeats; occasionally nonhomologous	1, 10, 109
Type II topoisomerase recombination (in vitro)	DNA gyrase, T4 DNA topoisomerase	Deletions and fusions by nonhomologous recombination, sometimes at short repeats	13, 49
Site-specific recombination (type I topoisomerases) (*E. coli*, *S. typhimurium*)	Site-specific recombinases (e.g., phage integrases, TnpR resolvase, Hin invertase, cassette integrase) and accesory proteins (e.g., IHF, FIS)	Insertions, excisions/deletions, inversions by concerted or successive cleavage-ligation reactions at short sequence repeats; tolerates mismatches	33, 42, 57, 95, 113

Continued on following page

TABLE 2 (Continued)

Genetic engineering system	Functions involved	DNA changes	References
Transposable elements (many species)	Transposases, accessory proteins (e.g., MuB, TnsD, E)	Insertions, transpositions, replicon fusions, adjacent deletions/excisions, adjacent inversions by ligation of 3′OH transposon ends to 5′ PO$_4$ groups from staggered cuts at nonhomologous target sites	14, 15, 43, 67, 82
DNA uptake (transformation competence) (*B. subtilis*)	Competence pheromones, Com signal transduction system and proteins involved in assembly of type IV pilus-related structure	Uptake of single strand independent of sequence	16, 36
DNA uptake (transformation competence) (*H. influenzae*)	cAMP, Crp, PtsI, and multiple Com proteins	Uptake of double-stranded DNA carrying species identifier sequence	18, 37, 93, 94

spond to the infecting type (28). *N. gonorrhoeae* also controls the synthesis of other surface proteins by Rec-independent unequal crossing-over or replication slippage between pentanucleotide repeats in the coding sequence (97). The occurrence of similar kinds of repeats in adhesin-coding sequences in the *Helicobacter pylori*, *Mycoplasma genitalium* and *Mycoplasma pneumoniae* genomes has led to the proposal that gene conversion and Rec-independent unequal crossing-over or replication slippage also play roles in antigenic variation in these species (26, 47, 100).

Multiphasic antigenic variation in *Borrelia hermsii* and *Borrelia burgdorferi* occurs by recombination between silent, promoterless *vmp* and *vls* sequences and telomeric expression sites on linear minichromosomes (3, 26, 114). The Vmp and Vls lipoproteins are the major antigenic determinants on the bacterial surface. Traces of these events can also be found by PCR analysis of field isolates (48). In addition, it appears that *Borrelia* spp. use postrecombination gene conversion events to further diversify their antigenic repertoire (25, 76).

Autotransporting (AT) virulence determinants in gram-negative bacteria evolve by fusion of an AT domain to a variety of virulence factors (60).

Investigation of the genetic basis of bacterial pathogenicity has indicated that different strains became pathogens by the acquisition of episomes carrying determinants for different kinds of virulence factors. These episomes include phages (35, 106), plasmids (64, 71), and extended chromosomal insertions termed "pathogenicity islands" (PAIs) (38). Examination of the boundaries of these PAIs (Fig. 2) (34, 38) clearly indicates that most of them arrived at their chromosomal sites by known natural genetic engineering mechanisms, either site-specific recombination similar to temperate phage integration (UPEC 536 and J96 and *Vibrio cholerae*), by the mediation of IS elements (*Yersinia pestis*), or by one of these two mechanisms, both of which generate flanking oligonucleotide direct repeats (*Dichelobacter nodosus* and *H. pylori*). The choice of

stable RNA loci for integration (EPEC, UPEC, *S. enterica* and *Yersinia enterocolitica*) is also reminiscent of temperate phage integration (12). Comparing the Cag PAIs of some strains of *H. pylori* also reveals further action of IS elements (100).

In recent years, concerns about enhancing bioremediation activities have directed attention to xenobiotic degradation loci in soil bacteria. Patterns of modular rearrangements have been observed in combining "upper" and "lower" pathway determinants to endow single species with the capacity to mineralize aromatic hydrocarbons (110). Many of the catabolic determinants for complete or partial degradation pathways are carried on transposons or are flanked by IS elements (75, 103, 112). Selection for simple modification of a haloaromatic degradation pathway often results in extensive DNA rearrangements (50), and comparison of toluene and chlorotoluene degradation operons reveals the same kinds of coding sequence rearrangements described above for *luxR* and *luxI* homologs (103).

ADAPTIVE MUTATION, ENVIRONMENTAL INPUTS, AND THE EPISODIC NATURE OF NATURAL GENETIC ENGINEERING

It has been known for several decades that many kinds of environmental factors have dramatic influences on mutation frequencies in bacterial cultures. Generally, as in the case of the SOS response (107), these mutagenic influences have been seen as by-products of repair processes. However, knowledge about natural genetic engineering systems now makes it possible to see DNA change as a useful cellular response to stress, frequently called "adaptive mutation" (19, 78, 90). Three cases of DNA change regulated by culture conditions have been well documented.

1. In *Alcaligenes eutrophus* strains, an extremely high frequency of both plasmid and chromosomal mutations has been found in the survivors of incubation at 37°C on medium containing methionine, cysteine, or serine (102). Up to 80% of the survivors carry mu-

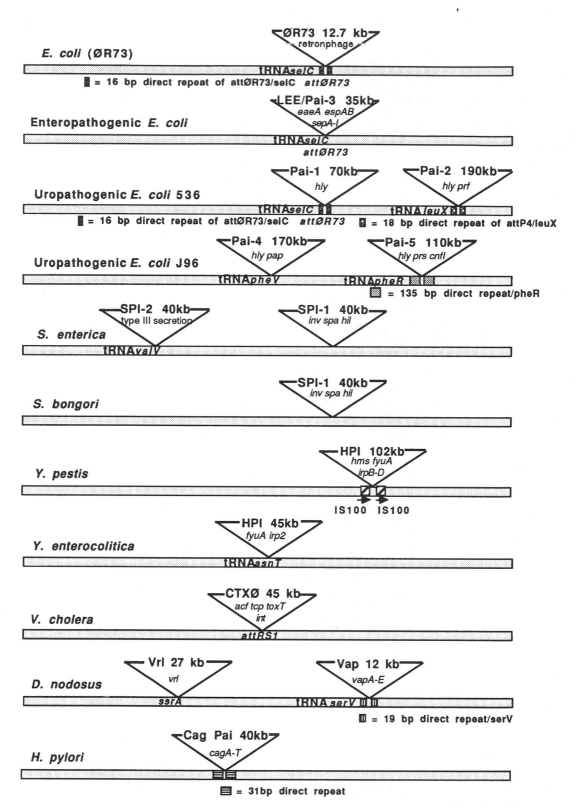

FIGURE 2 Pathogenicity islands (PAIs) in the chromosomes of different bacterial species. The internal lettering indicates some of the virulence functions encoded by each PAI. Based on references 34 and 38.

tations affecting many phenotypes (Lys⁻, Thr⁻, loss of autotrophy, pigment excretion, inability to utilize nitrate or ammonia as nitrogen sources, sensitivity to heavy metals, etc.), and many mutants carry multiple lesions (65). Many of the "survivors" retain thermosensitivity on rich medium, indicating that their ability to grow on the selection medium was not the result of a stable mutation. Some phenotypes, such as lysine or threonine auxotrophy, appear to be specific to "temperature-induced mutagenesis and mortality" (TIMM) because they cannot be recovered by penicillin selection after growth at 30°C. Examination of plasmids carrying TIMM-induced mutations reveals IS element insertion and excision events as well as extensive rearrangements that may be IS related (99). It appears that *A. eutrophus* strains possess two traits that can lead to rapid environmentally triggered genome modification: (i) the ability of some cells to enter a transient state in which they can proliferate at 37°C on enriched medium and (ii) a control system for derepressing IS element activity at 37°C. This fascinating example of regulatable hypermutation apparently involving IS elements merits further attention.

2. The best-known case of adaptive mutation is reversion of the *lac33* frameshift in a *lacI-lacZ* fusion on an F'*lac* plasmid (9). A particular class of −1 frameshift reversion events occurs at high frequencies on selective medium but not during normal growth (22, 79). Detailed studies have shown that Rec functions (24, 44, 45), F *tra* functions (23, 29, 73), and Dna polymerase II (21) are all required for adaptive frameshifts to occur. Thus, the underlying events involve a complex set of protein factors. Among these, the F *tra* functions are known to be regulated by the host Arc (aerobic respiration control) function (92) and activated by the conditions prevailing during selection: dense, highly aerobic cells unable to proliferate (70). Moreover, additional plasmid and chromosomal mutations are stimulated by the Lac selection and are found among the *lac33* pseudorevertants at frequencies that indicate that they did not arise in independent events (20, 101). Thus, the Lac selection appears to induce a hypermutable state of the kind postulated by Hall (41). In other words, the underlying processes creating these additional unselected mutations must be activated by aerobic starvation.

3. Aerobic starvation is also known to be responsible for activating the DNA rearrangements in the first clearly documented adaptive mutation system, the formation of *araB-lacZ* coding sequences fusions (62, 66, 85). This is one example of the general Casadaban method developed for fusing any N-terminal coding region to *lacZ* (11). The Casadaban method serves as an experimental model for the creation in vivo of multi-domain coding sequences. In Casadaban's original conception, the transposable Mu prophage served simply as mobile homology for inserting a decapitated *lacZ* into many genomic locations (Fig. 3), but our work showed that Mu sequences and transposition functions play an active role in fusion formation (Fig. 4) (61, 90, 91). The remarkable initial observation was that *araB-lacZ* fusions never occurred during normal bacterial growth (<10⁻¹⁰/CFU) but could be recovered at high frequencies (~10⁻⁵/CFU) after a few weeks incubation on selection plates or following prolonged starvation (62, 85). Studies of the genetic requirements for fusion formation have identified a number of essential cellular regulatory functions: IHF and HU (91), ClpXP protease (88; Maenhaut-Michel and Shapiro, unpublished), RpoS (30), and Crp (Shapiro and Maenhaut-Michel, unpublished). Taking advantage of Mu genetics and the thermosensitive Mu*cts62* repressor in this system, it has been established that the triggering of fusion formation by starvation includes two experimentally separable effects: (i) prophage derepression in stationary phase to permit Mu A transposase expression and (ii) activation of strand transfer and subsequent DNA processing steps to complete fusion formation (Fig. 4) (61; Shapiro et al., unpublished). Studies of Mu*cts62* derepression using a *pE-lacZ* reporter system (105) have shown

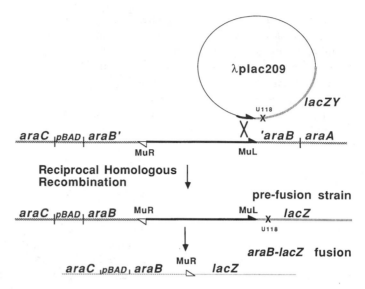

FIGURE 3 The Casadaban (11) system for producing *araB-lacZ* coding sequence fusions. The short MuL homology in λ*plac*209 allows the phage to integrate into an *araB*::Mu*cts62* prophage. The *lac* operon cannot be expressed because it lacks a promoter, and *lacZ* also carries the U118 *ochre* mutation at codon 17. To grow on lactose as a carbon source with arabinose as inducer on AraLac medium, an in-frame fusion must occur joining *araB* to a region of *lacZ* between codon 17 and codon 28. These fusions always carry an inverted segment of the MuR terminus (62).

that ClpPX and RpoS but not Crp play a role in stationary phase derepression (S. Lamrani, C. Ranquet, M.-J. Gama, J. Shapiro, G. Maenhaut-Michel, and A. Toussaint, unpublished). Thus, it may be hypothesized that starvation effect (ii) requires activation of one or more Crp-dependent operons under stress conditions.

Each adaptive mutation system has its own molecular mechanism: IS element movements in TIMM; Rec-, Tra-, and PolII-dependent frameshifting in *lac-33* reversion; and Mu A-mediated rearrangements in *araB-lacZ* fusions. What all three systems (and other examples of adaptive mutation) have in common is the activation of one or more natural genetic engineering systems capable of mediating DNA change in response to a particular kind of physiological stress. As seen in the *araB-lacZ* system, this genetic response to stress involves the control circuits that condition all bacterial responses to stress (46).

SIGNIFICANCE FOR THINKING ABOUT EVOLUTIONARY MECHANISMS

Bacteria continue to provide the most thoroughly documented examples of evolution occurring under our eyes. They also provided the molecular evidence to confirm McClintock's discovery of transposable elements and cellular functions capable of restructuring the genome (8, 63). These two aspects of bacterial genetics complement and illuminate each other. As we observe bacteria filling specific ecological niches, we discover the essential roles played by intracellular DNA rearrangements involving transposable elements, cassettes and integrons, and pathogenicity islands, as well as by intercellular DNA transfer systems involving DNA uptake systems, plasmids, phages, and conjugative transposons. We have also found evidence for the assembly of major functional systems, such as catabolic pathways, adhesion systems, and protein translocation machinery, by the rearrangement and joining of sequences encoding components used in a variety of contexts. From all this data, it is hard to escape the conclusion that natural genetic engineering plays a major role in what we may call bacterial "meso-evolution" (i.e., those evolutionary events that create functional complexes that confer new abilities on distinct strains within recognizable species boundaries) as distinguished from more limited "microevolutionary" events that alter a single protein or regulatory response (cf. reference 58). Given

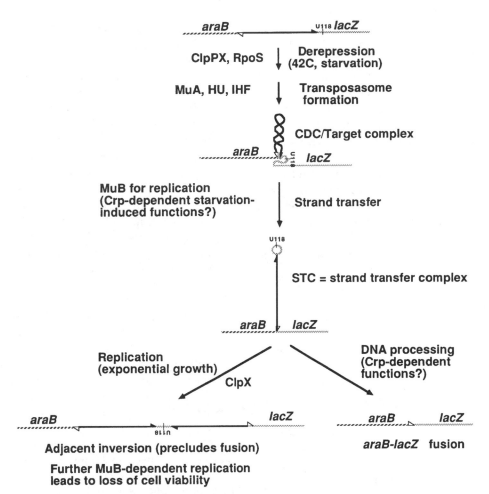

FIGURE 4 The different stages in *araB-lacZ* fusion formation. Inactivation of the Mu*cts62* repressor protein can occur either by incubation at high temperature or by prolonged aerobiosis at low temperature after growth has stopped. Stationary-phase derepression at low temperature requires ClpPX protease and RpoS. Derepression permits Mu A expression and subsequent transposasome formation. During active growth, Mu B protein facilitates the ligation of 3′ OH transposon ends in the transposasome to 5′ phosphate groups at the target site, thereby creating the strand transfer complex (STC). Mu prophage replication normally initiates after STC formation and removal of complexed Mu A protein by ClpX and other factors. Complete Mu prophage replication is incompatible with fusion formation, and further rounds of STC formation and replication are lethal to the cell. In the absence of Mu B protein, no STC appears to be formed under growth conditions after derepression, and the later steps leading to fusion formation appear to occur only under starvation conditions on the selective medium. Since the Crp protein is required for fusion formation in the presence of Mu B protein but is not essential for stationary phase derepression at low temperature, we hypothesize that it may control functions that inhibit Mu B activity and provide an alternative pathway to STC formation. Based on references 43, 62, 67, 90, and 91.

the requisite biochemical capabilities in bacterial cells (Table 2), rearrangement and diversification of basic genetic modules is a far more attractive hypothesis to explain the data than independent evolution of homologous determinants in each regulon.

Bacterial "macroevolution" into distinct genera and species still remains largely mysterious. Genetic mapping and whole genome sequencing have revealed many differences in the genomes of bacteria and archaea. The most notable involve the organization of distinct functional determinants (clustered or dispersed) and the repetitive genome components, which differ in identity, abundance, and distribution. Although we do not know the biological effects of many repetitive elements, it would be an error to assume they are noncoding. Not knowing how the sequence-specific *Haemophilus influenzae* transformation system operates, for example, we might conclude that the thousands of species identifier repeats distributed throughout the genome of this species were meaningless "junk DNA" (18, 93, 94). Similarly, if we did not know about RecBCD-mediated recombination, we would conclude the same about the 8-bp Chi sequences distributed throughout the *E. coli* genome (which, incidentally, are not even the most frequent octamer repeats) (5). Again, it seems far more reasonable to conclude that cellular natural genetic engineering capacities were involved in genome reorganizations and the spread of repetitive sequence elements during episodes of macroevolutionary change than that genomes diverged slowly by accumulating independent point mutations. While experimental tests of these ideas are extremely difficult because it is so hard to rule out contamination as the source of a new organism, there is an extensive older literature growing out of vaccine development on major phenotypic changes in bacterial cultures (39). It would be quite useful to revisit some of these examples of "microbic dissociation" with molecular technology.

The major mystery in evolution is the origin of novel biological adaptations, ranging from new protein functions to the formation of new structures with multiple interacting parts. Recognizing the modular, hierarchical nature of genome organization has provided a way of thinking about this problem. The reassortment of discrete genetic elements can lead to novel functions quite rapidly. The question then remains of how multiple discrete components can be integrated into workable interactive systems. A possible answer lies in two interrelated features of natural genetic engineering systems: their nonrandomness and their connections to signal transduction networks. Figure 2 illustrates, for example, that many phages and PAIs insert preferentially next to tRNA and other stable RNA coding sequences. In yeast, Ty elements demonstrate a similar preference, and it is known that the Ty insertion machinery associates with RNA polymerase III transcription factors (52). The phenomenon of adaptive mutation shows that the timing and frequency of DNA changes are definitely linked to cellular physiology via signal transduction functions. Perhaps, as with Ty elements, there are also connections influencing the location of rearrangement sites. If so, then natural genetic engineering has the capacity for nonrandom, biologically influenced genome reorganization that could assemble novel functional systems. We should recall that cellular signal transduction networks are computational, decision-making systems (6, 7). Extending these information-processing capabilities to genome reorganization opens an entire new world to evolutionary theory.

ACKNOWLEDGMENTS

I owe a deep debt of gratitude to my collaborators on Mu-based systems, Genevieve Maenhaut-Michel, Pat Higgins, David Leach, Ariane Toussaint, and their associates. My research on Mu-mediated genome rearrangements has been supported by the National Science Foundation. I am also grateful for many stimulating ideas to colleagues who attended an NSF- and ONR-sponsored workshop in October, 1997, "Cellular Computation and Decision-Making."

REVIEWS AND KEY PAPERS

Arber, W. 1993. Evolution of prokaryotic genomes. *Gene* **135**:49–56.

Berg, D. E., and M. M. Howe (ed.). 1989. *Mobile DNA*. American Society for Microbiology, Washington, D.C.

Echols, H. 1986. Multiple DNA-protein interactions governing high-precision DNA transactions. *Science* **233**:1050–1056.

Foster, P. L. 1993. Adaptive mutation: the uses of adversity. *Annu. Rev. Microbiol.* **47**:467–504.

Groisman, E., and H. Ochman. 1996. Pathogenicity islands: bacterial evolution in quantum leaps. *Cell* **87**:791–794.

Hacker, J., G. Blum-Oehler, I. Muhldorfer, and H. Tschape. 1997. Pathogenicity islands of virulent bacteria: structure, function and impact on microbial evolution. *Mol. Microbiol.* **23**:1089–1097.

Hall, R. M. 1997. Mobile gene cassettes and integrons: moving antibiotic resistance genes in gram-negative bacteria. *CIBA Found. Symp.* **207**:192–202.

Lawrence, J. G. 1997. Selfish operons and speciation by gene transfer. *Trends Microbiol.* **5**:355–359.

McClintock, B. 1984. Significance of responses of the genome to challenge. *Science* **226**:792–801.

Reznikoff, W. S. 1992. The lactose operon-controlling elements: a complex paradigm. *Mol. Microbiol.* **6**:2419–2422.

Salmond, G. P. C., B. W. Bycroft, G. S. A. B. Stewart, and P. Williams. 1995. The bacterial "enigma": cracking the code of cell-cell communication. *Mol. Microbiol.* **16**:615–624.

Shapiro, J. A. 1984. Observations on the formation of clones containing *araB-lacZ* cistron fusions. *Mol. Gen. Genet.* **194**:79–90.

Shapiro, J. A. 1997. Genome organization, natural genetic engineering, and adaptive mutation. *Trends Genet.* **13**:98–104.

Torkelson, J., R. S. Harris, M.-J. Lombardo, J. Nagendran, C. Thulin, and S. M. Rosenberg. 1997. Genome-wide hypermutation in a subpopulation of stationary-phase cells underlies recombination-dependent adaptive mutation. *EMBO J.* **16**:3303–3311

van der Meer, J. R. 1997. Evolution of novel metabolic pathways for the degradation of chloroaromatic compounds. *Antonie van Leeuwenhoek* **71**:159–178.

REFERENCES

1. Albertini, A. M., M. Hofer, M. P. Calos, T. D. Tlsty, and J. H. Miller. 1983. Analysis of spontaneous deletions and gene amplification in the lac region of Escherichia coli. *Cold Spring Harbor Symp. Quant. Biol.* **47**:841–850.

2. Arber, W. 1993. Evolution of prokaryotic genomes. *Gene* **135**:49–56.

3. Barbour, A. G. 1993. Linear DNA of Borrelia species and antigenic variation. *Trends Microbiol.* **1**:236–239.

4. Berg, D. E., and M. M. Howe (ed.). 1989. *Mobile DNA*. American Society for Microbiology, Washington, D.C.

5. Blattner, F. R., G. Plunkett, C. A. Bloch, N. T. Perna, V. Burland, M. Riley, J. Collado-Vides, J. D. Glasner, C. K. Rode, G. F. Mayhew, J. Gregor, N. W. Davis, H. A. Kirkpatrick, M. A. Goeden, D. J. Rose, B. Mau, and Y. Shao. 1997. The complete genome sequence of Escherichia coli K-12. *Science* **277**:1453–1474.

6. Bray, D. 1990. Intracellular signalling as a parallel distributed process. *J. Theor. Biol.* **143**:215–231.

7. Bray D. 1995. Protein molecules as computational elements in living cells. *Nature* **376**:307–12.

8. Bukhari, A. I., J. A. Shapiro, and S. L. Adhya (ed.). 1977. *DNA Insertion Elements, Plasmids, and Episomes*. Cold Spring Harbor Laboratory, Cold Spring Harbor, N.Y.

9. Cairns, J., and P. L. Foster. 1991. Adaptive reversion of a frameshift mutation in Escherichia coli. *Genetics* **128**:695–701.

10. Calos, M. P., D. Galas, and J. H. Miller. 1978. Genetic studies of the lac repressor. VIII. DNA sequence change resulting from an intragenic duplication. *J. Mol. Biol.* **126**:865–869.

11. Casadaban, M. J. 1976. Transposition and fusion of the lac genes to selected promoters in Escherichia coli using bacteriophages lambda and Mu. *J. Mol. Biol.* **104**:541–555.

12. Cheetham, B. F., and M. E. Katz. 1995. A role for bacteriophages in the evolution and transfer of bacterial virulence determinants. *Mol. Microbiol.* **18**:201–208.

13. Chiba, M., H. Shimizu, A. Fujimoto, H. Nashimoto, and H. Ikeda. 1989. Common sites for recombination and cleavage mediated by bacteriophage T4 DNA topoisomerase *in vitro*. *J. Biol. Chem.* **264**:12785–12790.

14. Craig, N. L. 1995. Unity in transposition reactions. *Science* **270**:253–254.

15. Craig, N. L. 1996. V(D)J recombination and transposition: closer than expected. *Science* **271**:1512.

16. Dubnau, D. 1997. Binding and transport of transforming DNA by Bacillus subtilis: the role of type-IV pilin-like proteins—a review. *Gene* **192**:191–198.

17. Echols, H. 1986. Multiple DNA-protein interactions governing high-precision DNA transactions. *Science* **233**:1050–1056.

18. Fleischmann, R. D., M. D. Adams, O. White, R. A. Clayton, E. F. Kirkness, A. R. Kerlavage, C. J. Bult, J. F. Tomb, B. A. Dougherty, and J. M. Merrick. 1995. Whole-genome random sequencing and assembly of *Haemophilus influenzae* Rd. *Science* **269**:496–512.

19. Foster, P. L. 1993. Adaptive mutation: the uses of adversity. *Annu. Rev. Microbiol.* **47**:467–504.

20. Foster, P. L. 1997. Nonadaptive mutations occur on the F' episome during adaptive mutation conditions in *Escherichia coli*. *J. Bacteriol.* **179**:1550–1554.

21. Foster, P. L., G. Gudmundsson, J. M. Trimarchi, H. Cai, and M. F. Goodman. 1995. Proofreading-defective DNA polymerase II increases adaptive mutation in *Escherichia coli*. *Proc. Natl. Acad. Sci. USA* **92**:7951–7955.

22. Foster, P. L., and J. M. Trimarchi. 1994. Adaptive reversion of a frameshift mutation in *Escherichia coli* by simple base deletions in homopolymeric runs. *Science* **265**:407–409.

23. Foster, P. L., and J. M. Trimarchi. 1995. Adaptive reversion of an episomal frameshift mutation in *Escherichia coli* requires conjugal functions but not actual conjugation. *Proc. Natl. Acad. Sci. USA* **92**:5487–5490.

24. Foster, P. L., J. M. Trimarchi, and R. Maurer. 1996. Two enzymes, both of which process recombination intermediates, have opposite effects on adaptive mutation in *Escherichia coli*. *Genetics* **142**:25–37.

25. Fraser, C. M., S. Casjens, W. M. Huang, G. G. Sutton, R. Clayton, R. Lathigra, O. White, K. A. Ketchum, R. Dodson, E. K. Hickey, M. Gwinn, B. Dougherty, J. F. Tomb, R. D. Fleischmann, D. Richardson, J. Peterson, A. R. Kerlavage, J. Quackenbush, S. Salzberg, M. Hanson, R. van Vugt, N. Palmer, M. D. Adams, J. Gocayne, and J. C. Venter. 1997. Genomic sequence of a Lyme disease spirochaete, *Borrelia burgdorferi*. *Nature* **390**:580–586.

26. Fraser, C. M., J. D. Gocayne, O. White, M. D. Adams, R. A. Clayton, R. D. Fleischmann, C. J. Bult, A. R. Kerlavage, G. Sutton, and J. M. Kelley. 1995. The minimal gene complement of *Mycoplasma genitalium*. *Science* **270**:397–403.

27. Fuqua C., S. C. Winans, and E. P. Greenberg. 1996. Census and consensus in bacterial ecosystems: the LuxR-LuxI family of quorum-sensing transcriptional regulators. *Annu. Rev. Microbiol.* **50**:727–751.

28. Fussenegger, M., T. Rudel, R. Barten, R. Ryll, and T. F. Meyer. 1997. Transformation competence and type-4 pilus biogenesis in *Neisseria gonorrhoeae*—a review. *Gene* **192**:125–134.

29. Galitski, T., and J. R. Roth. 1995. Evidence that F plasmid transfer replication underlies apparent adaptive mutation. *Science* **268**:421–23.

30. Gómez-Gómez, J. M., J. Blázquez, F. Baquero, and J. L. Martinez. 1997. H-NS and RpoS regulate emergence of LacAra⁺ mutants of *Escherichia coli* MCS2. *J. Bacteriol.* **179**:4620–4622.

31. Gralla, J. D., and J. Collado-Vides. 1996. Organization and function of transcription regulatory elements, p. 1232–1245. *In* F. C. Neidhardt, R. Curtiss III, J. L. Ingraham, E. C. C. Lin, K. B. Low, Jr., B. Magasanik, W. S. Reznikoff, M. Riley, M. Schaechter, and H. E. Umbarger (ed.), *Escherichia coli and Salmonella: Cellular and Molecular Biology*, 2nd ed. American Society for Microbiology, Washington, D.C.

32. Gray, K. M. 1997. Intercellular communication and group behavior in bacteria. *Trends Microbiol.* **5**:184–188.

33. Grindley, N. D. 1997. Site-specific recombination: synapsis and strand exchange revealed. *Curr. Biol.* **7**:R608–R612.

34. Groisman, E., and H. Ochman. 1996. Pathogenicity islands: bacterial evolution in quantum leaps. *Cell* **87**:791–794.

35. Groman, N. B. 1984. Conversion by corynephages and its role in the natural history of diphtheria. *J. Hyg.* (London) **93**:405–417.

36. Grossman, A. D. 1995. Genetic networks controlling the initiation of sporulation and the development of genetic competence in *Bacillus subtilis*. *Annu. Rev. Genet.* **29**:477–508.

37. Gwinn, M. L., D. Yi, H. O. Smith, and J. F. Tomb. 1996. Role of the two-component signal transduction and the phosphoenolpyruvate: carbohydrate phosphotransferase systems in competence development of *Haemophilus influenzae* Rd. *J. Bacteriol.* **178**:6366–6368.

38. Hacker, J., G. Blum-Oehler, I. Muhldorfer, and H. Tschape. 1997. Pathogenicity islands of virulent bacteria: structure, function and impact on microbial evolution. *Mol. Microbiol.* **23**:1089–1097.

39. Hadley, P. 1927. Microbic dissociation. *J. Infect. Dis.* **40**:1–312.

40. Hagemann, A. T., and N. L. Craig. 1993. Tn7 transposition creates a hotspot for homologous recombination at the transposon donor site. *Genetics* **133**:9–16.

41. Hall, B. G. 1990. Spontaneous point mutations that occur more often when advantageous than when neutral. *Genetics* **126**:5–16.

42. Hall, R. M. 1997. Mobile gene cassettes and integrons: moving antibiotic resistance genes in gram-negative bacteria. *CIBA Found. Symp.* **207**:192–202.

43. **Haniford, D. B., and G. Chaconas.** 1992. Mechanistic aspects of DNA transposition. *Curr. Opin. Genet. Dev.* **2:**698–704.

44. **Harris, R. S., S. Longerich, and S. M. Rosenberg.** 1994. Recombination in adaptive mutation. *Science* **264:**258–260.

45. **Harris, R. S., K. J. Ross, and S. M. Rosenberg.** 1996. Opposing roles of the Holliday junction processing systems of *Escherichia coli* in recombination-dependent adaptive mutation. *Genetics* **142:**681–691.

46. **Hengge-Aronis, R.** 1996. Back to log phase: sigma S as a global regulator in the osmotic control of gene expression in *Escherichia coli. Mol. Microbiol.* **21:**887–893.

47. **Himmelreich, R., H. Hilbert, H. Plagens, E. Pirkl, B. C. Li, and R. Herrmann.** 1996. Complete sequence analysis of the genome of the bacterium *Mycoplasma pneumoniae. Nucleic Acids Res.* **24:**4420–4449.

48. **Hinnebusch, B. J., A. G. Barbour, B. I. Restrepo, and T. G. Schwan.** 1998. Population structure of the relapsing fever spirochete *Borrelia hermsii* as indicated by polymorphism of two multigene families that encode immunogenic outer surface lipoproteins. *Infect. Immun.* **66:**432–440.

49. **Ikeda, H., K. Aoki, and A. Naito.** 1982. Illegitimate recombination mediated *in vitro* by DNA gyrase of *Escherichia coli*: structure of recombinant DNA molecules. *Proc. Natl. Acad. Sci. USA* **79:**3724–3728.

50. **Jeenes, D. J., and P. A. Williams.** 1982. Excision and integration of degradative pathway genes from TOL plasmid pWW0. *J. Bacteriol.* **150:**188–194.

51. **Kaneko, T., S. Sato, H. Kotani, A. Tanaka, E. Asamizu, Y. Nakamura, N. Miyajima, M. Hirosawa, M. Sugiura, S. Sasamoto, T. Kimura, T. Hosouchi, A. Matsuno, A. Muraki, N. Nakazaki, K. Naruo, S. Okumura, S. Shimpo, C. Takeuchi, T. Wada, A. Watanabe, M. Yamada, M. Yasuda, and S. Tabata.** 1996. Sequence analysis of the genome of the unicellular cyanobacterium *Synechocystis* sp. strain PCC6803. II. Sequence determination of the entire genome and assignment of potential protein-coding regions. *DNA Res.* **3:**109–136.

52. **Kirchner, J., C. M. Connolly, and S. B. Sandmeyer.** 1995. Requirement of RNA polymerase III transcription factors for *in vitro* position-specific integration of a retroviruslike element. *Science* **267:**1488–1491.

53. **Kleerebezem, M., L. E. Quadri, and O. P. Kuipers de Vos.** 1997. Quorum sensing by peptide pheromones and two component signal-transduction systems in Gram-positive bacteria. *Mol. Microbiol.* **24:**895–904.

54. **Kolter, R., D. A. Siegele, and A. Tormo.** 1993. The stationary phase of the bacterial life cycle. *Annu. Rev. Microbiol.* **47:**855–874.

55. **Kowalczykowski, S. C., D. A. Dixon, A. K. Eggleston, S. D. Lauder, and W. M. Rehrauer.** 1994. Biochemistry of homologous recombination in *Escherichia coli. Microbiol. Rev.* **58:** 401–465.

56. **Kunst, F., N. Ogasawara, I. Moszer, A. M. Albertini, G. Alloni, V. Azevedo, M. G. Bertero, P. Bessieres, A. Bolotin, S. Borchert, R. Borriss, L. Boursier, A. Brans, M. Braun, S. C. Brignell, S. Bron, S. Brouillet, C. V. Bruschi, B. Caldwell, V. Capuano, N. M. Carter, S. K. Choi, J. J. Codani, I. F. Connerton, and A. Danchin.** 1997. The complete genome sequence of the gram-positive bacterium *Bacillus subtilis. Nature* **390:**249–256.

57. **Landy, A.** 1990. Dynamic, structural and regulatory aspects of λ site-specific recombination. *Annu. Rev. Biochem.* **58:**913–949.

58. **Lawrence, J. G.** 1997. Selfish operons and speciation by gene transfer. *Trends Microbiol.* **5:**355–359.

59. **Loewen, P. C., and R. Hengge-Aronis.** 1994. The role of the sigma factor sigma S (KatF) in bacterial global regulation. *Annu. Rev. Microbiol.* **48:**53–80.

60. **Loveless, B. J., and M. H. Saier.** 1997. A novel family of channel-forming, autotransporting, bacterial virulence factors. *Mol. Membr. Biol.* **14:**113–123.

61. **Maenhaut-Michel, G., C. E. Blake, D. R. F. Leach, and J. A. Shapiro.** 1997. Different structures of selected and unselected *araB-lacZ* fusions. *Mol. Microbiol.* **23:**1133–146.

62. **Maenhaut-Michel, G., and J. A. Shapiro.** 1994. The roles of starvation and selective substrates in the emergence of *araB-lacZ* fusion clones. *EMBO J.* **13:**5229–5239.

63. **McClintock, B.** 1984. Significance of responses of the genome to challenge. *Science* **226:**792–801.

64. **Menard, R., C. Dehio, and P. J. Sansonetti.** 1996. Bacterial entry into epithelial cells: the paradigm of *Shigella. Trends Microbiol.* **4:**220–226.

65. **Mergeay, M., A. Sadouk, L. Diels, M. Faelen, J. Gerits, J. Denecke, and B. Powell.** 1986. High level spontaneous mutagenesis revealed by survival at non–optimal temperature in *Alcaligenes eutrophus* CH34. *Arch. Int. Physiol. Biochim.* **95:**36.

66. **Mittler, J., and R. E. Lenski.** 1990. Further experiments on excisions of Mu from *Escherichia coli* MCS2 cast doubt on directed mutation hypothesis. *Nature* **344:**173–175.

67. **Mizuuchi, K.** 1992. Transpositional recombination: mechanistic insights from studies of Mu

and other elements. *Annu. Rev. Biochem.* **61:** 1011–1051.

68. **Naas, T., M. Blot, W. M. Fitch, and W. Arber.** 1995. Dynamics of IS-related genetic rearrangements in resting *Escherichia coli* K-12. *Mol. Biol. Evol.* **12:**198–207.

69. **Pesci, E. C., and B. H. Iglewski.** 1997. The chain of command in *Pseudomonas* quorum sensing. *Trends Microbiol.* **5:**132–134.

70. **Peters, J. E., and S. A. Benson.** 1995. Redundant transfer of F′ plasmids occurs between *Escherichia coli* cells during nonlethal selection. *J. Bacteriol.* **177:**847–850.

71. **Portnoy, D. A., and R. J. Martinez.** 1985. Role of a plasmid in the pathogenicity of *Yersinia* species. *Curr. Top. Microbiol. Immunol.* **118:**29–51.

72. **Ptashne, M. 1986.** *A Genetic Switch.* Cell/Blackwell, Cambridge, Mass.

73. **Radicella, J. P., Park P. U., and Fox M. S.** 1995. Adaptive mutation in *Escherichia coli:* a role for conjugation. *Science* **268:**418–420.

74. **Recchia, G. D., and R. Hall.** 1995. Gene cassettes: a new class of mobile element. *Microbiology* **141:**3015–3027.

75. **Reddy, B. R., L. E. Shaw, J. R. Sayers, and P. A. Williams.** 1994. Two identical copies of IS1246, a 1275 base pair sequence related to other bacterial insertion sequences, enclose the *xyl* genes on TOL plasmid pWW0. *Microbiology* **140:**2305–2307.

76. **Restrepo, B. I., and A. G. Barbour.** 1994. Antigen diversity in the bacterium *B. hermsii* through "somatic" mutations in rearranged *vmp* genes. *Cell* **78:**867–876.

77. **Reznikoff, W. S.** 1992. The lactose operon-controlling elements: a complex paradigm. *Mol. Microbiol.* **6:**2419–2422.

78. **Rosenberg, S. M., R. S. Harris, and J. Torkelson.** 1995. Molecular handles on adaptive mutation. *Mol. Microbiol.* **18:**185–189.

79. **Rosenberg, S. M., S. Longerich, P. Gee, and R. S. Harris.** 1994. Adaptive mutation by deletion in small mononucleotide repeats. *Science* **265:**405–407.

80. **Saier, M. H., Jr., T. M. Ramseier, and J. Reizer.** 1996. Regulation of carbon utilization, p. 1325–1343. *In* F.C. Neidhardt, R. Curtiss, III, J. L. Ingraham, E. C. C. Lin, K. B. Low, Jr., B. Magasanik, W. S. Reznikoff, M. Riley, M. Schaechter, and H. E. Umbarger (ed.), *Escherichia coli and Salmonella: Cellular and Molecular Biology,* 2nd ed. American Society for Microbiology, Washington, D.C.

81. **Salmond, G. P. C., B. W. Bycroft, G. S. A. B. Stewart, and P. Williams.** 1995. The bacterial "enigma": cracking the code of cell-cell communication. *Mol. Microbiol.* **16:**615–624.

82. **Shapiro, J.** 1979. A molecular model for the transposition and replication of bacteriophage Mu and other transposable elements. *Proc. Natl. Acad. Sci. USA.* **76:**1933–1937.

83. **Shapiro, J. A.** 1982. Mobile genetic elements and reorganization of prokaryotic genomes, p. 9–32. *In* Y. Ikeda and T. Beppu (ed.), *Genetics of Industrial Microorganisms.* Kodansha, Tokyo.

84. **Shapiro, J. A. (ed.).** 1983. *Mobile Genetic Elements.* Academic Press, New York.

85. **Shapiro, J. A.** 1984. Observations on the formation of clones containing *araB-lacZ* cistron fusions. *Mol. Gen. Genet.* **194:**79–90.

86. **Shapiro, J. A.** 1991. Genomes as smart systems. *Genetica* **84:**3–4.

87. **Shapiro, J. A.** 1992. Natural genetic engineering in evolution. *Genetica* **86:**99–111.

88. **Shapiro, J. A.** 1993. A role for the Clp protease in activating Mu-mediated DNA rearrangements. *J. Bacteriol.* **175:**2625–2631.

89. **Shapiro, J. A.** 1995. The discovery and significance of mobile genetic elements, p. 1–17. *In* D. J. Sherratt (ed.), *Mobile Genetic Elements—Frontiers in Molecular Biology.* IRL Press, Oxford.

90. **Shapiro, J. A.** 1997. Genome organization, natural genetic engineering, and adaptive mutation. *Trends Genet.* **13:**98–104.

91. **Shapiro, J. A., and D. Leach.** 1990. Action of a transposable element in coding sequence fusions. *Genetics* **126:**293–299.

92. **Silverman, P. M., S. Rother, and H. Gaudin.** 1991. Arc and Sfr functions of the *Escherichia coli*K-12 *arcA* gene product are genetically and physiologically separable. *J. Bacteriol.* **173:**5648–5652.

93. **Sisco, K. L., and H. O. Smith.** 1979. Sequence-specific DNA uptake in *Haemophilus* transformation. *Proc. Natl. Acad. Sci. USA* **76:**972–976.

94. **Smith, H. O., J. F. Tomb, B. A. Dougherty, R. D. Fleischmann, and J. C. Venter.** 1995. Frequency and distribution of DNA uptake signal sequences in the *Haemophilus influenzae* Rd genome. *Science* **269:**538–540.

95. **Stark, W. M., M. R. Boocock, and D. J. Sherratt.** 1989. Catalysis by site-specific recombinases. *Trends Genet.* **8:**432–439.

96. **Stock, J. B., A. M. Stock, and J. M. Mottonen.** 1990. Signal transduction in bacteria. *Nature* **344:**395–400.

97. **Swanson, J., and J. M. Koomey.** 1989. Mechanisms for variation of pili and outer membrane protein II in *Neisseria gonorrhoeae*, p. 743–762. *In* D. E. Berg and M. M. Howe (ed.), *Mobile DNA.*

American Society for Microbiology, Washington, D.C.

98. **Swift, S., N. J. Bainton, and M. K. Winson.** 1994. Gram-negative bacterial communication by N-acyl homoserine lactones: a universal language? *Trends Microbiol.* **2:**193–198.

99. **Taghavi, S., M. Mergeay, and D. van der Lelie.** 1997. Genetic and physical maps of the *Alcaligenes eutrophus* CH34 megaplasmid pMOL28 and its derivative pMOL50 obtained after temperature-induced mutagenesis and mortality. *Plasmid* **37:**22–34.

100. **Tomb, J. F., O. White, A. R. Kerlavage, R. A. Clayton, G. G. Sutton, R. D. Fleischmann, K. A. Ketchum, H. P. Klenk, S. Gill, B. A. Dougherty, K. Nelson, J. Quackenbush, L. Zhou, E. F. Kirkness, S. Peterson, B. Loftus, D. Richardson, R. Dodson, H. G. Khalak, A. Glodek, K. McKenney, L. M. Fitzegerald, N. Lee, M. D. Adams, and J. C. Venter.** 1997. The complete genome sequence of the gastric pathogen *Helicobacter pylori. Nature* **388:**539–547.

101. **Torkelson, J., R. S. Harris, M.-J. Lombardo, J. Nagendran, C. Thulin, and S. M. Rosenberg.** 1997. Genome-wide hypermutation in a subpopulation of stationary-phase cells underlies recombination-dependent adaptive mutation. *EMBO J.* **16:**3303–3311.

102. **van der Lelie, D., A. Sadouk, A. Ferhat, S. Taghavi, A. Toussaint, and M. Mergeay.** 1992. Stress and survival in *Alcaligenes eutrophus* CH34: effects of temperature and genetic rearrangements, p. 27–32. *In* M. J. Gauthier (ed.), *Gene Transfers and Environment.* Springer Verlag, Heidelberg.

103. **van der Meer, J. R.** 1997. Evolution of novel metabolic pathways for the degradation of chloroaromatic compounds. *Antonie van Leeuwenhoek* **71:**159–178.

104. **Villarejo, M., P. J. Zamenhof, and I. Zabin.** 1972. Beta-galactosidase. In vivo α-complementation. *J. Biol. Chem.* **247:**2212–2216.

105. **Vogel, J. L., Z. J. Li, M. M. Howe, A. Toussaint, and N. P. Higgins.** 1991. Temperature-sensitive mutations in the bacteriophage Mu *c* repressor locate a 63-amino-acid DNA-binding domain. *J. Bacteriol.* **173:**6568–6577.

106. **Waldor, M. K., and J. J. Mekalanos.** 1996. Lysogenic conversion by a filamentous phage encoding cholera toxin. *Science* **272:**1910–1914.

107. **Walker, G.** 1996. The SOS response of *Escherichia coli*, p. 1400–1416. *In* F. C. Neidhardt, R. Curtiss III, J. L. Ingraham, E. C. C. Lin, K. B. Low, Jr., B. Magasanik, W. S. Reznikoff, M. Riley, M. Schaechter, and H. E. Umbarger (ed.), *Escherichia coli and Salmonella: Cellular and Molecular Biology*, 2nd ed. American Society for Microbiology, Washington, D.C.

108. **Watanabe, T.** 1963. Infective heredity of multiple drug resistance in bacteria. *Bacteriol. Rev.* **27:**87–115.

109. **Whoriskey, S. K., V. H. Nghiem, P. M. Leong, J. M. Masson, and J. H. Miller.** 1987. Genetic rearrangements and gene amplification in *Escherichia coli:* DNA sequences at the junctures of amplified gene fusions. *Genes Dev.* **1:**227–237.

110. **Williams, P. A., and J. R. Sayers.** 1994. The evolution of pathways for aromatic hydrocarbon oxidation in *Pseudomonas. Biodegradation* **5:**195–217.

111. **Wirth, R., A. Muscholl, and G. Wanner.** 1996. The role of pheromones in bacterial interactions. *Trends Microbiol.* **4:**96–103.

112. **Wyndham, R. C., A. E. Cashore, C. H. Nakatsu, and M. C. Peel.** 1994. Catabolic transposons. *Biodegradation* **5:**323–342.

113. **Yang, W., and K. Mizuuchi.** 1997. Site-specific recombination in plane view. *Structure* **5:**1401–1406.

114. **Zhang, J. R., J. M. Hardham, A. G. Barbour, and S. J. Norris.** 1997. Antigenic variation in Lyme disease borreliae by promiscuous recombination of VMP-like sequence cassettes. *Cell* **89:**275–285.

MULTIDRUG RESISTANCE TRANSPORTERS IN *ESCHERICHIA COLI*

Eitan Bibi, Rotem Edgar, Oded Béjà,
Yael Meller-Harel, and Iris Hillel

22

TRANSPORT-MEDIATED MULTIDRUG RESISTANCE

Multidrug resistance occurs when eukaryotic or prokaryotic cells become simultaneously resistant to a large number of both structurally and functionally unrelated cytotoxic compounds. One major form of multidrug resistance is caused by the overexpression of membrane transport proteins termed Mdr. Recently, a variety of multidrug resistance efflux systems have been found to be widely distributed in bacteria, including some pathogenic species (19, 20, 31, 36, 37). These resistance systems are associated with four different families of transport proteins: the major facilitator superfamily (MFS) (27), the resistance-nodulation-division (RND) family (41), the SMR family (38), and one Mdr protein from *Lactococcus lactis* (45) that belongs to the ATP-binding cassette (ABC) superfamily (16) and is probably driven by ATP hydrolysis. Proteins from the SMR and RND families were identified only in prokaryotes, and RND proteins are found exclusively in gram-negative species. The transporters of the MFS, RND, and SMR groups are usually driven by the transmembrane proton electrochemical gradient as demonstrated with intact cells using ionophores (7, 11, 14, 22, 23). All Mdr proteins except those of the RND family apparently function as independent cytoplasmic transport units, although functional reconstitution of purified proteins has been performed in only a limited number of cases (15, 46). In general, the broad substrate specificity and ability of the prokaryotic multidrug resistance transporters to extrude a variety of unrelated drugs from the cell is similar to P-glycoprotein-mediated multidrug resistance in mammalian systems (12, 13); both recognize lipophilic compounds, many of which tend to be positively charged under physiological conditions. However, many of the bacterial Mdr proteins also interact with neutral drugs, some of which are relatively hydrophilic, and there are transporters that most probably export lipophilic anionic drugs (32). Therefore, in addition to their potential clinical importance, the multispecific Mdr proteins pose intriguing questions concerning their transport mechanism.

There are still no conclusive descriptions regarding some major aspects of the transport-related multidrug resistance phenomenon. As previously described, each Mdr protein can

Eitan Bibi, Rotem Edgar, Oded Béjà, Yael Meller-Harel, and Iris Hillel, Department of Biological Chemistry, Weizmann Institute of Science, Rehovot 76100, Israel.

Microbial Ecology and Infectious Disease, Edited by Eugene Rosenberg
©1999 American Society for Microbiology, Washington, D.C.

handle an extremely broad spectrum of chemically unrelated species, a property that cannot be found in many non-Mdr solute transport systems. Putative models have been designed that attempt to explain this unusual property of Mdr proteins (8, 43), such as the obvious suggestion that their drug-binding pocket is flexible in structure or conformation and thus able to accommodate several structurally different compounds. However, this and many other explanations are still unproven. Moreover, the mechanism of action of multidrug transporters in general remains largely not understood, especially concerning the driving force and how is it coupled stoichiometrically to the export process (43). With several Mdr proteins that are able to export both positively charged and neutral drugs, this issue becomes even more complicated because the transport process may be electrogenic with one substrate and electroneutral with the other or, alternatively, if the Mdr protein is a proton/drug antiporter, it may exchange one substrate for more protons than the other substrate. To understand these questions fully, it is essential to analyze the transport process with purified Mdr proteins reconstituted into liposomes. In addition to these mechanistic questions, the normal functions of Mdr proteins and their physiological substrates are still generally unknown, although recent studies may support the concept that some Mdr proteins may exhibit preferences toward distinct physiological substrates (30). However, since knockout experiments in bacteria usually did not reveal clear phenotypes, studying this aspect is like searching for a needle in a haystack. Recent phylogenetic evaluations have indicated that Mdr proteins have evolved through only a few primordial systems, relatively early in evolution. Since then, these proteins have been subjected to frequent modulations that have primarily affected their substrate recognition patterns (40). These results are more consistent with the proposal that the physiological role of Mdr proteins may indeed be related to drug resistance, i.e., protection against toxic materials in the environment.

MULTIDRUG TRANSPORTERS IN *E. COLI*

A homology search of the *Escherichia coli* genome with known drug translocator genes has led to identification of 29 putative drug transporters (40), of which only 10 were tested and proved to be single-drug transporters (11, 33, 36, 40). Moreover, this group of characterized *E. coli* drug transporters contains only seven members, which so far have been shown to confer multidrug resistance and belong to either (i) the SMR family: EmrE (28, 39, 42), (ii) the RND family: AcrB and AcrF (17, 25), or (iii) the MFS family: EmrB, Bcr, EmrD, and MdfA (5, 11, 24, 29). Involvement of the two putative *E. coli* Mdr proteins of the ABC superfamily in multidrug efflux has not been shown. Proteins of the RND family are probably different from the other Mdr transporters in *E. coli*, because they require helper periplasmic and outer membrane proteins for proper in vivo function (10). Together, the *E. coli* Mdr proteins cover a wide spectrum of drugs including many known and clinically useful antibiotics.

Some transporters are more specific and recognize, under physiological conditions, only lipophilic cations (EmrE) (46), uncharged compounds, or weak acids (EmrB, EmrD) (21). Others recognize both neutral and positively charged drugs and, to a lesser extent, hydrophilic compounds (MdfA) (11); unexpectedly, some of the transporters confer resistance against both positive and negative lipophilic ions (AcrB) (32). An intriguing phenomenon is the ability of the RND complex AcrAB to confer resistance to β-lactam antibiotics that do not normally enter the cytoplasm and execute their antibiotic activity in the periplasmic space. However, it is important to obtain direct evidence for the β-lactam efflux by the purified AcrB transporter reconstituted into liposomes to demonstrate active extrusion of these compounds from the cytosol or the membrane bilayer (32). Theoretically, there is also an interesting, purely speculative possibility that the Acr system may be able to remove these drugs from the periplasm and export them across the outer membrane.

The physiological role of the *E. coli* Mdr proteins and Mdr proteins in general is frequently questioned and was discussed in detail in a recent review by Neyfakh (30). One possible way to test their role is by studying *mdr* knockout mutants. However, in a limited number of cases in which knockout mutants have been studied, the deleted strains that became somewhat more susceptible to drugs were otherwise indistinguishable from their wild-type counterpart parent. Mutation in the *acr* locus renders *E. coli* supersensitive to large lipophilic agents such as acriflavine (25). Moreover, a null mutation in another *E. coli* RND complex, the *acrEF* locus, does not reveal any specific phenotypes (26). Knockout of the *mdfA* gene (Edgar, Hillel, and Bibi, unpublished data) led to ethidium sensitivity, but this is the only apparent phenotype of the deleted strain.

Another approach to studying the physiological role of Mdr proteins is to identify the mechanism by which their expression is regulated. More specifically, if the expression of a single Mdr protein is induced by a variety of agents that are also substrates of the transporter, this supports the notion that multidrug resistance is its primary physiological role. In some cases, it was demonstrated that this was so, and the expression of several Mdr proteins in *E. coli* is regulated and influenced by the corresponding drugs or their consequent toxicity. For example, expression of the uncoupler resistance protein EmrD can be induced by a low-energy shock caused by adding uncouplers (29), and experiments with the grampositive bacterium *Bacillus subtilis* have clearly demonstrated overlapping profiles of substrate specificities between the Mdr protein (Bmr) and its expression activator BmrR (1). In fact, certain strategies of multidrug resistance in *E. coli* are also induced by global regulatory systems, of which the *marRAB* locus is also of particular relevance to the transport-mediated multidrug resistance phenomenon in *E. coli* (9).

Finally, recent observations have suggested that other transport proteins in *E. coli*, not belonging to the three major families previously described, may also be able to confer multidrug resistance. The TehA protein, originally identified as a tellurite-resistance determinant together with TehB, was found to be able to confer substantial levels of resistance to a few unrelated lipophilic cations (44). TehA was modeled as a 10-transmembrane-segment (TMs) protein, but the C-terminal three TMs are not required for the multidrug resistance function of TehA. The TehA Mdr activity may possibly be explained by the borderline homology between the central part of the protein (TMs 2–5) with Mdr proteins of the SMR family such as EmrE (21.8% with long gaps). However, this seems unlikely because another protein in *E. coli*, SugE, which exhibits higher homology with EmrE (40% with no gaps), does not confer resistance to a variety of toxic compounds (Edgar and Bibi, unpublished data). Moreover, the expression of TehA causes methyl viologen sensitivity, whereas EmrE confers resistance to this compound (46). Anyway, the TehA-mediated multidrug resistance reflects other modes by which bacteria can extend their drug resistance capabilities.

STRUCTURAL ASPECTS OF MULTIDRUG RESISTANCE PROTEINS IN *E. COLI*

Although representatives of all three groups of *E. coli* Mdr proteins (see above) exhibit similar transport activities that are similarly driven by the proton electrochemical potential and possess overlapping substrate recognition profiles, they have different primary and secondary structures. The larger proteins are AcrB and AcrF, which contain 1,049 and 1,034 residues, respectively. Their membrane topology has not yet been analyzed experimentally, but predictions based on their hydropathy profiles and sequence alignments suggest that they cross the membrane 12 times with two very long and hydrophilic periplasmic domains connecting TM1-2 and TM7-8 (36). Since

AcrB and AcrF both require periplasmic proteins for their function (MFP proteins) (10), these periplasmic loops possibly interact with the periplasmic subunits. As already mentioned, we can speculate that these loops may interact with some drugs (e.g., β-lactams), thus presenting them to the outer membrane export pathway. Since, with the exception of these loops, the organization of AcrB and AcrF in the membrane is similar to proteins of the MFS, the membrane segments possibly compose the active domain that removes toxic compounds from the cytosol or from the lipid bilayer to the periplasmic domains.

As previously mentioned, four characterized Mdr proteins in *E. coli* belong to the MFS, three of which (Bcr, EmrD, and MdfA) exhibit 12 putative TMs, and only one (EmrB) having two additional TMs, which for sequence similarity considerations probably presents a single evolutionary event through which two foreign TMs were inserted in the middle of a 12-TM transporter. Note that the actual topology of the MFS-related Mdr proteins in *E. coli* has not yet been analyzed experimentally. The 12-TM model is based on the hydrophobicity plot and the limited similarity with some better-characterized specific drug transporters (such as TetA from pBR322, reference 2), and the 14-TM structure of EmrB is based both on its hydrophobicity and its similarity to the *Staphylococcus aureus* Mdr protein QacA, which probably has 14 TMs (35). It is not known whether the additional TM pair in EmrB (and the other 14-TM proteins) is important for active transport, since sequence alignment revealed similarity only between the rest of the protein and the 12-TM Mdr proteins.

EmrE, which represents the third type of *E. coli* Mdr proteins, is unique among transport systems in general and Mdr proteins in particular. It is only 110 amino acid residues long and is proposed to cross the membrane four times (similar to its close homolog QacC, reference 34), with about 80% of its polypeptide chain α-helical and embedded in the lipid bilayer (3). An important structurally related question is what is the oligomeric organization of functional EmrE, because it is very small and, like certain ion channels, may form an oligomeric drug pathway. Results of dominant-negative experiments support an oligomeric organization (47), possibly with a trimeric structure, which may lead to a 12-TM-like transporter, but this proposal remains to be proven. It is interesting that the 12-TM motif seems to return in one version or another in all three groups of *E. coli* Mdr proteins.

Finally, there is nothing special in the primary or secondary structures of the Mdr proteins (except for a very short signature [36]) compared with other solute transport proteins, and it appears that their unusually broad substrate recognition profiles is due to a distinct three-dimensional organization that may have similar properties in different Mdr proteins.

FUNCTIONAL ASPECTS OF MULTIDRUG RESISTANCE PROTEINS IN *E. COLI*

Among all *E. coli* Mdr proteins, only EmrE has been purified, reconstituted in liposomes, and shown to be solely capable of mediating H^+/drug antiport activity across the lipid bilayer (46). For functional analysis, it is important to accomplish similar studies with the MFS-related Mdr proteins, but even more crucial to perform such studies with AcrB and AcrF, where periplasmic components may have a role in transport. From experiments with intact cells expressing Mdr proteins, it can be concluded that all of the characterized *E. coli* proteins are probably driven by the proton electrochemical gradient. With the RND-related transport complex AcrAB, Ma et al. (25) compared acriflavin uptake by intact wild-type cells and cells carrying an *acr* mutation (N43) and tested the effect of carbonyl cyanide *m*-chlorophenylhydrazone (CCCP), which dissipates the proton electrochemical gradient, on acriflavin accumulation. Prior to adding CCCP, the mutated strain accumulated acriflavin to a level about 10-fold higher than the wild-type cells. CCCP abolished this difference and increased acriflavin uptake in both cell types to a similar level, indicating the presence of an alternative acriflavin export system(s) in *E. coli*.

With the MFS-related Mdr transporters of *E. coli*, only MdfA was shown to utilize the proton electrochemical gradient as an energy source for drug export. Chloramphenicol accumulation in cells expressing MdfA is substantially lower than that in control cells with an insertless vector, and the uncoupler CCCP caused a rapid increase in chloramphenicol uptake in both cell types (33). As with AcrAB, the most probable explanation for the effect of CCCP is that *E. coli* has, in addition to MdfA, another chloramphenicol export system(s) also driven by the proton electrochemical potential. To investigate in detail the driving force of the transport activity of MdfA, the effect of several energy sources on drug efflux was analyzed (11). In these experiments, ethidium bromide transport experiments were conducted using an *unc⁻* derivative of *E. coli* UTL2 (4) that lacks a functional F_1-F_0-ATPase (6). It was shown that glucose is unable to energize ethidium efflux in *unc⁻* cells. By contrast, addition of the nonfermentable carbon sources D-lactate or succinate sufficed to energize the ethidium bromide efflux, as expected if ATP is not required for active efflux by MdfA. Moreover, inhibition of respiration by cyanide (which blocks the generation of the proton electrochemical gradient, but does not affect ATP production in *unc⁻* cells) abrogates efflux activity completely. Overall, although these experiments clearly indicated that MdfA is driven by the proton electrochemical potential, it is essential to reconstitute the purified protein into liposomes for direct demonstration and analysis of requirements for pH gradient and/or electrical potential.

Such an analysis has been performed with EmrE, the *E. coli* representative of the small Mdr translocators (46). First it was shown that liposomes reconstituted with EmrE in the presence of NH_4Cl and DNA are able to accumulate ethidium bromide when diluted into NH_4Cl-free buffer and that this function is abolished upon ΔpH depletion by nigericin. Second, the transport of radiolabeled methyl viologen into the proteoliposomes against a concentration gradient also depended on ΔpH. In conclusion, these studies have confirmed that EmrE is a proton/drug antiporter, and for analyzing the exact stoichiometry, the protein has to be purified to homogeneity and reconstituted into liposomes.

As stated above, one of the most puzzling properties of Mdr transporters is their ability to handle a variety of structurally dissimilar compounds. Therefore, an important research program would be to search for amino acid residues located in the drug translocation pathway of Mdr proteins. In *E. coli*, such a detailed study has so far been described only with EmrE. In this study, Lebendiker and Schuldiner (18) performed cysteine accessibility assays (using sulfhydryl-reactive agents) and proposed that there is a drug-specific translocation pathway in EmrE and that the cysteine residues at positions 41 and 95 are oriented toward the pathway. A few point mutations that abrogated transport activity were also generated in EmrE (47). Among these point mutations, Glu-14 is particularly interesting because it is the only charged residue inside the membrane-embedded sequence of EmrE. Moreover, since a negative charge at this position is conserved in all SMR proteins, it may have an important role. Indeed, although the mutant E14C of EmrE is expressed at a level similar to that of wild type, it is unable to confer resistance to various drugs or to affect drug accumulation, suggesting that E14 is essential. Recently, we have noticed that other drug transporters also have a negatively charged residue at a similar position inside putative TM 1 (Edgar and Bibi, unpublished data). In fact, in the MFS protein MdfA, this residue (E26) is also the only charged residue inside the proposed membrane-embedded segments of the protein. Unlike EmrE, MdfA recognizes both positively charged drugs (e.g., ethidium) and neutral drugs (e.g., chloramphenicol), so it is important to compare the effect of a mutation at this position on the transport of these drugs. In conclusion, our understanding of the broad specificity exhibited by the *E. coli* Mdr proteins is still very vague, and in addition to structural information, extensive molecular biological and biochemical investigation is required.

ACKNOWLEDGMENT

Research in our laboratory is supported by the MINERVA Foundation, Munich, Germany, and by the Israel Cancer Research Fund.

REVIEWS AND KEY PAPERS

Bolhuis, H., H. W. van Veen, B. Poolman, A. J. M. Driessen, and W. N. Konings. 1997. Mechanisms of multidrug transporters. *FEMS Microbiol. Rev.* **21:**55–84.

Gottesman, M. M., I. Pastan, and S. V. Ambudkar. 1996. P-Glycoprotein and multidrug resistance. *Curr. Opin. Genet. Dev.* **6:**610–617

Hancock, R. E. W. 1997. The bacterial outer membrane as a drug barrier. *Trends Microbiol.* **5:** 37–42.

Levy, S. B. 1992. Active efflux mechanisms for antimicrobial resistance. *Antimicrob. Agents Chemother.* **36:**695–703.

Neyfakh, A. A. 1997. Natural functions of bacterial multidrug transporters. *Trends Microbiol.* **5:**309–313.

Nikaido, H. 1996. Multidrug efflux pumps of gram-negative bacteria. *J. Bacteriol.* **178:**5853–5859.

Paulsen, I. T., M. H. Brown, and R. A. Skurray. 1996. Proton-dependent multidrug efflux systems. *Microbiol. Rev.* **60:**575–608.

Paulsen, I. T., R. A. Skurray, R. Tam, M. H. Saier, Jr., R. J. Turner, J. H. Weiner, E. B. Goldberg, and L. L. Grinius. 1996. The SMR family: a novel family of multidrug efflux proteins involved with the efflux of lipophilic drugs. *Mol. Microbiol.* **19:**1167–1175.

Saier, M. H., Jr., I. T. Paulsen, M. K. Sliwinski, S. S. Pao, R. A. Skurray, and H. Nikaido. 1998. Evolutionary origins of multidrug and drug-specific efflux pumps in bacteria. *FASEB J.* **12:** 265–274.

Schuldiner, S., M. Lebendiker, and H. Yerushalmi. 1997. EmrE, the smallest ion-coupled transporter, provides a unique paradigm for structure-function studies. *J. Exp. Biol.* **200:**335–341.

REFERENCES

1. Ahmed, M., C. M. Borsch, S. S. Taylor, N. Vazquez-Laslop, and A. A. Neyfakh. 1994. A protein that activates expression of a multidrug efflux transporter upon binding the transporter substrates. *J. Biol. Chem.* **269:**28506–28513.

2. Allard, J. D., and K. P. Bertrand. 1992. Membrane topology of the pBR322 tetracycline resistance protein. TetA-PhoA gene fusions and implications for the mechanism of TetA membrane insertion. *J. Biol. Chem.* **267:**17809–17819.

3. Arkin, I., W. Russ, M. Lebendiker, and S. Schuldiner. 1996. Determining the secondary structure and orientation of EmrE, a multi-drug transporter, indicates a transmembrane four-helix bundle. *Biochemistry* **35:**7233–7238.

4. Béjà, O., and E. Bibi. 1996. Functional expression of mouse Mdr1 in a membrane permeability mutant of *Escherichia coli. Proc. Natl. Acad. Sci. USA* **93:**5969–5964.

5. Bentley, J., L. S. Hyatt, K. Ainley, J. H. Parish, R. B. Herbert, and G. R. White. 1993. Cloning and sequence analysis of an *Escherichia coli* gene conferring bicyclomycin resistance. *Gene* **15:**117–120.

6. Bibi, E., R. Edgar, and O. Béjà. 1998. Expression of eukaryotic ABC proteins in *Escherichia coli. Methods Enzymol.* **292:**370–382.

7. Bolhuis H., H. W. van Veen, J. R. Brands, M. Putman, B. Poolman, A. J. M. Driessen, and W. N. Konings. 1996. Energetics and mechanism of drug transport mediated by the lactococcal multidrug transporter LmrP. *J. Biol. Chem.* **271:**24123–24128.

8. Bolhuis, H., H. W. van Veen, B. Poolman, A. J. M. Driessen, and W. N. Konings. 1997. Mechanisms of multidrug transporters. *FEMS Microbiol. Rev.* **21:**55–84.

9. Cohen, S. P., H. Hachler, and S. B. Levy. 1993. Genetic and functional analysis of the multiple antibiotic resistance (*mar*) locus in *Escherichia coli. J. Bacteriol.* **175:**1484–1492.

10. Dinh, T., I. T. Paulsen, and M. H. Saier, Jr. 1994. A family of extracytoplasmic proteins that allow transport of large molecules across the outer membranes of gram-negative bacteria. *J. Bacteriol.* **176:**3825–3831.

11. Edgar, R., and E. Bibi. 1997. MdfA, an *Escherichia coli* multidrug resistance protein with an extraordinary broad spectrum of drug recognition. *J. Bacteriol.* **179:**2274–2280.

12. Gottesman, M. M., and I. Pastan. 1993. Biochemistry of multidrug resistance mediated by the multidrug transporter. *Annu. Rev. Biochem.* **62:**385–427.

13. Gottesman, M. M., I. Pastan, and S. V. Ambudkar. 1996. P-Glycoprotein and multidrug resistance. *Curr. Opin. Genet. Dev.* **6:**610–617.

14. **Grinius, L., G. Dreguniene, E. B. Goldberg, C. H. Liao, S. J. Projan.** 1992. A staphylococcal multidrug resistance gene product is a member of a new protein family. *Plasmid* **27:**119–129.

15. **Grinius, L. L., and E. B. Goldberg.** 1994. Bacterial multidrug resistance is due to a single membrane protein which functions as a drug pump. *J. Biol. Chem.* **269:**29998–30004.

16. **Higgins, C. F.** 1992. ABC transporters: from microorganisms to man. *Annu. Rev. Cell Biol.* **8:** 67–113.

17. **Klein, J. R., B. Henrich, and R. Plapp.** 1991. Molecular analysis and nucleotide sequence of the envCD operon of *Escherichia coli. Mol. Gen. Genet.* **230:**230–240.

18. **Lebendiker, M., and S. Schuldiner.** 1996. Identification of residues in the translocation pathway of EmrE, a multidrug antiporter from *Escherichia coli. J. Biol. Chem.* **271:**21193–21199.

19. **Levy, S. B.** 1992. Active efflux mechanisms for antimicrobial resistance. *Antimicrob. Agents Chemother.* **36:**695–703.

20. **Lewis, K.** 1994. Multidrug resistance pumps in bacteria: variations on a theme. *Trends Biochem. Sci.* **19:**119–123.

21. **Lewis, K., V. Naroditskaya, A. Ferrante, and I. Fokina.** 1994. Bacterial resistance to uncouplers. *J. Bioenerg. Biomembr.* **20:**639–646.

22. **Li, X. Z., D. Ma, D. M. Livermore, and H. Nikaido.** 1994. Role of efflux pump(s) in intrinsic resistance of *Pseudomonas aeruginosa*: active efflux as a contributing factor to beta-lactam resistance. *Antimicrob. Agents Chemother.* **38:**1742–1752.

23. **Littlejohn, T. G., I. T. Paulsen, M. T. Gillespie, J. M. Tennent, M. Midgley, I. G. Jones, A. S. Purewal, and R. A. Skurray.** 1992. Substrate specificity and energetics of antiseptic and disinfectant resistance in *Staphylococcus aureus. FEMS Microbiol. Lett.* **15:**259–265.

24. **Lomovskaya, O., and K. Lewis.** 1992. Emr, an *Escherichia coli* locus for multidrug resistance. *Proc. Natl. Acad. Sci. USA* **89:**8938–8942.

25. **Ma, D., D. N. Cook, M. Alberti, N. G. Pon, H. Nikaido, and J. E. Hearst.** 1993. Molecular cloning and characterization of acrA and acrE genes of *Escherichia coli. J. Bacteriol.* **175:**6299–6313.

26. **Ma, D., D. N. Cook, J. E. Hearst, and H. Nikaido.** 1994. Efflux pumps and drug resistance in Gram-negative bacteria. *Trends Microbiol.* **2:** 489–493.

27. **Marger, M. D., and M. H. Saier, Jr.** 1993. A major superfamily of transmembrane facilitators that catalyse uniport, symport and antiport. *Trends Biochem. Sci.* **18:**13–20.

28. **Morimoyo, M., E. Hongo, H. Hama-Inaba, and I. Machida.** 1992. Cloning and characterization of the mvrC gene of *Escherichia coli* K-12 which confers resistance against methyl viologen toxicity. *Nucleic Acids Res.* **20:**3159–3165.

29. **Naroditskaya, V., M. J. Schlosser, N. Y. Fang, and K. Lewis.** 1993. An *E. coli* gene emrD is involved in adaptation to low energy shock. *Biochem. Biophys. Res. Commun.* **196:**803–809.

30. **Neyfakh, A. A.** 1997. Natural functions of bacterial multidrug transporters. *Trends Microbiol.* **5:** 309–313.

31. **Nikaido, H.** 1994. Prevention of drug access to bacterial targets: permeability barriers and active efflux. *Science* **264:**382–388.

32. **Nikaido, H.** 1996. Multidrug efflux pumps of gram-negative bacteria. *J. Bacteriol.* **178:**5853–5859.

33. **Nilsen, I. W., I. Bakke, A. Vader, Ø. Olsvik, and M. R. El-Gewely.** 1996. Isolation of cmr, a novel *Escherichia coli* chloramphenicol resistance gene encoding a putative efflux pump. *J. Bacteriol.* **178:**3188–3193.

34. **Paulsen, I. T., M. H. Brown, S. J. Dunstan, and R. A. Skurray.** 1995. Molecular characterization of the staphylococcal multidrug resistance export protein QacC. *J. Bacteriol.* **177:**2827–2833.

35. **Paulsen, I. T., M. H. Brown, T. G. Littlejohn, B. A. Mitchell, and R. A. Skurray.** 1996. Multidrug resistance proteins QacA and QacB from *Staphylococcus aureus*: membrane topology and identification of residues involved in substrate specificity. *Proc. Natl. Acad. Sci. USA* **93:**3630–3635.

36. **Paulsen, I. T., M. H. Brown, and R. A. Skurray.** 1996. Proton-dependent multidrug efflux systems. *Microbiol. Rev.* **60:**575–608.

37. **Paulsen, I. T., and R. A. Skurray.** 1993. Topology, structure and evolution of two families of proteins involved in antibiotic and antiseptic resistance in eukaryotes and prokaryotes—an analysis. *Gene* **124:**1–11.

38. **Paulsen, I. T., R. A. Skurray, R. Tam, M. H. Saier, Jr., R. J. Turner, J. H. Weiner, E. B. Goldberg, and L. L. Grinius.** 1996. The SMR family: a novel family of multidrug efflux proteins involved with the efflux of lipophilic drugs. *Mol. Microbiol.* **19:**1167–1175.

39. **Purewal, A. S.** 1991. Nucleotide sequence of the ethidium efflux gene from *Escherichia coli. FEMS Microbiol. Lett.* **82:**229–232.

40. **Saier, M. H., Jr., I. T. Paulsen, M. K. Sliwinski, S. S. Pao, R. A. Skurray, and H. Nikaido.** 1998. Evolutionary origins of multi-

drug and drug-specific efflux pumps in bacteria. *FASEB J.* **12**:265–274.

41. **Saier, M. H., Jr., R. Tam, A. Reizer, and J. Reizer.** 1994. Two novel families of bacterial membrane proteins concerned with nodulation cell division and transport. *Mol. Microbiol.* **11:** 841–847.

42. **Schuldiner, S., M. Lebendiker, and H. Yerushalmi.** 1997. EmrE, the smallest ion-coupled transporter, provides a unique paradigm for structure-function studies. *J. Exp. Biol.* **200:** 335–341.

43. **Stein, W. D.** 1997. Kinetics of the multidrug transporter (P-glycoprotein) and its reversal. *Physiol. Rev.* **77:**545–590.

44. **Turner, R. J., D. E. Taylor, and J. H. Weiner.** 1997. Expression of *Escherichia coli* TehA gives resistance to antiseptics and disinfectants

similar to that conferred by multidrug resistance efflux pumps. *Antimicrob. Agents Chemother.* **41:** 440–444.

45. **van Veen, H. W., K. Venema, H. Bolhuis, I. Oussenko, J. Kok, B. Poolman, A. J. Driessen, and W. N. Konings.** 1996. Multidrug resistance mediated by a bacterial homolog of the human multidrug transporter MDR1. *Proc. Natl. Acad. Sci. USA* **93:**10668–10672.

46. **Yerushalmi, H., M. Lebendiker, and S. Schuldiner.** 1995. EmrE, an *Escherichia coli* 12-kDa multidrug transporter, exchanges toxic cations and H+ and is soluble in organic solvents. *J. Biol. Chem.* **270:**6856–6863.

47. **Yerushalmi, H., M. Lebendiker, and S. Schuldiner.** 1996. Negative dominance studies demonstrate the oligomeric structure of EmrE, a multidrug antiporter from *Escherichia coli*. *J. Biol. Chem.* **271:**31044–31048.

COMPLEX PATTERN FORMATION AND COOPERATIVE ORGANIZATION OF BACTERIAL COLONIES

David L. Gutnick and Eshel Ben-Jacob

23

The ability of microbes to colonize surfaces endows these organisms with important ecological advantages. It is not surprising, therefore, that there are few sterile surfaces (either biological or nonbiological) in nature. For example, the ability to grow on and quickly spread across a surface provides the population with a protected environment. In addition, adherent microbial populations are frequently more resistant to toxic elements such as heavy metals, xenobiotics, and antibiotics. This ability of microorganisms to distribute themselves over a surface is often reflected in the development of complex multicellular structures such as biofilms, microbial mats, or dense aggregates of heterogeneous populations (which, under appropriate conditions, often form unique patterns (see reference 52 and other chapters in this volume).

Pattern formation (55) has been observed in the development of various bacterial colonies, which display a rich variety of intricate morphologies and shapes, suggesting a level of organization and cellular communication that transcends the well-studied behavior of the individual cells. Although they have not yet been investigated in this context, such processes are likely to play major roles in various pathogenic processes, particularly in view of the importance of adhesion and growth at surfaces, which is frequently a key phase in microbial infection.

Here we describe results of complex patterning during growth of bacterial colonies under relatively "hostile" conditions of low nutrient levels and relatively hard agar surfaces; conditions in which classical bacterial chemotaxis is rarely observed. Under such conditions, which are frequently found in various natural ecosystems, complex colonial patterns have been observed (7–9, 14, 16, 19, 34, 44–50). By analogy with patterning in nonliving systems, pattern formation during colonial development can be viewed as a diffusion-limited process resulting from the low levels of growth substrate available to the growing cells. Indeed, for some conditions, bacterial colonies can develop patterns reminiscent of those observed during growth of diffusion limitation in nonliving systems, such as snowflake formation, electrochemical deposition, growth in a Hele-Shaw cell, etc. (5,

David L. Gutnick, Department of Molecular Microbiology and Biotechnology, George S. Wise Faculty of Life Sciences, Tel Aviv University, Tel Aviv 69978, Israel. *Eshel Ben-Jacob*, School of Physics and Astronomy, Raymond and Beverly Sackler Faculty of Exact Sciences, Tel Aviv University, Tel Aviv 69978, Israel.

Microbial Ecology and Infectious Disease, Edited by Eugene Rosenberg
©1999 American Society for Microbiology, Washington, D.C.

9, 12). It is commonly accepted that pattern formation in abiotic systems results in large part from a competition between the drive of the diffusion field on the one hand and a stabilizing counterforce operating at the microscopic scale (such as surface tension) on the other.

However, bacteria can exhibit richer behavior than that observed in abiotic patterning, which most likely reflects the additional levels of complexity involved. This may result in part from the development of sophisticated processes of communication and signal transduction that have been shown to play major roles not only in the physiological responses of the individual cell, but in the behavior of the population as a whole (35, 36, 39, 43, 51, 52, 56, and this volume). In bacterial pattern formation, the cells themselves are autonomous self-replicating organisms, each with its own self-interest and internal degrees of freedom. Nevertheless, efficient adaptation to adverse conditions most likely requires the kind of cooperative interactions that generate complex patterns such as those illustrated in Fig. 1. To study such processes, we have combined approaches from microbiology and microbial physiology, with a generic modeling approach designed to serve as a research tool. As we show below, the models suggest the interplay of several modes of cell-cell communication and chemotaxis that modulate the cellular dynamics, growth, and morphology of the colony.

MORPHOTYPES

Three patterns with different geometrical characteristics are shown in Fig. 1. The first shows a branching pattern. The second pattern also exhibits branching characteristics, but the branches are much thinner, and all have a twist with the same handedness. In the third pattern, every branch has a droplet of fluid at its tip and exhibits a whirlpool, or vortex, morphology. The droplet of fluid contains large numbers of cells frequently seen to rotate around a common center at many cell-lengths per second. When examined under the mi-

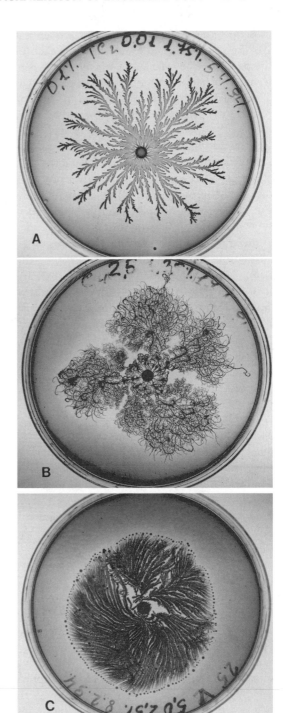

FIGURE 1 Representative examples of the colonial patterns generated by three morphotypes: T, C, V (Fig. 1A, B, C, respectively). (A) T (tip-splitting) morphotype, characteristic branching morphology. (B) C (chiral) morphotype; branched pattern showing thin branches, all twisted with the same handedness. (C) V (vortex) morphotype, each branch has a leading droplet composed of many cells moving in a correlated motion around the center.

croscope, the dynamics of cellular movement are also seen to be quite different for each of the patterns. We refer to the characteristic patterning properties of a microbial population as a *morphotype*. The patterns in Fig. 1 are representative patterns of the tip-splitting (T), chiral (C), and vortex (V) morphotypes, respectively. Different bacterial species can exhibit similar morphotype characteristics, although not necessarily under the same conditions. Moreover, as we show below, a strain can undergo a transition from one morphotype to another. This transition occurs under a specific set of conditions and requires an adaptation period of about 2 days. Once the new morphotype emerges from the pattern, it is genetically stable. Both pattern formation and morphotype transition appear to require modes of organized intercellular communication and cooperative interactions that are characteristic features of other cell-density-dependent phenomena currently under investigation in microbial physiology (see Greenberg, this volume).

MORPHOTYPE ORIGIN

The pattern-forming morphotypes shown in Fig. 1 were initially picked as very rare isolates from cultures of *Bacillus subtilis* strain 168 that were plated on thin hard agar surfaces (16, 19). Nevertheless, a variety of nutritional and biochemical characterizations demonstrated that these strains, although motile, aerobic, and spore forming, were in fact much different from *B. subtilis*. For example, the morphotypes exhibited resistance to a variety of antibiotics effective against *B. subtilis*. In addition, unlike strain 168, these strains were not auxotrophic for tryptophan. Moreover, molecular studies using RAPD (random amplified polymorphic DNA) analysis (Friedkin, unpublished) as well as Southern analysis using *B. subtilis* DNA as a probe showed that the strains were quite different. Finally, 16S RNA sequence analysis in combination with a number of phenotypic and biochemical characterizations including fatty acid analysis was used to place the strains within the genus *Paenibacillus*.

The latter were formerly considered to be strains of *Bacillus* but have recently been reclassified (53). All of the morphotypes fall within this cluster, exhibiting similarity values between 89 and 98%. In addition to the T, C, and V morphotypes, two additional morphotypes, LN (for "loooped network," otherwise referred to as the "spaghetti" morphotype) and SV (for "spiral vortex") were also located within the *Paenibacillus* cluster (Fig. 2). Since both the T and C morphotypes exhibit branched patterns, we recommend that they be assigned to a new species, *Paenibacillus dendritiformis*, (from the Greek word for branching). The T and C morphotypes may in fact be variants of this species. The vortex morphotype has been assigned the species name *P. vortex*. Although the pattern formation of *P. vortex* resembles colonial morphology previously reported for *Bacillus circulans* (33, 54, 59), we were not able to observe the morphology with isolates of this strain obtained from the Bacillus Genetics Stock Center. Interestingly, many of the closely related species such as *P. thiaminolyticus*, *P. alvei*, and *P. polymyxa* have now been shown to exhibit characteristics of both the T and C morphotypes, albeit under different conditions (M. Tcherpakov, in press). These results are compatible with those recently reported by Rudner et al. (50a), although the strains in this case were assigned to the genus *Bacillus* rather than *Paenibacillus*.

T AND C MORPHOTYPES: DYNAMICS AND MODELING

The results of close microscopic and macroscopic examination of the relevant pattern-forming characteristics of the T, C, and V morphotypes led to the development of a generic modeling approach (3, 4, 16). While modeling of a biological process can be limited to finding a suitable formulation for process simulation, we have sought to develop a generic model that not only leads to numerical simulation, but also incorporates biological features experimentally. In addition, ideally, the model should enable us to make predictions to account for unanticipated experimen-

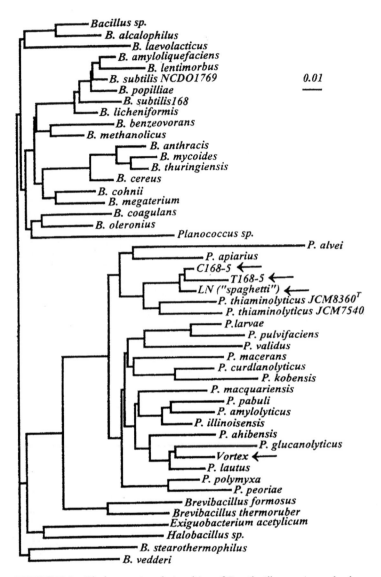

FIGURE 2 Phylogenetic relationships of *Paenibacillus* species and other closely related bacteria based on 16S rDNA gene sequences. The tree was generated by the neighbor-joining method. Bar, 0.01 nucleotide substitutions per site. The arrows show the relative positions of several of the morphotypes.

tal observations. The characteristics of the particular morphotype and its dynamics were subsequently incorporated into such a generic model. We use the models as research tools to predict various aspects of the dynamics, interactions, and cellular signaling leading to formation of such intricate morphologies (9).

T Morphotype

The patterns exhibited by tip-splitting *P. dendritiformis* (T morphotype) vary widely as the conditions are varied. Under the microscope, cells were seen to swim in a characteristic random walk-like fashion, while transmission electron microscopy clearly demonstrated the presence of peritrichous flagella (Fig. 3A). This swimming was confined to a fluid that seemed to be produced by the cells in a growth-associated fashion, although the fluid might also have been extracted by the cells from the semisolid growth media. Isolated cells spotted on the agar surface failed to move. The boundary of the fluid thus defines a local boundary for the branch of the developing colony. Branching occurs via random colli-

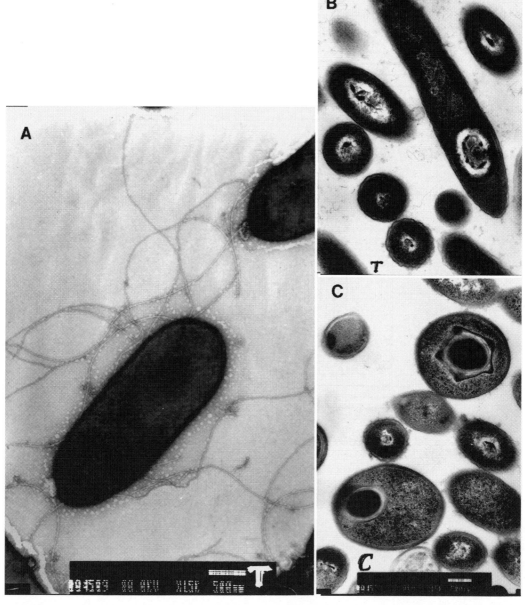

FIGURE 3 Transmission electron micrography illustrating (A) the presence of peritrichous flagella associated with the swimming T morphotype; (B) spores present in nonmotile cells of T morphotype; and (C) spores present in nonmotile cells of C morphotype.

sions of the confined cells at various points along the boundary of the fluid. Colonial development involves propagation of the boundary as a result of cellular movement, growth, and production of additional wetting fluid. Observations also revealed that the cells were more active at the outer parts of the colony; closer to the center, they no longer move, and some were shown to sporulate (Fig. 3B and C).

The resulting patterns developed by the colonies were shown to vary with both agar concentration and energy (in this case peptone) levels. The branching patterns exhibited for the T morphotype are characteristically observed at high agar concentrations (>1.5% agar). Under these conditions, and at substrate concentrations above 1% peptone, the patterns were found to be very compact. In a range between 0.5 and 1.0% peptone, the patterns exhibited radial symmetry characterized by dense "fingers," with each finger being wider than the distance between fingers. At intermediate peptone levels (0.3–0.5%), the branches become thinner; a condition in which branch width is smaller than the distance between branches. At even lower peptone levels, the colonies exhibit a more organized structure in which the fine branches come together to form a radial-type structure. A closer look at an individual branch reveals density variation within the branch, giving rise to a three-dimensional structure consisting of cell aggregates that accumulate in layers (Fig. 4). The aggregates form spots, layers, and even ridges, occasionally giving rise to a structure resembling a leaf vein. These cellular aggregates within the branches consist of motile cells, and their thickness and cell density appear to be part of the overall dynamics of collective cellular movement.

Morphotype Transition and Formation of the Chiral Morphotype (Fig. 5)

When plated on soft agar (concentrations of about 1% or less), colonies of *P. dendritiformis* var. *dendron* develop with characteristic T morphology for a period of about 48 h, after which a morphotype transition may occur, leading to a burst of new colonial growth, the chiral, or C, morphotype. Once isolated, cells of this chiral morphotype, termed *P. dendritiformis*, repeatedly give rise to this new form of colonial morphology in which the branches all twist with the same handedness (Fig. 6). Chirality, initially discovered by Pasteur, is a property well recognized throughout nature (2, 11). In addition to the enormous difference in morphology between the genetically similar morphotypes, microscopic observations indicated that the cells of the C morphotype are longer and more closely aligned with each other than those of the T morphotype. Moreover, it became clear from the electron microscopic observations that the chiral structure of the colonial branches was not reflected in a twisting of the cells themselves. Rather, the twisting branches arise from the collective biased movement of the strongly aligned cells within the wetting fluid. One possibility to explain chirality may have to do with the specific handedness associated with flagellar rotation (11, 31). Ben-Jacob et al. have proposed that it is this property of flagellar handedness, coupled with strong cell-cell orientation interactions which accounts for the observed chirality (15).

As in the case of the T morphotype, members of the C morphotype also exhibit a morphology diagram with a profusion of complex patterns (6, 9, 11). In addition, they also produce a wetting fluid. Interestingly, colonial development with var. *chirales* was found to propagate faster with about two orders of magnitude fewer cells than the T morphotype. It was proposed that the colonial growth velocity (the rate of spreading) was responsible for the selection pressure leading to these T to C morphotype transitions. If this hypothesis is correct, one would expect to observe the reverse transition from C to T under growth conditions favoring the growth of the T morphotype (a harder agar surface). Indeed such reverse transitions are observed when cells of the C morphotype are spotted on harder agar,

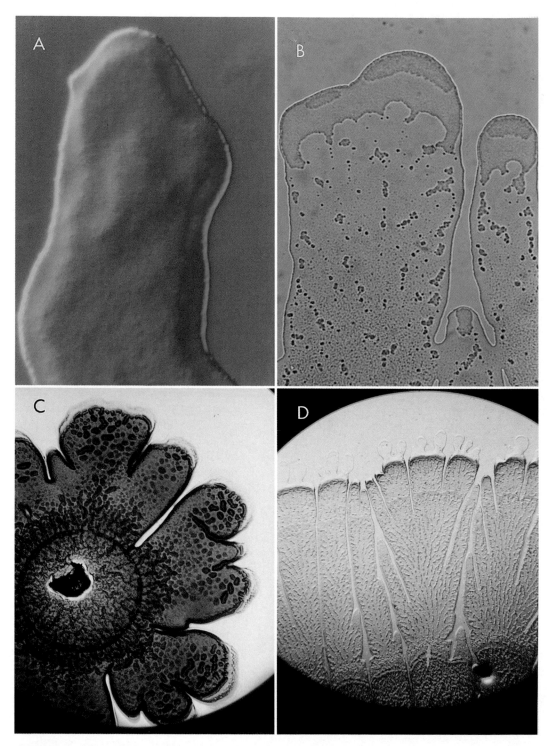

FIGURE 4 (A) A closer look at colonies of the T morphotype. (B) The cells swim within an envelope of wetting fluid that forms a well-defined boundary. (C) Within the branch, cellular aggregates frequently accumulate (darker regions). (D) The distribution of aggregates varies markedly during the growth of the colony. Note the leaf vein-like arrangement resulting from formation of three-dimensional cellular aggregates.

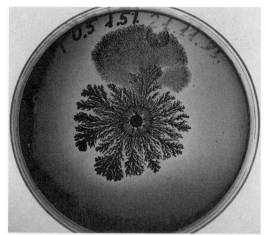

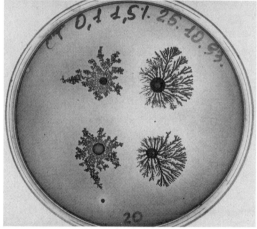

FIGURE 5 Morphotype transition from T to C. The transition was obtained by spotting cells from the T morphotype onto soft agar (1%). (A) An example of a morphotype transition from T to C. (B) Examples of isolated populations of T and C morphotypes. Cells were picked from the regions of T and the burst of C, respectively. Individual colonies were purified through several cycles of restreaking under conditions where the morphotype characteristics are normally not observed. Individual colonies were then spotted onto a plate containing 1.5% agar and 0.1% peptone. As illustrated here, the morphotypes retain their specific characteristics even after several such cycles of growth under "nonselective" conditions.

on which T morphotype spreads faster than the C. The T to C transitions are quite frequent. About 60% of T colonies give rise to the chiral morphology after about 2 days. The question arose as to whether this was a true morphotype transition, or whether the C was simply present as a small minority within the T population. Recent findings using strains marked with antibiotic resistance markers have demonstrated that under the specific conditions, the cells undergo an actual morphotype transition (Tcherpakov et al., in preparation). Moreover, morphotype transition appears to be a more general phenomenon. For example, at least two different isolates of *P. thiaminolyticus* from various collections have also been shown to exhibit characteristics representing both T and C morphotypes, albeit under slightly different conditions of nutrient and agar concentration. In addition, these strains also undergo the same mode of morphotype transition in which chiral morphology is "selected" at a lower agar concentration (Tcherpakov et al., in preparation).

Morphotype Mixing

Studies of morphotype transition have demonstrated that the C morphotypes burst out from a T pattern when the T cells are inoculated on plates containing low agar concentrations. The fact that this morphotype transition occurs only under a specific set of conditions suggests the possibility that there is selection for the population that yields the fastest-growing colony. Surprisingly, however, when a mixed population of 99.9% C and 0.1% T cells was plated under conditions that favored the growth of C cells, a pattern with mixed colonial morphology was obtained. The initial growth was chiral, followed by a tip-splitting morphology, which gave rise to chiral patterns. The question arises then as to the origin of the patterns; do they arise by morphotype transition or is the T morphotype simply "preserved" within the original mixture?

Studies on this question are currently in progress using mixtures of populations carrying different antibiotic resistance markers. Initial mixing experiments were carried out with cells of the C morphotype carrying resistance to nalidixic acid and T cells resistant to rifampin (at ratios of 10^3 to 10^4:1, respectively),

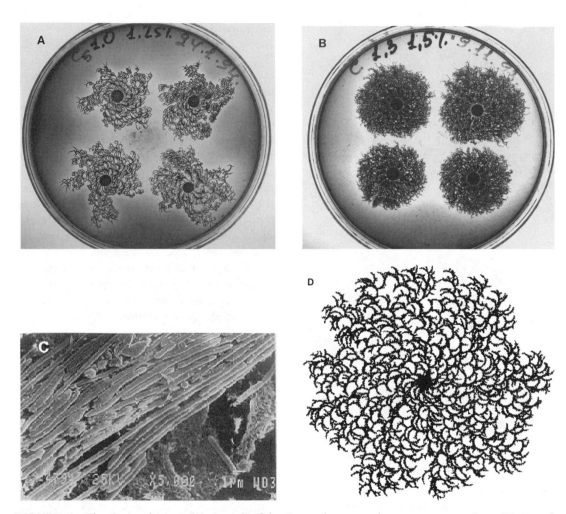

FIGURE 6 The C morphotype. (A) Growth of the C morphotype on low agar concentrations. (B) Growth of the C morphotype on higher agar concentrations. (C) Scanning electron micrograph of C cells. Note that the while the branches twist with the same handedness, there is no twisting of the individual cells. (D) Simulation of the model of the C morphotype. Details of the model are presented in the text.

which were spotted on soft agar. The colonial morphology was as described above, namely, an initial ring of chiral growth, followed by a branched or T-like morphology from which bursts of C cells emerged. Once the pattern was formed, the cells were replica plated to plates containing either rifampin (the minority input T population) or nalidixic acid (the majority C population). Surprisingly, there was only a tiny group of cells remaining at the site of the inoculum that retained the original nalidixic acid marker, even though they repre-

sented the vast majority of the original inoculum. Essentially the entire pattern consisted only of cells that were rifampin resistant. Thus, despite the appearance of distinct morphotypes, they all appear to arise from a single population of cells. This pattern was obtained with mixtures that were prepared from stationary-phase cells of the two morphotypes. However, when the cells were spotted from an exponential-phase population, at very low ratios of T, the pattern obtained was exclusively that of the population of C morphotype, and the cells were all resistant to nalidixic acid, as would be expected. The results of these experiments suggest that in addition to the external conditions governing morphotype expression, the physiological state of the cells at the time of inoculation plays a major role in the mode of colonial development with these strains.

Modeling of T and C Morphotypes

The "communicating walkers model" was developed to model colonial development of the T and C morphotypes (16, 17, 19). In the model, the bacteria are represented by particles (termed "walkers") that represent about 10^2 to 10^4 bacterial cells. Two features specify the walker: its position relative to the boundary of the wetting fluid and its metabolic state (referred to as its "internal energy"). For high concentrations of the energy source, the consumption of food is greater than its utilization, and the internal energy increases until a threshold level is reached, at which point the walker divides. When the food source is limiting, the walker consumes only the available amount, which may be less than required for maximum cellular activity. As the energy level drops to zero, the walkers become nonmotile and remain in their "prespore" state. As the walkers consume the growth substrate, the concentration decreases in front of the colony and additional nutrient diffuses toward the colony, generating diffusion-limited growth.

Experimental observations have demonstrated that the bacteria swim within the lubrication fluid. In the model, the walkers perform a random walk. At each time step, each of the active (motile) walkers moves a step at a random angle. The walkers are confined within an envelope (defined by a tridiagonal lattice) that represents the boundary of the lubricating fluid. In the event that the "step" taken by a walker would lead to movement outside the boundary, the step is not performed, and a counter on the appropriate segment of the envelope is increased by one. When a segment counter reaches a threshold value of N_c, the segment of the envelope propagates, adding additional lattice area to the colony. The requirement for N_c hits represents colonial growth through unoccupied areas. This feature reflects the local cooperativity in the behavior of the bacterial cells. To a first approximation, the value of N_c reflects the concentration of the agar, since more hits would be required to "push" the envelope on a harder surface (Fig. 7).

The model for the C morphotype (Fig. 6D) assumes that branch twisting arises from the flagellar handedness as well as from the strong orientation interaction owing to the increased size of the cells (5, 6, 9, 11). To represent the cellular orientation, each walker is assigned an angle. The model thus takes into account not only the position of the walker relative to the boundary, but its orientation angle as well. Every time step, each of the active walkers performs a rotation to a new orientation that is derived from its previous one. Once oriented, the walker advances a step either in the forward or reverse direction (an actual experimental observation).

Chemosignaling and Cooperative Cellular Organization

Although the model as described above captures certain aspects of morphotype patterning, it is insufficient to describe the remarkable spectrum of colonial morphologies observed as conditions are varied. We assume that this level of cellular organization is mediated by an interplay of signaling networks involving cell-cell communication and signal transduction.

Chemotaxis is the best-studied and most-prevalent signal transduction system in motile bacteria (32, 37). This process involves changes in the movement of the cell in response to a gradient of certain chemical fields (1, 20, 21, 24, 41). The movement is biased along the gradient, in either the forward (in the direction of the gradient) or the reverse direction. Thus, chemotaxis enables microbial cells in a variety of natural environments to exploit chemoattraction and chemorepulsion to obtain a more favorable situation such as movement toward a nutrient, escape from

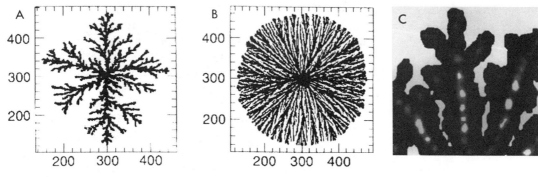

FIGURE 7 Simulations of the communicating walkers model for the T morphotype. (A) Growth at low peptone levels in the absence of chemorepulsion signaling. (B) Growth under the same conditions in the presence of long-range chemorepulsion. (C) Modeling the density variations within a branch by including the short-range chemoattraction.

predation, movement toward specific surfaces, or protection by cellular aggregation. Usually chemotaxis implies a response to an externally produced field such as attraction toward supplemented nutrients. However, self-generated bacterial chemosignaling by the excretion of amino acids and peptides has also been demonstrated (25–27, 60). In the case of *Escherichia coli* and *Salmonella typhimurium*, this mode of chemoattraction involves membrane receptors such as the Tar receptor for chemotaxis as well as a new receptor system involving chemoattraction on rich medium (25). In gram-negative bacteria, at least 50 different gene products are involved in governing the mode by which microbes employ the chemotactic system to modulate their movement. The cell "senses" the concentration of the chemoattractant (or repellent) by measuring the fraction of receptors occupied by the signaling molecules. Thus, at very high concentrations, the chemotactic response vanishes because of receptor saturation—the "receptor law." At the lower limit of attractant, the response is also negligible, since it is "masked" by noise in the system. Swimming bacteria perform chemotaxis by modulating the time gap between tumbling events. Increasing (or decreasing) this time gap when swimming up the gradient or attractant (or repellent) bias generates movement toward (or away from) favorable (unfavorable) locations.

Ben-Jacob et al. have assumed (5, 9, 28) that for adaptive self-organization, the T morphotype employs three modes of chemotactic signaling. One is the nutritional chemotaxis toward an externally supplied energy source mentioned above. We would expect this type of signaling to be dominant for an intermediate range of nutrient levels. The two other types of chemotaxis are generated by the cells themselves operating on different length scales. One mode of chemotactic response, short-range chemoattraction, is assumed to regulate the dynamics within the branches, while the other, long-range chemorepulsion, regulates the organization of the branches. Chemoattraction has been shown to account for cellular aggregation and pattern formation in *E. coli* (26, 27) and *S. typhimurium* (25, 60). As can be seen in Fig. 6, incorporation of short-range chemoattractant into the model for the T morphotype can lead to formation of three-dimensional structures that closely resemble structures observed experimentally.

In Fig. 6 we also demonstrate the dramatic effect obtained when long-range chemorepulsive signaling is incorporated into the model under conditions of nutritional deprivation. Under these conditions, we assume that a chemorepellent is excreted by the stressed walkers. The pattern becomes much denser with a smooth circular envelope, while the branches are thinner and radially oriented. This structure enables the colony to spread over the same distance with fewer walkers, thereby providing the developing colony with a distinct biological advantage under certain condition of nutrient stress.

VORTEX (V) MORPHOTYPE

Observations of complex patterning during colony development by *B. circulans* on a hard agar surface were reported more than 50 years ago (59). The observed phenomena include "turbulent like" collective flow, complicated eddy (vortex) dynamics, merging and splitting of vortices, rotating "bagels," and more. This behavior is not unique to *B. circulans*. During studies of complex bacterial patterning, we isolated new strains exhibiting similar behavior (7–9, 19). We refer to the new morphotype produced by these strains as the vortex (V) morphotype (Fig. 8). This strain has also been shown to be a member of the genus *Paenibacillus* (Tcherpakov et al., submitted).

A wide variety of branching patterns is exhibited by each of the vortex-forming strains as the growth conditions are varied. Some representative patterns are shown in Fig. 8. Each branch is produced by a leading droplet of cells and emits side branches, each with its own leading droplet. Microscopic observations revealed that each leading droplet consists of hundreds to millions of cells that circle a common center (hence the term vortex) at a cell speed of about 10 μm/s. Both the size of a vortex and the speed of the cells can vary

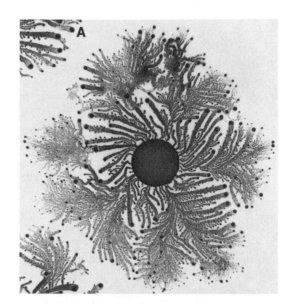

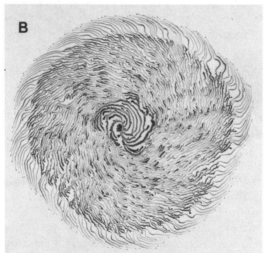

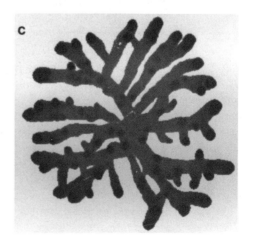

FIGURE 8 Vortex morphotypes. (A) Colony of the V morphotype. Note the droplets of fluid located at the tip of each branch. These droplets contain many cells rotating around a common center (the vortex). (B) Colony of the SV morphotype. Droplets of fluid and vortices are present at the tips of the branches, but the overall structure and morphology of the colony is different. (C) Results of numerical simulation of the vortex model, which includes rotational, short-range chemoattractive, long-range chemorepulsive, and nutritional chemotaxis. Note the similarity between panels A and C.

depending on the growth conditions and the location of the specific vortex in the colony. Within a given colony, both clockwise and anticlockwise rotating vortices are observed. The vortices in a colony can also consist of either a single or multiple layers of cells. We occasionally observed vortices with an empty core, which we refer to as "bagel" shaped. After formation, the number of cells in the vortex increases, and the vortex expands and is translocated as a unit.

The speed of the vortices is slower than the speed of the individual cells circulating around its center. Bacterial cells are also contained in the trails left behind the leading vortices. Some of these cells are immobile, while others move, swirling with complex dynamics. The migrating groups of cells are very reminiscent of the "worm" motion of slime mold or schools of multicellular organisms. The whole intricate dynamics are confined to the trail of the leading vortex, and neither a single cell nor a group of moving cells can pass out of the boundary of the trail. Only vortices formed in the trails can break out of the trail and create a new branch.

Microscopic observations of the V morphotype also reveal that the bacterial motion is performed in a fluid on the agar surface. As is the case with the other morphotypes, this wetting fluid is also assumed to be excreted by the cells and/or extracted by the cells from the agar. We do not observe tumbling motion or movement forward and backward. Rather, the motion is exclusively forward along the long axis of the cell. Moreover, the cells tend to move in the same direction and with the same speed as the surrounding neighboring cells, in what appears to be a synchronized group movement. Electron microscopic observations show that the bacteria have flagella, which suggests that the motility is likely to be swarming. Close inspection of these observations enables construction of a model for colonial development of swarming bacteria, which is also applicable to gliding bacteria.

The model is inspired by the communicating walkers model. Here the cells are represented by "swarmers." Each swarmer has a forward propulsive force. The balance of this force and friction forces tends to set the swarmer's speed to a specific value. In keeping with microscopic investigations demonstrating the synchrony of the movement of strongly aligned cells, we also include velocity-velocity interactions that tend to set the swarmer's velocity to the mean velocity of its neighbors (7). In addition, we assume that the swarmers produce an extracellular "wetting" fluid that they secrete during colonial growth. This extracellular slime also influences bacterial motion. In the model, the swarmers can move only if the level of the wetting fluid is above a threshold value. The above features, which are derived directly from the observations, suffice to describe the collective migration of bacteria.

However, an additional feature has to be considered to explain the emergence of vortices. We propose a rotational chemotaxis that differs from the chemotaxis normally employed by tumbling bacteria (7). We propose that each individual cell modulates its propulsive force according to the local concentration of a chemotactic signaling material. In a group of cells, such a response creates a propulsion force gradient. Together with the velocity-velocity interaction, this imposes a torque on the average motion of the cells. Therefore, a swarmer moving at an angle to the chemical gradient is subjected to a torque that causes the swarmer to twist toward the direction of the local gradient of the chemoattractant. This new chemotactic element can account for the ability of the cells to rotate around a common center, despite the fact that they can only move forward. We have shown that chemomodulation can indeed lead to formation of stationary vortices (fixed in size and at a fixed locations, and rotating "bagels." All these elements are of a length comparable to, or smaller than, an individual branch of a colony. During colonial development, these elements are organized to form the observed global pattern.

UNSOLVED QUESTIONS AND FUTURE RESEARCH

In this chapter we describe an interdisciplinary approach to study the mode and dynamics of pattern formation and cooperative organization leading to complex pattern formation in bacteria. Employing concepts from studies of patterning in nonliving systems coupled with detailed morphotype characterization has led to the development of a generic modeling approach that has been incorporated into the study. The models introduced here do not represent the only approach to simulating complex pattern formation, but they do incorporate elements that allow us to make experimentally testable predictions. For example, our models incorporate the notions of new cell-generated signaling molecules involved in chemorepulsion or vortex generation. The existence, nature, chemical composition, and mode of action of such hypothetical materials remains a subject of intense investigation in our laboratories. In addition and central to the models is the concept of the wetting fluid that generates the boundary or "communal envelope." What is the nature of such materials, how are they generated and elaborated? Clearly, many open questions remain to be answered in the future. For example, given the enormous biodiversity in the microbial world, the question of variety, distribution, and prevalence of morphotypes in various natural environments presents a formidable challenge to the microbial ecologist. In this regard, it will be important to determine the extent and significance of complex patterning as it relates to colonial development in these environments. Moreover, in our view, major new insights should emerge as we begin to unravel the genetic basis of cooperative morphotype behavior. It is not unlikely, for example, that different strains with similar morphotype characteristics may in fact use alternative physiological and genetic strategies to generate similar patterns. Will the generic models developed here be applicable in such circumstances? It is clear that both pattern formation and morphotype transition may pro-vide an additional mode of multicellular behavior in the microbial world. At least in some cases, microbial populations can become transformed from a herd of individual cells to an organized community of mutual interest.

REVIEWS AND KEY PAPERS

Ben-Jacob, E., and I. Cohen. 1997. From snow-flake formation to the growth of bacterial colonies. II. Cooperative formation of complex patterns. *Contemp. Phys.* **38:**205–241.

Ben-Jacob, E., I. Cohen, and D. L. Gutnick. 1998. Cooperative organization of bacterial colonies; from genotype to morphotype. *Annu. Rev. Microbiol.* **52,** in press.

Ben-Jacob, E., O. Shochet, A. Tenenbaum, I. Cohen, A. Czirok, and T. Viksek. 1994. Generic modelling of cooperative growth patterns in bacterial colonies. *Nature* **368:**46–49.

Fuqua, W. C., S. C. Winans, and E. P. Greenberg. 1996. Census and consensus in bacterial ecosystems: the LuxR-LuxI family of quorum-sensing transcriptional regulators. *Annu. Rev. Microbiol.* **50:**727–751.

Kaiser, D., and R. Losick. 1993. How and why bacteria talk to each other. *Cell* **73:**873–887.

Losick, R., and D. Kaiser. 1997. Why and how bacteria communicate. *Sci. Am.* **276:**52–57.

Matsuyama, T., and M. Matsushita. 1993. Fractal morphogenesis by a bacterial cell population. *Crit. Rev. Microbiol.* **19:**117–135.

Shapiro, J. A. 1988. Bacteria as multicellular organisms. *Sci. Am.* **258**(6):62–69.

Shapiro, J. A., and M. Dworkin (ed.). 1997. *Bacteria as Multicellular Organisms.* Oxford University Press, New York.

REFERENCES

1. **Adler, J.** 1969. Chemoreceptors in bacteria. *Science* **166:**1588–1597.
2. **Avetisov, V. A., V. I. Goldanskii, and V. V. Kuzmin.** 1991. Handedness, origin of life and evolution, *Phys. Today* **July 1991:**33–41.
3. **Ben-Jacob, E.** 1993. From snowflake formation to the growth of bacterial colonies. Part I: Diffusive patterning in non-living systems. *Contemp. Phys.* **34:**247–273.
4. **Ben-Jacob, E., and I. Cohen.** 1997. From snowflake formation to the growth of bacterial colonies. II. Cooperative formation of complex colonial patterns. *Contemp. Phys.* **38:**205–241.
5. **Ben-Jacob, E., and I. Cohen.** 1997. Cooperative formation of bacterial patterns, p. 394–416. *In* J. A. Shapiro and M. Dworkin (ed.), *Bacteria*

as Multicellular Organisms. Oxford University Press, New York.

6. **Ben-Jacob, E., I. Cohen, and A. Czirok.** 1996. Smart bacterial colonies, p. 307–324. *In* H. Flyvbjerg, J. Hertz, M. H. Jensen, O. G. Mauritsen, and K. Sneppen (ed.), *Physics of Biological Systems: From Molecules to Species.* Springer, Berlin.

7. **Ben-Jacob, E., I. Cohen, A. Czirok, T. Vicsek, and D. L. Gutnick.** 1997. Chemomodulation of cellular movement and collective formation of vortices by swarming bacteria and colonial development. *Physica A* **238:**181–197.

8. **Ben-Jacob, E., I. Cohen, and D. L. Gutnick.** 1998. Chemotaxis based self-organization during colonial morphogenesis. *Comm. Mol. Cell. Biophys.,* in press.

9. **Ben-Jacob, E., I. Cohen, and D. L. Gutnick.** 1998. Cooperative organization of bacterial colonies; from genotype to morphotype. *Annu. Rev. Microbiol.* **51,** in press.

10. **Ben-Jacob, E., I. Cohen, O. Shochet, I. Aranson, H. Levine, and L. Tsimiring.** 1995. Complex bacterial patterns. *Nature* **373:**566–567.

11. **Ben-Jacob, E., I. Cohen, O. Shochet, A. Czirok, and T. Vicsek.** 1995. Cooperative formation of chiral patterns during growth of bacterial colonies. *Phys. Rev. Lett.* **75**(15):2800–2902.

12. **Ben-Jacob, E., and P. Garik.** 1990. The formation of patterns in non-equilibrium growth. *Nature* **343:**523–530.

13. **Ben-Jacob, E., P. Garik, T. Muller, and D. Grier.** 1988. Characterization of morphology transitions in diffusion-controlled systems. *Phys. Rev. A* **38:**1370.

14. **Ben-Jacob, E., H. Shmueli, O. Shochet, and A. Tenenbaum.** 1992. Adaptive self-organization during growth of bacterial colonies. *Physica A* **187:**378–424.

15. **Ben-Jacob, E., O. Shochet, I. Cohen, A. Tenenbaum, A. Czirok, and T. Vicsek.** 1995. Cooperative strategies in formation of complex bacterial patterns. *Fractals* **3:**849–868.

16. **Ben-Jacob, E., O. Shochet, A. Tenenbaum, I. Cohen, A. Czirok, and T. Viksek.** 1994. Generic modelling of cooperative growth patterns in bacterial colonies. *Nature* **368:**46–49.

17. **Ben-Jacob, E., O. Shochet, A. Tenenbaum, I. Cohen, A. Czirok, and T. Vicsek.** 1994. Communication, regulation and control during complex patterning of bacterial colonies. *Fractals* **2**(1):15–44.

18. **Ben-Jacob, E., O. Shochet, A. Tenenbaum, I. Cohen, A. Czirok, and T. Vicsek.** 1996. Response of bacterial colonies to imposed anisotropy. *Phys. Rev. E* **53:**1835–1845.

19. **Ben-Jacob, E., A. Tenenbaum, O. Shochet, and O. Avidan.** 1994. Holotransformations of bacterial colonies and genome cybernetics. *Physica A* **202:**1–47.

20. **Berg, H. C.** 1993. *Random Walks in Biology.* Princeton University Press, Princeton, N.J.

21. **Berg, H. C., and E. M. Purcell.** 1977. Physics of chemoreception. *Biophys. J.* **20:**193–219.

22. **Berg, H. C., and P. M. Tedesco.** 1975. Transient response to chemotactic stimuli in *Escherichia coli. Proc. Natl. Acad. Sci. USA* **72**(8):3235–3239.

23. **Bischoff, D. S., and G. W. Ordal.** 1992. *Bacillus subtilis* chemotaxis: a deviation from the *Escherichia coli* paradigm. *Mol. Microbiol.* **6:**23–28.

24. **Blair, D. F.** 1995. How bacteria sense and swim. *Annu. Rev. Microbiol.* **49:**489–522.

25. **Blat, Y., and M. Eisenbach.** 1995. Tar-dependent and –independent pattern formation by *Salmonella typhimurium. J. Bacteriol.* **177:**1683–1691.

26. **Budrene, E. O., and H. C. Berg.** 1991. Complex patterns formed by motile cells of *Esherichia coli. Nature* **349:**630–633.

27. **Budrene, E. O., and H. C. Berg.** 1995. Dynamics of formation of symmetrical patterns by chemotactic bacteria. *Nature* **376:**49–53.

28. **Cohen, I., A. Czirok, and E. Ben-Jacob.** 1996. Chemotactic-based adaptive self organization during colonial development. *Physica A* **233:**678–698.

29. **Czirok, A., E. Ben-Jacob, I. Cohen, and T. Vicsek.** 1996. Formation of complex bacterial colonies via self-generated vortices. *Phys. Rev. E* **54:**1791–1801.

30. **Dukler, A.** 1993. Isolation and characterization of bacteria growing in patterns on the surface of solid agar. Senior research project in the laboratory of David Gutnick, Tel-Aviv University, unpublished data.

31. **Eisenbach, M.** 1990. Functions of the flagellar modes of rotation in bacterial motility and chemotaxis. *Mol. Microbiol.* **4**(2):161–167.

32. **Eisenbach M.** 1996. Control of bacterial chemotaxis. *Mol. Microbiol.* **20:**903–910.

33. **Ford, W. W.** 1916. Studies on aerobic spore-bearing non-pathogenic bacteria. 2. Miscellaneous cultures. *J. Bacteriol.* **1:**518–526.

34. **Fujikawa, H., and M. Matsushita.** 1989. Fractal growth of *Bacillus subtilis* on agar plates. *J. Phys. Soc. Jpn.* **58:**3875–3878.

35. **Fuqua, W. C., S. C. Winans, and E. P. Greenberg.** 1994. Quorum sensing in bacteria: the LuxR-LuxI family of cell density-responsive transcriptional regulators. *J. Bacteriol.* **176:**269–275.

36. **Fuqua, W. C., S. C. Winans, and E. P. Greenberg.** 1996. Census and consensus in bac-

terial ecosystems: the LuxR-LuxI family of quorum-sensing transcriptional regulators. *Annu. Rev. Microbiol.* **50:**727–751.

37. **Garrity, L. F., and G. W. Ordal.** 1995. Chemotaxis in *Bacillus subtilis*: how bacteria monitor environmental signals. *Pharmacol. Ther.*, p. 87–104.

38. **Harshey, R. M.** 1994. Bees aren't the only ones: swarming in gram-negative bacteria. *Mol. Microbiol.* **13:**389–394.

39. **Kaiser, D., and R. Losick.** 1993. How and why bacteria talk to each other. *Cell* **73:**873–887.

40. **Kitsunezaki, S.** 1997. Interface dynamics for bacterial colony formation. *J. Phys. Soc. Jpn.* **66:**1544–1550.

41. **Lackiie, J. M. (ed.).** 1986. *Biology of the Chemotactic Response.* Cambridge University Press, New York.

42. **Langer, J. S.** 1989. Dendrites, viscous fingering and the theory of pattern formation. *Science* **243:**1150–1154.

43. **Losick, R., and D. Kaiser.** 1997. Why and how bacteria communicate. *Sci. Am.* **276:**52–57.

44. **MacNeil, S. D., A. Mouzeyan, and P. L. Hartzell.** 1994. Genes required for both gliding motility and development in *Myxococcus xanthus. Mol. Microbiol.* **14:** 785–795.

45. **Matsushita, M., and H. Fujikawa.** 1990. Diffusion-limited growth in bacterial colony formation. *Physica A* **168:**498–506.

46. **Matsushita, M., J. Wakita, H. Itoh, I. Rafols, T. Matsuyama, H. Sakaguchi, and M. Mimura.** 1998. Interface growth and pattern formation in bacterial colonies. *Physica A* **249:**517–524.

47. **Matsushita, M., J.-I. Wakita, and T. Matsuyama.** 1995. Growth and morphological changes of bacteria colonies, p. 609–618. *In* P. E. Cladis and P. Palffy-Muhoray (ed.) *Spatio-Temporal Patterns in Nonequilibrium Complex Systems*, Sante-Fe Institute Studies in the Sciences of Complexity. Addison-Wesley Publishing Co., Inc., Reading, Mass.

48. **Matsuyama, T., K. Kaneda, Y. Nakagawa, K. Isa, H. Hara-Hotta, and I. Yano.** 1992. A novel extracellular cyclic lipopeptide which promotes flagellum-dependent and -independent spreading growth of *Serratia marcescens J. Bacteriol.* **174:**1768–1776.

49. **Matsuyama, T., and M. Matsushita.** 1993. Fractal morphogenesis by a bacterial cell population. *Crit. Rev. Microbiol.* **19:**117–135.

50. **Mendelson, N. H., and B. Salhi.** 1996. Patterns of reporter gene expression in the phase diagram of *Bacillus subtilis* colony forms. *J. Bacteriol.* **178:**1980–1989.

50a.**Rudner, R., O. Martsinkevich, W. Leung, and E. Jarvis.** 1998. Classification and genetic characterization of pattern forming bacilli. *Mol. Microbiol.* **27:**687–703.

51. **Shapiro, J. A.** 1988. Bacteria as multicellular organisms. *Sci. Am.* **258**(6)**:**62–69.

52. **Shapiro, J. A., and M. Dworkin (ed.).** 1997. *Bacteria as Multicellular Organisms.* Oxford University Press, New York.

53. **Shida, O., H. Takagi, K. Kadowaki, I. K. Nakamura, and K. Komagata.** 1997. Transfer of *Bacillus alginolyticus, Bacillus chondroitinus, Bacillus curdlanolyticus*, Bacillus glucanolyticus, *Bacillus kobensis* and *Bacillus thiaminolyticus* to the genus *Paenibacillus* and emended description of the genus *Paenibacillus. Int. J. Syst. Bacteriol.* **47:**289–298.

54. **Smith, R. N., and F. E. Clark.** 1938. Motile colonies of *Bacillus alvei* and other bacteria. *J. Bacteriol.* **35:**59–60.

55. **Stevens, F. S.** 1974. *Pattern in Nature.* Little, Brown & Co., Boston.

56. **Stock, J. B., A. M. Stock, and M. Mottonen.** 1990. Signal transduction in bacteria. *Nature* **344:**395–400.

57. **Tsimiring, L., H. Levine, I. Aranson, E. Ben-Jacob, I. Cohen, O. Shochet, and W. N. Reynolds.** 1995. Aggregation patterns in stressed bacteria. *Phys. Rev. Lett.* **75:**1859–1862.

58. **Vicsek, T., A. Czirok, E. Ben-Jacob, I. Cohen, O. Shochet, and A. Tenenbaum.** 1995. Novel type of phase transition in a system of self-driven particles. *Phys. Rev. Lett.* **75:**1226–1229.

59. **Wolf, G. (ed.).** 1968. *Encyclopaedia Cinematographica.* Institut für Wissenschaftlichen Film, Göttingen, Germany.

60. **Woodward, D. E., R. Tyson, M. R., Myerscough, J. D. Murray, E. O. Budrene, and H. C. Berg.** 1995. Spatio-temporal patterns generated by *Salmonella typhimurium. Biophys. J.* **68:**2181–2189.

CELL BIOLOGY OF TRANSMISSIBLE SPONGIFORM ENCEPHALOPATHY PRIONS: DO PRIONS REPLICATE ON CHOLESTEROL-RICH MEMBRANE RAFTS?

Albert Taraboulos

24

INTRODUCTION

Prions

Prions are proteinaceous infectious agents that seem to propagate in the host without the help of autonomous nucleic acid genes. Instead, prions transmit their identity to their "progeny" by an "epigenetic" process that includes the pathological refolding of a host protein (for review, see, for instance, reference 35 and references therein). Here, the focus is on the interaction of these pathogens with the host cell and especially on their relationship with specialized microdomains of cell membranes, or "rafts." While prions were first postulated as infectious pathogens of mammals, prionlike phenomena have recently been found in several microorganisms as well (see below and Table 1). It is thus conceivable that microbiologists will become very interested in this novel phenomenon in the near future.

The discovery of prions is linked to a category of fatal encephalopathies of humans and animals known as the transmissible spongiform encephalopathies (TSE). Diseases such as scrapie of sheep (long the TSE experimental prototype), as well as Creutzfeldt-Jakob disease (CJD) and kuru of humans, have long been known for their peculiar characteristics. In particular, the infectious agent resisted procedures that inactivate nucleic acids (2), and CJD could either (i) appear as an infectious (transmissible) disease, (ii) appear as an autosomal dominant hereditary disorder in some families, or even (iii) pop up sporadically in the population at large. Most intriguingly, the brains of the genetic and sporadic patients (who had not been infected from exogenous sources) contained infectious material that could transmit the disease to experimental animals ("spontaneous prions"). Biochemical analysis of infectious fractions led to the discovery of the prion protein PrP^{Sc} (5, 31) and to the formulation of the prion hypothesis (34). Extensive work then led to the recognition that the TSEs (to which bovine spongiform encephalopathy [BSE] was added in 1986 [56]) are caused and transmitted by proteinaceous agents that may function without the involvement of nucleic acids.

Prion Proteins

The only known component of the TSE prion is the host-encoded protein PrP^{Sc}, which is an abnormal conformer of the nor-

Albert Taraboulos, Department of Molecular Biology, the Hebrew University-Hadassah Medical School, P.O. Box 12272, Jerusalem 91120, Israel.

Microbial Ecology and Infectious Disease, Edited by Eugene Rosenberg
©1999 American Society for Microbiology, Washington, D.C.

mal prion protein PrP^C. PrP^C is a small glycoprotein (M_r = ca. 26 kDa without the N-linked carbohydrates) that is attached to the surface of neurons and other cells through a glycophosphatidyl inositol (GPI) moiety. The normal function of PrP^C is unclear (9). The two PrP isoforms differ enormously in their properties: in contrast to PrP^C, the abnormal isoform PrP^{Sc} is insoluble in detergents, possesses a protease-resistant core denominated PrP27-30, and tends to form amyloidic fibrils called prion "rods" (27, 29). Considerable effort was invested in deciphering the structural features that might underlie these vast biochemical differences. It is now clear that the two PrP isoforms possess the same amino acid sequence and identical covalent modifications but differ considerably in their tertiary structure. The linear organization of PrP is shown in Fig 1. Spectroscopic studies have demonstrated that PrP^{Sc} is rich in α-helices and devoid of β-sheets, whereas PrP^{Sc} is highly enriched in β-sheets (15, 32, 33). PrP^{Sc} is formed posttranslationally (6), probably from PrP^C (7, 13).

All these findings are incorporated into a simple and elegant, but not yet proven, "protein only" model of prion replication, that stipulates that TSE prions are composed of PrP^{Sc} and that PrP^{Sc} is able to "coerce" PrP^C molecules of the host into its own aberrant conformation. In a propitious environment, these properties would then lead to a proteinaceous reaction such as

$$PrP^C + PrP^{Sc} \rightarrow 2PrP^{Sc} \qquad (1)$$

This is supposed to require direct physical interaction between "substrate" PrP^C and "seed" PrP^{Sc}. This simple protein-only model incorporates most of the existing data about the infectious particle (e.g., its resistance to nucleic acid inactivating procedures). However, at least one property of prions, the existence of isolates or "strains," is not easily accounted for by this simple model. When inoculated to identical animals, prions of different strains give rise to diseases that are clinically and pathologically disparate, and these properties "breed true" upon successive passages in experimental animals. There is now evidence that strains may after all be specified by alternative PrP^{Sc} conformations (39), a model that would be in line with the protein-only paradigm. Nevertheless, existing data do not completely preclude the involve-

TABLE 1 Prions and prion analogs

Prion	Reference	Organism	Phenotype	Protein base	Cellular accessory factors
TSE	35	Mammals	Neuronal death	PrP	Protein X and others
[URE3]	55	Saccharomyces cerevisiae	N_2 catabolic enzymes depressed	ure2p	hsp104
[PSI]	25	S. cerevisiae	Increased readthrough of termination codons	Sup35p	hsp104
[HET-s★]	18	Podospora anserina	Altered heterokaryon incompatibility reaction	het-s	?

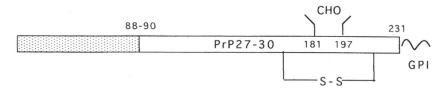

FIGURE 1 Map of mature PrP. PrP covalent modifications: (i) the C-terminal GPI moiety, (ii) two N-linked carbohydrates (CHO), and (iii) a disulfide bridge between two cysteines. PrP27-30 is the protease-resistant core of PrP^{Sc}.

ment of molecules other than PrP within the prion particle.

The exact details of how reaction 1 proceeds are not known. Based on the observed formation of fibrils by amyloidogenic peptides in vitro, a seeding-polymerization model for prion propagation was proposed (17). In this model, the active "catalytic" prion (i.e., the particle that imposes its tertiary structure on PrP^C) is a large amyloidic fibrillar PrP^{Sc} polymer, akin to the prion rods, that works by accreting PrP^C monomers. However, data on UV inactivation of prion infectivity, as well as ultrafiltration data, suggest that the infectious agent may be as small as a PrP dimer, indicating that large amyloidic fibrils are not needed as a catalytic prion. Rather, reaction 1 might involve heterodimers of interacting PrP^C and PrP^{Sc} (35). Attempts to mimic reaction 1 in the test tube have been partially successful. When PrP^C was mixed with excess PrP^{Sc} (22) or PrP synthetic peptides (21), PrP^C acquired prionlike properties such as partial resistance to proteolysis. However, whether bona fide infectious prions were produced in these reactions remains to be determined.

Research in the field of prion analogs in yeast and fungi (Table 1) has profited from the concepts developed for the TSE prions. The three fungal prions appear to employ self-propagating conformational switches similar to that proposed by the protein-only paradigm, and their phenotypes are probably related to the loss of the normal function of their protein base.

Cell Biology of Prions: Where Do Prions Replicate?

Prions "replicate" in permissive cells. In the framework of the protein-only model, under-

standing the cell biology of prions is essentially reduced to deciphering the cellular metabolism of the PrP isoforms.

Very few cell lines have been reproducibly infected in culture. Most data in this field were obtained in the N2a neuroblastoma cell line model. Infection of N2a cells with mouse prions (RML strain) has resulted in establishment of a persistently infected line, ScN2a, many subclones and variants of which now exist in several laboratories. These cells produce both PrP^{Sc} and prion infectivity (10).

Experiments usually involve N2a and ScN2a cells or other pairs of infected and uninfected cells. The existing PrP antibodies do not differentiate between PrP^C and PrP^{Sc}. Thus, to study each of these isoforms separately in ScN2a cells, one must first separate them from each other by taking advantage of their disparate properties. For instance, proteinase K is routinely used to digest away PrP^C from cell lysates while converting PrP^{Sc} to PrP27-30 (the protease-resistant core). Resulting PrP27-30 must then be denatured (usually with chaotropic salts) before it can be recognized by PrP antibodies (40, 51). A monoclonal antibody (MAb) that recognizes PrP^{Sc} specifically has now been described, but it has not yet been used in cell biological investigations (23).

The metabolism of PrP^C and PrP^{Sc} in cultured cells has been delineated through the work of many investigators. Its salient points are summarized in Fig. 2. Scrapie-infected mouse neuroblastoma ScN2a cells contain both PrP^C and PrP^{Sc}, while only PrP^C is found in uninfected cells. PrP^C is synthesized in the endoplasmic reticulum (ER) and is exported

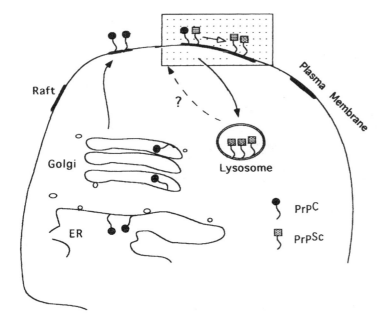

FIGURE 2 Cell biology of PrP. Whether PrP^{Sc} is formed on the plasma membrane (grey box) is not known. See text for other details.

to the cell surface within 15 min of its synthesis. Plasma membrane PrP^C seems to recycle to the interior of the cell with a period of about 1 h, maybe through clathrin-coated pits (41). Two mutually exclusive metabolic fates await PrP^C in ScN2a cells. While most PrP^C molecules are degraded with a $t_{1/2}$ of ca. 6 h in a two-step pathway (14, 50), about 5% of the PrP^C molecules escape degradation and acquire the characteristics of PrP^{Sc}.

The first step of PrP^C degradation is very interesting in that it appears to remove amino acid sequences that are absolutely essential for the ability of PrP^C to form PrP^{Sc}. The endoprotease that is involved in PrP^C processing thus exerts a protective antiprion effect, and in this sense it behaves like the α-secretase of Alzheimer's disease, which severs the amyloid precursor protein (APP) in the middle of the amyloidogenic sequences and thereby prevents formation of the beta amyloid. N-linked glycosylation is not needed for the efficient conversion of PrP^C into PrP^{Sc} (48). Whether PrP^{Sc} is formed on the plasma membrane or during internalization of PrP^C is unknown (7). Because brefeldin A completely inhibits conversion of nascent PrP^C into PrP^{Sc}, we have hypothesized that PrP^{Sc} formation takes place

in a compartment of the endomembrane system that is distal to the ER-Golgi (47). About 1 h after acquiring protease resistance, most PrP^{Sc} molecules are N-terminally trimmed in an acidic compartment (47) and accumulate primarily in lysosomes (28). PrP carrying some of the pathogenic mutations (that cause prion disease in humans) have intrinsic prionlike properties even in the absence of exogenous infection (24), but they do not form bona fide PrP^{Sc} in cultured cells (in contrast to their ability to initiate prion disease in transgenic mice (20).

We are trying to determine the exact subcellular compartments where PrP^{Sc} is formed and where other steps in PrP metabolism take place. In the protein-only model, these sites could be considered to be the "replication grounds" of prions in the host cell.

GPI Proteins and Cholesterol and Sphingolipid Rafts

Most, if not all, GPI-anchored proteins become largely insoluble in cold TX-100 while traversing the Golgi complex. Brown and Rose (8) demonstrated that GPI-anchored proteins owe this insolubility to their association with membrane complexes highly enriched in cholesterol and sphingolipids. The existence of such microdomains, or rafts, of specialized lipid composition had previously been hypothesized (43) to explain the sorting of lipids in polarized epithelial cells. In polarized cells, GPI anchors act as a sorting signal that functions in concert with rafts. It is now clear that rafts may serve not only as sorting platforms for resident molecules (such as GPI proteins) but also as the site where other cellular activities take place. These activities possibly include the transduction of signals through the plasma membrane, the endocytosis of folate (potocytosis)(4), and other processes as well (reviewed in reference 42). Experiments performed on model membranes in vitro suggest that rafts may consist of laterally separated phases within cellular membranes and include lipids of high T_m such as sphingolipids, with the properties of the liquid-ordered phase (1).

Rafts are related to caveolae, a novel subcompartment of eukaryotic membranes that has seen revived interest over the past decade (reviewed in reference 3). In contrast to rafts, which are amorphous, caveolae have a well-defined morphology. They appear in the electron microscope as small (50 nm) saccules that hang beneath the plasma membrane of some cell types. In some cases, they can be internalized. GPI proteins have a clear affinity for caveolae as well, but the details of this association are unclear and disputed (26).

Because the PrP isoforms both possess a GPI moiety (45), the question arose whether rafts of caveolae might be involved in PrP metabolism in general and in the formation of PrP^{Sc} in particular.

RAFTS CONTROL PRION FORMATION

Because N2a cells, like neurons, have no or few caveolae, we focused our efforts on the rafts found in these cells. These domains are most easily detected through their insolubility in a variety of nonionic detergents such as Triton X-100. When cells are lysed in such detergents, rafts and their resident molecules remain insoluble and form buoyant complexes that can be separated in suitable density gradients (8). To characterize the role of rafts in the metabolism of PrP in N2a and ScN2a cells, we asked the following questions (30): Are both PrP isoforms found in rafts? Are they in the *same* rafts? Is PrP^{Sc} still formed if PrP is removed from rafts by manipulating the GPI anchoring sequences of PrP? What happens to the metabolism of PrP if the lipid composition of rafts is altered by pharmacological agents? Our findings are summarized below.

Both PrP Isoforms Are In Rafts

To determine if the PrP isoforms associate with rafts, we used flotation density gradients as well as related assays. We determined that both PrP isoforms associate with TX-100-insoluble rafts. The association of PrP with rafts was also demonstrated by Vey and colleagues (54), who used a detergent-free method originally developed for the isolation of caveolae. That PrP^C is found in rafts was not unexpected, since most if not all GPI proteins are bound to these domains. In contrast, there was no a priori reason to assume that PrP^{Sc} would be found in these domains as well. Although PrP^{Sc} possesses a GPI tail, whether it is anchored to membranes through this moiety has not been determined. Unlike PrP^C and most other GPI proteins, PrP^{Sc} cannot be detached from cellular membranes with the GPI-specific phospholipase PIPLC.

Our finding thus suggests that PrP^{Sc} is indeed attached to membranes through its GPI anchor. The finding that the substrate PrP^C of reaction 1, as well as its "catalyst" and product PrP^{Sc}, is found in rafts strongly suggests that the proteinaceous prion process takes place in these membrane microdomains.

PrP^C and PrP^{Sc} Mostly Reside on Disparate Rafts

Since PrP^C is primarily a cell-surface molecule, while PrP^{Sc} is found mainly in lysosomes, it was reasonable to assume that the rafts in which these proteins reside might possess different properties. We thus looked for experimental conditions that would separate these putatively disparate rafts. We indeed found that when the TX-100 cell lysates were incubated at 37°C (rather than 4°C) prior to the flotation gradient, PrP^C migrated to low-density fractions (light [L] rafts), whereas PrP^{Sc} was found primarily in heavier regions of the gradient (heavy [H] rafts) (30). However, some PrP^{Sc} was still found in L-rafts, and further studies will be needed to determine if catalytic fractions of PrP^{Sc} are found in overlapping L-rafts.

Removing PrP from Rafts Prevents PrP^{Sc} Formation

To disconnect PrP from rafts, we replaced the GPI anchoring signal at the carboxy terminus of the PrP gene with the transmembrane (TM) and cytoplasmic sequences from mouse CD4. The resulting chimeric gene (which was epitopically tagged) was then transfected into ScN2a cells, which provided endogenous prions to drive reaction 1. We determined that the transgene was expressed in these cells and formed chimeric PrP^C-CD4 and that PrP^C-CD4 was absent from TX-100-insoluble, buoyant fractions of the gradient, and thus was not in rafts. Most interestingly, chimeric PrP^C-CD4 did not acquire protease resistance in these cells, i.e., was unable to form PrP^{Sc} (49). This finding again suggests (but does not prove) that being in rafts is essential for PrP^C molecules to form PrP^{Sc}. An obvious caveat of this approach is that adding a rigid TM tail to PrP might prevent the subsequent conformational changes that are required for the formation of PrP^{Sc}. Additional constructs with other TM sequences, all originating from nonraft proteins, subsequently failed to form PrP^{Sc} in ScN2a cells. However, there are now several known TM-anchored (non-GPI) proteins that reside in rafts (38), and it will be interesting to see if PrP fused to such raft TM sequences is able to form PrP^{Sc}.

Modifying Cellular Cholesterol and Sphingolipids Modulates PrP^{Sc} Synthesis

We reasoned that if reaction 1 indeed takes place on rafts (or is controlled by them), then the lipid composition of these domains might modulate the formation of PrP^{Sc}. Indeed, several functions that have been assigned to rafts have been shown to depend on normal levels of cholesterol and sphingolipids, the two major lipid constituents of rafts. For instance, folate potocytosis was vastly reduced both when compactin was used to deplete cellular cholesterol (16) and when fumonisin B$_1$ (46) was used to reduce the level of cellular sphingolipids.

We used a similar pharmacological approach to study the role of rafts in the formation of PrP^{Sc}. When cells were depleted of cholesterol by use of either lovastatin or β-cyclodextrin, PrP^{Sc} synthesis was vastly reduced (30). With sphingolipids, the situation was more complex and more interesting. Depending on the type of sphingolipid targeted in the experiment, PrP^{Sc} levels could be either decreased or increased (N. Naslavsky and A. Taraboulos, unpublished data). Thus, cholesterol and sphingolipids play distinguishable roles in the metabolism of PrP^{Sc}.

RAFTS

GPI proteins tend to associate with cholesterol- and glycolipid-rich membranal rafts. Both PrP^C and PrP^{Sc} possess a GPI moiety, and our results strongly suggest that their metabolism takes place in rafts. Thus rafts may be the replicating site of TSE prions.

How do rafts encourage the formation of prions? An attractive possibility is that rafts might help crowd the PrP isoforms laterally on the plane of the membrane, thereby fostering their interaction and facilitating reaction 1. Putative accessory molecules that have been hypothesized to facilitate formation of PrP^{Sc} in the cell might also be made more available by such lateral clustering. Direct measurements will be needed to verify whether the PrP isoforms are indeed found in high lateral density within the cell membrane.

Rafts could also control PrP^{Sc} formation through entirely different mechanisms. For instance, there is growing evidence that rafts and caveolae are associated with specific internalization pathways. Thus, being in rafts, the PrP could gain access to subcellular compartments that are propitious for the formation of PrP^{Sc}.

Prion diseases present very interesting parallels with a more widespread amyloidosis of the brain, Alzheimer's disease. In both cases, a normal membrane protein precursor is transformed into an abnormal product that subsequently precipitates into amyloidic structures. Cholesterol- and glycolipid-rich rafts now add another interesting twist to this similarity. Simons and his colleagues have recently shown that depleting cellular cholesterol prevents the formation of the pathologic Aβ in cultured neurons (44). Thus, in addition to their growing list of activities, rafts are now clearly involved in the development of two important neurodegenerative diseases.

The finding that PrP^C is associated primarily with H-rafts is intriguing. Since PrP^{Sc} accumulates mainly in secondary lysosomes (28), these results indicate that rafts exist in the late endocytic compartments of these cells (30). It will be interesting to determine whether the presence of H-rafts in lysosomes is a pathological feature specific to cells infected with prions. Whether abnormal accumulation of lipids in such pathological rafts could play a role in the pathogenicity of prions remains to be determined.

Four prionlike phenomena have now been described (Table 1). In contrast to the TSE prion, which is based on a cell-surface glycoprotein, the fungal prions are based on soluble, cytosolic proteins. Thus, while rafts do exist in yeast, it is plausible that they will play little or no role in the biogenesis of the fungal prions.

UNRESOLVED QUESTIONS

As the prion concept is gaining wide acceptance, efforts will be made to decipher details of the structure, mechanisms, and biology of the TSE prion. Conceivably, cell culture systems infected with prions will help answer questions about the interaction of prions with their host cell, as well as questions of more general scope. Some open questions that can

be approached in cell culture systems are listed below.

Cell Biology of Prions

1. What exact subcellular compartments are visited by the PrP isoforms? Where is PrP^{Sc} formed? How does lysosomal PrP^{Sc} gain access to cell-surface PrP^C?

2. How do rafts intervene in the formation of PrP^{Sc}?

3. What proteases are involved in PrP^C degradation?

4. How are prions (and PrP^{Sc}) transmitted from cell to cell?

5. Why are most cell lines resistant to infection with prions, and why is prion infection so unstable in most permissive cells? Can one establish new and better cell culture systems for prions?

6. What is the membranal topology of PrP^{Sc}?

7. What are the mechanisms of prion pathogenicity? This has been studied in GT-1 cells, which display profound cytopathic effects upon infection with prions (37).

8. Does PrP^{Sc} formation require interaction of PrP^C with cellular components such as protein X (53) or other PrP-binding proteins (36)?

Some General Questions That Can Be Addressed in Cultured Cells

1. Are there structural molecules other than PrP^{Sc} in TSE prions? What are they?

2. Are there metabolic intermediates between PrP^C and PrP^{Sc} in cells infected with prions?

3. What is the structural basis of prion strains?

4. How do the pathogenic mutations in PrP cause the familial prion diseases? For example, Harris and his colleagues have shown that PrP^C molecules carrying any of several pathogenic mutations spontaneously acquire prionlike properties when expressed in uninfected CHO cells (24).

5. Is prion formation modulated by chaperones (52)?

6. Infected cells can be used to screen for candidate antiprion molecules such as Congo red (11, 12), polyene antibiotics (19, 57), and others.

ACKNOWLEDGMENTS

This paper is dedicated to the memory of Dan Serban, an unforgettable friend and an excellent colleague and mentor, who passed away on May 22, 1998. I am grateful to him for many stimulating and fruitful discussions over the years. This work was supported by generous grants from the Israel Center for the Study of Emerging Diseases and from the Israel Academy of Sciences.

REVIEWS AND KEY PAPERS

Gabizon, R., and A. Taraboulos. 1997. Of mice and (mad) cows—transgenic mice help to understand prions. *Trends Genet.* **13**:264–269.

Harris, D. A., A. Gorodinsky, S. Lehmann, K. Moulder, and S. L. Shyng. 1996. Cell biology of the prion protein. *Curr. Top. Microbiol. Immunol.* **207**:77–93.

Lindquist, S. 1997. Mad cows meet psi-chotic yeast: the expansion of the prion hypothesis. *Cell* **89**: 495–498.

Prusiner, S. B. 1982. Novel proteinaceous infectious particles cause scrapie. *Science* **216**:136–144.

Prusiner, S. B., M. R. Scott, S. J. DeArmond, and F. E. Cohen. 1998. Prion protein biology. *Cell* **93**:337–348.

REFERENCES

1. **Ahmed, S. N., and D. A. Brown.** 1997. On the origin of sphingolipid/cholesterol-rich detergent-insoluble cell membranes: physiological concentrations of cholesterol and sphingolipids induce formation of a detergent-insoluble, liquid-ordered phase in model membranes. *Biochemistry* **36**:10944–10953.

2. **Alper, T., D. A. Haig, and M. C. Clarke.** 1978. The scrapie agent: evidence against its dependence for replication on intrinsic nucleic acid. *J. Gen. Virol.* **41**:503–516.

3. **Anderson, R. G.** 1993. Caveolae: where incoming and outgoing messengers meet. *Proc. Natl. Acad. Sci. USA* **90**:10909–10913.

4. **Anderson, R. G. W., B. A. Kamen, K. G. Rothberg, and S. W. Lacey.** 1992. Potocytosis: sequestration and transport of small molecules by caveolae. *Science* **255**:410–411.

5. **Bolton, D. C., M. P. McKinley, and S. B. Prusiner.** 1982. Identification of a protein that purifies with the scrapie prion. *Science* **218**:1309–1311.

6. **Borchelt, D. R., M. Scott, A. Taraboulos, N. Stahl, and S. B. Prusiner.** 1990. Scrapie and cellular prion proteins differ in their kinetics of synthesis and topology in cultured cells. *J. Cell Biol.* **110**:743–752.

7. **Borchelt, D. R., A. Taraboulos, and S. B. Prusiner.** 1992. Evidence for synthesis of scrapie prion proteins in the endocytic pathway. *J. Biol. Chem.* **267**:16188–16199.

8. **Brown, D. A., and J. K. Rose.** 1992. Sorting of GPI-anchored proteins to glycolipid-enriched membrane subdomains during transport to the apical cell surface. *Cell* **68**:533–544.

9. **Büeler, H., M. Fischer, Y. Lang, H. Bluethmann, H.-P. Lipp, S. J. DeArmond, S. B. Prusiner, M. Aguet, and C. Weissmann.** 1992. Normal development and behaviour of mice lacking the neuronal cell-surface PrP protein. *Nature* **356**:577–582.

10. **Butler, D. A., M. R. D. Scott, J. M. Bockman, D. R. Borchelt, A. Taraboulos, K. K. Hsiao, D. T. Kingsbury, and S. B. Prusiner.** 1988. Scrapie-infected murine neuroblastoma cells produce protease-resistant prion proteins. *J. Virol.* **62**:1558–1564.

11. **Caspi, S., M. Halimi, A. Yanai, S. B. Sasson, A. Taraboulos, and R. Gabizon.** 1998. The anti-prion activity of congo red. Putative mechanism. *J. Biol. Chem.* **273**:3484–3489.

12. **Caughey, B., K. Brown, G. J. Raymond, G. E. Katzenstein, and W. Thresher.** 1994. Binding of the protease-sensitive form of PrP (prion protein) to sulfated glycosaminoglycan and Congo red. *J. Virol.* **68**:2135–2141. (Erratum, **68**:4107).

13. **Caughey, B., and G. J. Raymond.** 1991. The scrapie-associated form of PrP is made from a cell surface precursor that is both protease- and phospholipase-sensitive. *J. Biol. Chem.* **266**:18217–18223.

14. **Caughey, B., G. J. Raymond, D. Ernst, and R. E. Race.** 1991. N-terminal truncation of the scrapie-associated form of PrP by lysosomal protease(s): implications regarding the site of conversion of PrP to the protease-resistant state. *J. Virol.* **65**:6597–6603.

15. **Caughey, B. W., A. Dong, K. S. Bhat, D. Ernst, S. F. Hayes, and W. S. Caughey.** 1991. Secondary structure analysis of the scrapie-associated protein PrP 27-30 in water by infrared spectroscopy. *Biochemistry* **30**:7672–7680.

16. **Chang, W. J., K. G. Rothberg, B. A. Kamen, and R. G. Anderson.** 1992. Lowering the cholesterol content of MA104 cells inhibits receptor-mediated transport of folate. *J. Cell Biol.* **118**:63–69.

17. **Come, J. H., P. E. Fraser, and P. T. Lansbury, Jr.** 1993. A kinetic model for amyloid formation in the prion diseases: importance of seeding. *Proc. Natl. Acad. Sci. USA* **90:**5959–5963.

18. **Coustou, V., C. Deleu, S. Saupe, and J. Begueret.** 1997. The protein product of the het-s heterokaryon incompatibility gene of the fungus *Podospora anserina* behaves as a prion analog. *Proc. Natl. Acad. Sci. USA* **94:**9773–9778.

19. **Demaimay, R., K. T. Adjou, V. Beringue, S. Demart, C. I. Lasmezas, J. P. Deslys, M. Seman, and D. Dormont.** 1997. Late treatment with polyene antibiotics can prolong the survival time of scrapie-infected animals. *J. Virol.* **71:**9685–9689.

20. **Hsiao, K. K., D. Groth, M. Scott, S. L. Yang, H. Serban, D. Rapp, D. Foster, M. Torchia, S. J. Dearmond, and S. B. Prusiner.** 1994. Serial transmission in rodents of neurodegeneration from transgenic mice expressing mutant prion protein. *Proc. Natl. Acad. Sci. USA* **91:**9126–9130.

21. **Kaneko, K., D. Peretz, K. M. Pan, T. C. Blochberger, H. Wille, R. Gabizon, O. H. Griffith, F. E. Cohen, M. A. Baldwin, and S. B. Prusiner.** 1995. Prion protein (PrP) synthetic peptides induce cellular PrP to acquire properties of the scrapie isoform. *Proc. Natl. Acad. Sci. USA* **92:**11160–11164.

22. **Kocisko, D. A., J. H. Come, S. A. Priola, B. Chesebro, G. J. Raymond, P. T. Lansbury, Jr., and B. Caughey.** 1994. Cell-free formation of protease-resistant prion protein. *Nature* **370:**471–474.

23. **Korth, C., B. Stierli, P. Streit, M. Moser, O. Schaller, R. Fischer, W. Schulz-Schaeffer, H. Kretzschmar, A. Raeber, U. Braun, F. Ehrensperger, S. Hornemann, R. Glockshuber, R. Riek, M. Billeter, K. Wuthrich, and B. Oesch.** 1997. Prion (PrPSc)-specific epitope defined by a monoclonal antibody. *Nature* **390:**74–77.

24. **Lehmann, S., and D. A. Harris.** 1996. Mutant and infectious prion proteins display common biochemical properties in cultured cells. *J. Biol. Chem.* **271:**1633–1637.

25. **Lindquist, S.** 1997. Mad cows meet psi-chotic yeast: the expansion of the prion hypothesis. *Cell* **89:**495–498.

26. **Mayor, S., K. G. Rothberg, and F. R. Maxfield.** 1994. Sequestration of GPI-anchored proteins in caveolae triggered by cross-linking. *Science* **264:**1948–1951.

27. **McKinley, M. P., D. C. Bolton, and S. B. Prusiner.** 1983. Fibril-like structures in preparations of scrapie prions purified from hamster brain. *Proc. Electr. Microsc. Soc. Am.* **41:**802–803.

28. **McKinley, M. P., A. Taraboulos, L. Kenaga, D. Serban, S. J. DeArmond, A. Stieber, and S. B. Prusiner.** 1990. Ultrastructural localization of scrapie prion proteins in secondary lysosomes of infected cultured cells. *J. Cell Biol.* **111:**316a.

29. **Meyer, R. K., M. P. McKinley, K. A. Bowman, M. B. Braunfeld, R. A. Barry, and S. B. Prusiner.** 1986. Separation and properties of cellular and scrapie prion proteins. *Proc. Natl. Acad. Sci. USA* **83:**2310–2314.

30. **Naslavsky, N., R. Stein, A. Yanai, G. Friedlander, and A. Taraboulos.** 1997. Characterization of detergent-insoluble complexes containing the cellular prion protein and its scrapie isoform. *J. Biol. Chem.* **272:**6324–6331.

31. **Oesch, B., D. Westaway, M. Wälchli, M. P. McKinley, S. B. H. Kent, R. Aebersold, R. A. Barry, P. Tempst, D. B. Teplow, L. E. Hood, S. B. Prusiner, and C. Weissmann.** 1985. A cellular gene encodes scrapie PrP 27-30 protein. *Cell* **40:**735–746.

32. **Pan, K. M., M. Baldwin, J. Nguyen, M. Gasset, A. Serban, D. Groth, I. Mehlhorn, Z. Huang, R. J. Fletterick, F. E. Cohen, and S. B. Prusiner.** 1993. Conversion of alpha-helices into beta-sheets features in the formation of the scrapie prion proteins. *Proc. Natl. Acad. Sci. USA* **90:**10962–10966.

33. **Peretz, D., R. A. Williamson, Y. Matsunaga, H. Serban, C. Pinilla, R. B. Bastidas, R. Rozenshteyn, T. L. James, R. A. Houghten, F. E. Cohen, S. B. Prusiner, and D. R. Burton.** 1997. A conformational transition at the N terminus of the prion protein features in formation of the scrapie isoform. *J. Mol. Biol.* **273:**614–622.

34. **Prusiner, S. B.** 1982. Novel proteinaceous infectious particles cause scrapie. *Science* **216:**136–144.

35. **Prusiner, S. B., M. R. Scott, S. J. DeArmond, and F. E. Cohen.** 1998. Prion protein biology. *Cell* **93:**337–348.

36. **Rieger, R., F. Edenhofer, C. I. Lasmezas, and S. Weiss.** 1997. The human 37-kDa laminin receptor precursor interacts with the prion protein in eukaryotic cells (see comments). *Nat. Med.* **3:**1383–1388.

37. **Schätzl, H. M., L. Laszlo, D. M. Holtzman, J. Tatzelt, S. J. DeArmond, R. I. Weiner, W. C. Mobley, and S. B. Prusiner.** 1997. A hypothalamic neuronal cell line persistently infected with scrapie prions exhibits apoptosis. *J. Virol.* **71:**8821–8831.

38. **Scheiffele, P., M. G. Roth, and K. Simons.** 1997. Interaction of influenza virus haemagglutinin with sphingolipid-cholesterol membrane domains via its transmembrane domain. *EMBO J.* **16:**5501–5508.

39. **Scott, M. R., D. Groth, J. Tatzelt, M. Torchia, P. Tremblay, S. J. DeArmond, and S. B. Prusiner.** 1997. Propagation of prion strains through specific conformers of the prion protein. *J. Virol.* **71:**9032–9044.

40. **Serban, D., A. Taraboulos, S. J. De-Armond, and S. B. Prusiner.** 1990. Rapid detection of Creutzfeldt-Jakob disease and scrapie prion proteins. *Neurology* **40:**110–117.

41. **Shyng, S. L., J. E. Heuser, and D. A. Harris.** 1994. A glycolipid-anchored prion protein is endocytosed via clathrin-coated pits. *J. Cell Biol.* **125:**1239–1250.

42. **Simons, K., and E. Ikonen.** 1997. Functional rafts in cell membranes. *Nature* **387:**569–572.

43. **Simons, K., and G. van Meer.** 1988. Lipid sorting in epithelial cells. *Biochemistry* **27:**6197–6202.

44. **Simons, M., P. Keller, B. De Strooper, K. Beyreuther, C. G. Dotti, and K. Simons.** 1998. Cholesterol depletion inhibits the generation of beta-amyloid in hippocampal neurons. *Proc. Natl. Acad. Sci. USA* **95:**6460–64604.

45. **Stahl, N., D. R. Borchelt, K. Hsiao, and S. B. Prusiner.** 1987. Scrapie prion protein contains a phosphatidylinositol glycolipid. *Cell* **51:**229–240.

46. **Stevens, V. L., and J. Tang.** 1997. Fumonisin B1-induced sphingolipid depletion inhibits vitamin uptake via the glycophosphatidylinositol-anchored folate receptor. *J. Biol. Chem.* **272:**18020–18025.

47. **Taraboulos, A., A. J. Raeber, D. R. Borchelt, D. Serban, and S. B. Prusiner.** 1992. Synthesis and trafficking of prion proteins in cultured cells. *Mol. Cell Biol.* **3:**851–863.

48. **Taraboulos, A., M. Rogers, D. R. Borchelt, M. P. McKinley, M. Scott, D. Serban, and S. B. Prusiner.** 1990. Acquisition of protease resistance by prion proteins in scrapie-infected cells does not require asparagine-linked glycosylation. *Proc. Natl. Acad. Sci. USA* **87:**8262–8266.

49. **Taraboulos, A., M. Scott, A. Semenov, D. Avrahami, L. Laszlo, S. B. Prusiner, and D. Avraham.** 1995. Cholesterol depletion and modification of COOH-terminal targeting sequence of the prion protein inhibit formation of the scrapie isoform. *J. Cell Biol.* **129:**121–132. (Erratum, **130:**501).

50. **Taraboulos, A., M. Scott, A. Semenov, D. Avrahami, and S. B. Prusiner.** 1994. Biosynthesis of the prion proteins in scrapie-infected cells in culture. *Braz. J. Med. Biol. Res.* **27:**303–307.

51. **Taraboulos, A., D. Serban, and S. B. Prusiner.** 1990. Scrapie prion proteins accumulate in the cytoplasm of persistently infected cultured cells. *J. Cell Biol.* **110:**2117–2132.

52. **Tatzelt, J., J. Zuo, R. Voellmy, M. Scott, U. Hartl, S. B. Prusiner, and W. J. Welch.** 1995. Scrapie prions selectively modify the stress response in neuroblastoma cells. *Proc. Natl. Acad. Sci. USA* **92:**2944–2948.

53. **Telling, G. C., M. Scott, J. Mastrianni, R. Gabizon, M. Torchia, F. E. Cohen, S. J. DeArmond, and S. B. Prusiner.** 1995. Prion propagation in mice expressing human and chimeric PrP transgenes implicates the interaction of cellular PrP with another protein. *Cell* **83:**79–90.

54. **Vey, M., S. Pilkuhn, H. Wille, R. Nixon, S. J. DeArmond, E. J. Smart, R. G. W. Anderson, A. Taraboulos, and S. B. Prusiner.** 1996. Subcellular colocalization of the cellular and scrapie prion proteins in caveolar-like membranous domains. *Proc. Natl. Acad. Sci. USA* **93:**14945–14949.

55. **Wickner, R. B.** 1994. [URE3] as an altered URE2 protein: evidence for a prion analog in *Saccharomyces cerevisiae* (see comments). *Science* **264:**566–569.

56. **Wilesmith, J. W.** 1988. Bovine spongiform encephalopathy. *Vet. Rec.* **122:**614.

57. **Xi, Y. G., L. Ingrosso, A. Ladogana, C. Masullo, and M. Pocchiari.** 1992. Amphotericin B treatment dissociates *in vivo* replication of the scrapie agent from PrP accumulation. *Nature* **356:**598–601.

INDEX